Neuroprogression and
Staging in Bipolar Disorder

Neuroprogression and Staging in Bipolar Disorder

Edited by

Flavio Kapczinski

Professor of Psychiatry at Universidade Federal do Rio Grande do Sul; Director of the Laboratory of Molecular Psychiatry, Hospital de Clinicas de Porto Alegre; Visiting Professor of Psychiatry at the Department of Psychiatry and Behavioral Sciences at the University of Texas Health Science Center at Houston.

Eduard Vieta

Professor of Psychiatry, Head of Department and Director of the Bipolar Disorders Program, Hospital Clinic, University of Barcelona, IDIBAPS, CIBERSAM, Barcelona, Catalonia, Spain.

Pedro V. S. Magalhães

Professor of Psychiatry, Universidade Federal do Rio Grande do Sul, Hospital de Clínicas de Porto Alegre, Brazil.

Michael Berk

NHMRC Senior Principal Research Fellow, Alfred Deakin Professor of Psychiatry, School of Medicine, Deakin University, Australia; Director, IMPACT Strategic Research Centre (Innovation in Mental and Physical Health and Clinical Treatment), Deakin University, Australia; Professorial Research Fellow, The Florey Institute of Neuroscience and Mental Health, Orygen, The National Centre of Excellence in Youth Mental Health and the Department of Psychiatry, University of Melbourne, Australia.

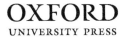

OXFORD
UNIVERSITY PRESS

OXFORD
UNIVERSITY PRESS

Great Clarendon Street, Oxford, OX2 6DP,
United Kingdom

Oxford University Press is a department of the University of Oxford.
It furthers the University's objective of excellence in research, scholarship,
and education by publishing worldwide. Oxford is a registered trade mark of
Oxford University Press in the UK and in certain other countries

© Oxford University Press 2015

The moral rights of the authors have been asserted

First Edition published in 2015
Impression: 1

Published in the United States of America by Oxford University Press
198 Madison Avenue, New York, NY 10016, United States of America

British Library Cataloguing in Publication Data
Data available

Library of Congress Control Number: 2014955851

ISBN 978-0-19-870999-2

Printed in Great Britain by
Clays Ltd, St Ives plc

Foreword

This beautiful book is the main delivery of the Task Force on Staging of the International Society of Bipolar Disorders (ISBD). As the internationally recognized forum the mission of the ISBD is to foster ongoing international collaboration on education and research with an objective to advance the treatment of all aspects of bipolar disorders, resulting in improvements in outcomes/quality of life for those with bipolar disorder and their significant others.

This aim is accomplished not only by holding every year the worldwide biggest international conference on bipolar disorder, but also by their many task forces: currently 8 completed and 12 ongoing. They represent the key research activities of the Society, each focusing on a separate topic and aiming to examine and synthesize evidence usually in the form of position statements and related publications.

The task force on Staging was started when - inspired by the early work of McGorry et al. (2006) on staging in schizophrenia - the first models for staging in bipolar disorder were developed by among others Berk et al. (2007) and Kapczinski et al. (2009) who each had a different approach, focusing on the development of and episodic course of the illness (Berk et al.) versus on the progress in inter-episode functional impairment (Kapczinski et al.). As with other Task Forces it was then immediately recognized that not only a staging model would help to better understand the development and consequences of the illness, but also that both models might complement each other. Therefore, this joint initiative to bring together both views in one Task Force was welcomed with great enthusiasm.

As past president of the ISBD we were involved in finding the right place for the (shortened) report of the Task Force: the publication in the Acta Psychiatrica Scandinavica (Kapczinski et al, 2014). And subsequently, we were very pleased and proud about this book, a real proof of international collaboration with 45 authors from 12 countries and

3 continents. The book not only presents the different approaches as indicated above, but also places the discussion in a broader perspective, with chapters on research and (potential) clinical implications, including cognition, neuroprogression, neuroprotection, biomarkers, imaging and stage-specific differences/indications for treatment. I want to thank all authors (see page ix–xii) and all members of the Task Force (see the reference of Kapczinski et al, 2014 below) for their efforts!

Willem A. Nolen
President ISBD, 2012–2014

References

Berk M, Hallam KT, McGorry PD. (2007) The potential utility of a staging model as a course specifier: a bipolar disorder perspective. J Affect Disord 100:279–281.

McGorry PD, Hickie IB, Yung AR, et al. (2006) Clinical staging of psychiatric disorders: a heuristic framework for choosing earlier, safer and more effective interventions. Aust NZ J Psychiat 40:616–622.

Kapczinski F, Dias VV, Kauer-Sant'Anna M, et al. (2009) Clinical implications of a staging model for bipolar disorders. Expert Rev Neurother 9:957–966.

Kapczinski F, Magalhães PV, Balanzá-Martinez V, Dias VV, Frangou S, Gama CS, Gonzalez-Pinto A, Grande I, Ha K, Kauer-Sant'Anna M, Kunz M, Kupka R, Leboyer M, Lopez-Jaramillo C, Post RM, Rybakowski JK, Scott J, trejilevitch S, Tohen M, Vazquez G, Yatham L, Vieta E, Berk M. (2014) Staging systems in bipolar disorder: an International Society for Bipolar Disorders Task Force Report. Acta Psychiatr Scand 130:354–363.

Contents

Contributors

Vicent Balanzá-Martínez,
Department of Medicine,
University of Valencia,
CIBERSAM, Valencia, Spain

Anusha Baskaran,
Centre for Neuroscience Studies,
Queen's University; Providence
Care, Mental Health Services,
Kingston, ON, Canada

Frank Bellivier,
INSERM U797, Pole de
Psychiatrie, CHU de Créteil,
Hôpital Henri Mondor & Paris 12
University, Créteil, France

Michael Berk,
NHMRC Senior Principal Research
Fellow, Alfred Deakin Professor
of Psychiatry, School of Medicine,
Deakin University, Australia;
Director, IMPACT Strategic
Research Centre (Innovation
in Mental and Physical Health
and Clinical Treatment), Deakin
University, Australia; Professorial
Research Fellow, The Florey
Institute of Neuroscience and
Mental Health, Orygen, The
National Centre of Excellence
in Youth Mental Health and
the Department of Psychiatry,
University of Melbourne, Australia

Caterina del Mar Bonnin,
IDIBAPS, Bipolar Disorders
Program, Hospital Clinic,
University of Barcelona,
CIBERSAM, Barcelona, Spain

Joana Bücker,
Laboratory of Molecular
Psychiatry and Bipolar Disorders
Program and INCT Translational
Medicine, Hospital de Clínicas
de Porto Alegre, Universidade
Federal do Rio Grande do Sul,
Porto Alegre, Brazil

Francesc Colom,
IDIBAPS, Bipolar Disorders
Program, Hospital Clinic,
University of Barcelona,
CIBERSAM, Barcelona, Spain

Aroldo A. Dargél,
Laboratory of Molecular
Psychiatry, INCT Translational
Medicine, Hospital de Clínicas
de Porto Alegre (HCPA), Porto
Alegre (RS), Brazil

Benicio N. Frey,
Associate Professor, Department of Psychiatry and Behavioural Neurosciences, McMaster University, Hamilton, ON, Canada

Gabriel R. Fries,
Laboratory of Molecular Psychiatry, Centro de Pesquisas Experimentais, Hospital de Clínicas de Porto Alegre, Porto Alegre, Brazil

Clarissa S. Gama,
Molecular Psychiatry Laboratory, Hospital de Clínicas de Porto Alegre/CPE, Porto Alegre, Brazil

Benjamin I. Goldstein,
Sunnybrook Research Institute, Sunnybrook Health Sciences Centre, Toronto, ON, Canada

Xenia Gonda,
Department of Clinical and Theoretical Mental Health, Faculty of Medicine, Semmelweis University, Budapest, Hungary

Iria Grande,
Bipolar Disorders Unit, Clinical Institute of Neurosciences, Hospital Clinic, University of Barcelona, IDIBAPS, CIBERSAM, Barcelona, Catalonia, Spain

Bartholomeus C.M. Haarman,
University Medical Center, Department of Psychiatry, Groningen, The Netherlands

Manon H. J. Hillegers,
UMC Utrecht Brain Center Rudolf Magnus, Utrecht, The Netherlands

Romain Icick,
CSAPA Espace Murger, Service de Psychiatrie d'Adultes, Groupe Hospitalier Saint-Louis—Lariboisiere—Fernand Widal, Assistance Publique—Hôpitaux de Paris, Paris, France

Esther Jiménez,
IDIBAPS, Bipolar Disorders Program, Hospital Clinic, University of Barcelona, CIBERSAM, Barcelona, Spain

Flavio Kapczinski,
Professor of Psychiatry at Universidade Federal do Rio Grande do Sul; Director of the Laboratory of Molecular Psychiatry, Hospital de Clinicas de Porto Alegre; Visiting Professor of Psychiatry at the Department of Psychiatry and Behavioral Sciences at the University of Texas Health Science Center at Houston

Marcia Kauer-Sant'Anna,
Laboratory of Molecular Psychiatry, Hospital de Clínicas de Porto Alegre, Porto Alegre, Brazil

Maurício Kunz,
Laboratório de Psiquiatria
Molecular, Centro de Pesquisas,
Hospital de Clínicas
de Porto Alegre,
Programa de Pós-Graduação
em Medicina Psiquiatria,
Universidade Federal do Rio
Grande do Sul, Porto Alegre,
Brazil

Ralph W. Kupka,
Altrecht Institute for Mental
Health Care and University
Medical Center Utrecht,
Utrecht, The Netherlands

María Lacruz,
Hospital Francesc de Borja,
Valencia, Spain

Marion Leboyer,
Université Paris-Est,
INSERM U955,
Psychiatrie Génétique,
Créteil, France

Pedro V. S. Magalhães,
Professor of Psychiatry,
Universidade Federal do
Rio Grande do Sul, Hospital
de Clínicas de Porto Alegre,
Brazil

Anabel Martinez-Aran,
IDIBAPS, Bipolar Disorders
Program, Hospital Clinic,
University of Barcelona,
CIBERSAM, Barcelona, Spain

Diego J. Martino,
Bipolar Disorders Program,
Department of Psychiatry,
Favaloro Foundation Neuroscience
Institute, Buenos Aires, Argentina

Roger McIntyre,
UHN—Toronto Western
Hospital, Toronto, ON, Canada

Luciano Minuzzi,
Department of Psychiatry and
Behavioural Neurosciences,
McMaster University, Hamilton,
ON, Canada

Robert M. Post,
Bipolar Collaborative Network,
Bethesda, MD, USA

María Reinares,
IDIBAPS, Bipolar Disorders
Program, Hospital Clinic,
University of Barcelona,
CIBERSAM, Barcelona, Spain

Aline André Rodrigues,
Hospital de Clínicas de Porto
Alegre, Porto Alegre, Brazil

Adriane R. Rosa,
Professor of Pharmacology,
Universidade Federal do Rio
Grande do Sul (UFRGS),
Hospital de Clinicas de Porto
Alegre, Porto Alegre, Brazil

Janusz K. Rybakowski,
Department of Adult Psychiatry,
Poznan University of Medical
Sciences, Poznan, Poland

Roberto B. Sassi,
Department of Psychiatry and
Behavioural Neurosciences,
McMaster University, Hamilton,
ON, Canada

Jan Scott,
Academic Psychiatry, Wolfson
Unit, Camous for Vitality &
Ageing, Newcastle upon Tyne,
UK

Brisa Solé,
IDIBAPS, Bipolar Disorders
Program, Hospital Clinic,
University of Barcelona,
CIBERSAM, Barcelona, Spain

Sergio A. Strejilevich,
Bipolar Disorders Program,
Department of Psychiatry,
Favaloro Foundation
Neuroscience Institute, Buenos
Aires, Argentina

Rafael Tabarés-Seisdedos,
Department of Medicine,
University of Valencia,
CIBERSAM, Valencia, Spain

Carla Torrent,
IDIBAPS, Bipolar Disorders
Program, Hospital Clinic,
University of Barcelona,
CIBERSAM, Barcelona, Spain

Imma Torres,
IDIBAPS, Bipolar Disorders
Program, Hospital Clinic,
University of Barcelona,
CIBERSAM, Barcelona, Spain

Gustavo H. Vázquez,
Department of Neuroscience,
University of Palermo, Buenos
Aires, Argentina

Eduard Vieta,
Professor of Psychiatry, Head
of Department and Director of
the Bipolar Disorders Program,
Hospital Clinic, University of
Barcelona, IDIBAPS, CIBERSAM,
Barcelona, Catalonia, Spain

Lakshmi N. Yatham,
Department of Psychiatry,
University of British Columbia,
Vancouver, BC, Canada

Chapter 1

Clinical staging in bipolar disorder: a historical perspective

Robert M. Post

Introduction

Kraepelin (1921) was among the first to implicitly stage the development and evolution of bipolar disorder. He did this in multiple ways. Based on his careful graphing of the longitudinal course of bipolar disorder, he saw that the recurrence of episodes tended to speed up over time and graphed this as a function of the increasingly shorter duration of well-intervals between successive episodes. This provided the basis for considering episode progression (what we have labelled episode sensitization), and the later identification of faster recurrences, such as rapid and ultra-rapid cycling. At the same time, based on his careful clinical observations, Kraepelin recognized that initial episodes were often precipitated by psychosocial stressors, but with multiple occurrences they could also occur with just the anticipation of stressors or none at all, yielding the idea of a later, more autonomous stage of illness.

Kraepelin also recognized that some subtypes of mania and depression, such as dysphoric mania (characterized by high levels of anxiety and irritability), ran a more difficult course and required more hospitalizations, especially in women. Thus, differences in the qualitative aspects of clinical presentation could also have prognostic significance.

All three of these observations of faster episode recurrence, the transition from precipitated to more spontaneous episode occurrence, and illness subtypes such as dysphoric mania have been widely replicated and set the stage for their incorporation into various implicit or explicit staging models.

Faster episode recurrences and cycle acceleration

Jules Angst and Paul Grof, among many others, also saw the general tendency for cycle acceleration as a function of number of prior episode, and initial reviews of the literature (Post 1992) supported this general, but not invariant, trend. In one of the largest and most cogent demonstrations, Lars Kessing et al. (1998) found that the number of prior hospitalizations for depression was the best predictor of subsequent recurrences (with a shorter latency) in either unipolar or bipolar depression, and that multiple potential confounders could not explain this effect. A similar effect was demonstrated for the number of prior manias and the vulnerability to relapse.

The number of prior episodes and frequency of their recurrence took on added importance in the modern era of psychopharmacology, where for example, it was observed that those with rapid cycling (four or more episodes/year) were less likely to respond to lithium (Dunner et al. 1979). Multiple studies replicated these findings, with few exceptions (Post et al. 2012). Moreover, greater number of prior episodes appeared to be a relative predictor of non-response to multiple agent and naturalistic treatment.

A continuum of cycle frequencies and faster patterns of recurrence are now widely recognized (Kupka et al. 2005), and attempts have been made to further categorize faster episode cut-offs, such as ultra-rapid cycling (four or more episodes/month) and ultra-ultra (or ultradian) cycling (where chaotic and dramatic mood fluctuations occur multiple times within a 24-hour period on 4 or more days/week) (Kramlinger and Post 1996). Patients with ultradian cycling patterns appear to respond especially well to the dihydropyridine L-type calcium channel blocker nimodopine (Davanzo et al. 1999; Pazzaglia et al. 1993; Post and Leverich 2008) but further work is required to delineate pharmacological responsiveness of this stage of illness, which tends to occur relatively late in the course illness in adults (Post and Leverich 2008) or very early in the youngest children with bipolar not otherwise specified (NOS) presentations (Birmaher et al. 2009; Geller et al. 1998).

Progression from triggered to spontaneous episodes

This general pattern of increasing autonomy of episodes as a function of the number of prior recurrences (stress sensitization) has been best documented in unipolar depression (Kendler et al. 2000, 2001; Slavich et al. 2011), but also appears to apply to patients with bipolar disorder as well (Post and Miklowitz 2010). However, in addition, in bipolar illness, there is also evidence of stress accumulation or stress generation in those with childhood adversity (Dienes et al. 2006), such that there may be both increasing number of stressors and sensitivity to them.

Dysphoric mania

Kraepelin's initial observations about the poor prognosis of dysphoric mania have been confirmed, and more modern pharmacological dissection suggests that lithium is more often effective in classic euphoric mania, while valproate may have some advantages in the dysphoric subtype (Post and Leverich 2008).

Sensitization and kindling as models of illness progression and staging

Based on the Kraepelinian observations of illness course, Post (1992) drew analogies to other behaviour syndromes in animals that also showed evidence of illness progression—kindling and sensitization. In kindling, the amygdala is stimulated once a day for one second, generating increasing behaviour responsivity (seizure stage evolution) that culminates in the development of full-blown seizures with rearing and falling. Following sufficient numbers of the electrically induced variety, seizures also begin to emerge spontaneously (Post 2007).

Thus, amygdala kindling has three general stages: (I) the initial or Development stage; (II) mid or Completed stage of full-blown triggered seizures; and (III) the late or Spontaneous stage (Fig. 1.1). The evolution and progression of these stages in kindled seizures are relatively invariant and of importance for their pathophysiological and pharmacotherapeutic implications.

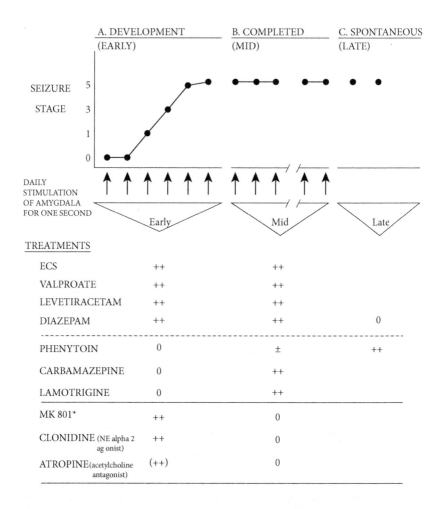

++ = highly effective; ± = ambiguous; 0 = not effective; ( ) = inconsistent data
* glutamate NMDA$_R$ antagonist

Fig. 1.1 Dissociation of Pharmagological Responsivity as a Function of Phase of Amygdala Kindling Evolution

In the Development stage of kindling, electrophysiological, biochemical, neuropeptide, and immediate early genes (transcription factors) progressively increase from no or minimal changes in neurobiology and behaviour to unilateral ones, and ultimately bilateral alterations. This reveals a dramatic anatomical evolution of neurobiological alterations in response to repetition of the same stimulation. As might be expected from this spatiotemporal progression of the amygdala-kindled 'memory trace', pharmacological interventions are differentially effective in the Development, Completed, and Spontaneous stages; some drugs work in one, but not another stage (Fig. 1.1).

We have postulated that the initial Developmental, mid-phase Pre-cipitated Episodes, and late Spontaneous Episodes of bipolar disorder might similarly be differentially responsive to different pharmacological and even some psychosocial interventions (Scott et al. 2013). There is some evidence that this might be the case, but this requires much further study (Fig. 1.2). A major caveat to consider here is that the specific drugs that are effective against different stages of amygdala-kindled seizures are likely to be dissimilar from the drugs that work in bipolar disorder (even though some are also anticonvulsants). The case is especially clear in considering lithium and the atypical antipsychotics, which are not anticonvulsants at all.

Interestingly, the local anaesthetics lidocaine and cocaine can also show a kindling-like progression of stages (from developing, to full-blown triggered, to spontaneous) in the development of both panic

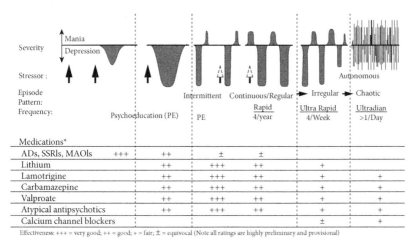

Medications*						
ADs, SSRIs, MAOIs	+++	++	±	±		
Lithium		++	+++	++	+	
Lamotrigine		++	+++	++	+	+
Carbamazepine		++	+++	++	+	+
Valproate		++	+++	++	+	+
Atypical antipsychotics		++	+++	++	+	+
Calcium channel blockers					±	+

Effectiveness: +++ = very good; ++ = good; + = fair; ± = equivocal (Note all ratings are highly preliminary and provisional)

Fig. 1.2 Does Pharmacology of Bipolar Disorder Vary as a Function of Phase of Illness Evolution?

attacks and seizures (in what may be viewed as pharmacological kindling). Similarly, repeated bouts of alcohol withdrawal (not intoxication) can kindle to increasingly severe behavioural (delirium tremens) and seizure endpoints (Ballenger and Post 1978). Thus, kindling is an indirect or non-homologous model for illness progression, as seizures do not accompany mood episodes in the affective disorders.

In contrast to kindling processes where seizures are the typical end point, behavioural sensitization typically refers to increasing hyperactivity and stereotypy responses to repetition of the same dose of psychomotor stimulant, such as amphetamine, cocaine, or methylphenidate. Evidence suggests that repeated stimulant use in humans also progresses through initial stages of relatively benign euphoria to more severe and dysphoric behavioural disruption, and ultimately to paranoid psychosis. Thus, episode sensitization in bipolar disorder may reflect increases in severity and type of manifestation, as well as an increased vulnerability to recurrence.

As in kindling, the initial Development stage of increasing behavioural reactivity to stimulants is again differentially responsive to pharmacological treatments compared to the later Expression phase (after the animal has already been sensitized). For example, antipsychotics block the development, but not the expression of stimulant-induced behavioural sensitization, and this may have relevance for antipsychotic responsiveness clinically (Post et al. 1987).

Responses to some intermittent stressors can also show sensitization in their behavioural or biochemical responses (rather than tolerance and down-regulation). Thus, we label these two phenomena of increasing responsivity to repetition of the same inducing stimulus as stimulant sensitization and stressor sensitization. There also appears to be cross-sensitization between the stressor- and stimulant-induced effects, and vice versa (Antelman et al. 1980; Kalivas and Stewart 1991).

If we refer to the findings that affective episodes tend to recur successively more rapidly as evidence of episode sensitization, we now have three types of intermittent recurrences that can sensitize or increase in their responsiveness: stressors, episodes, and abused substances.

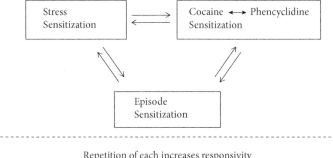

Fig. 1.3 Cross Sensitization Among Stressors, Drugs of Abuse, And Episodes

Both clinical and preclinical data suggest that each type of sensitization can show cross-sensitization to the other two, and thus create a vicious positive feedback cycle, with each element contributing to illness progression (Fig. 1.3). For example, recurrent stressors can cross sensitize to both affect episode recurrence and renewed use of substances.

Neurobiological consequences of episode, stress, and substance sensitization

Not only do mood episodes recur faster and more spontaneously, but greater numbers of affective episodes are associated with greater amounts of treatment resistance, cognitive deficits, and multiple brain and somatic pathological changes (Post et al. 2012). Duration of illness and number of episodes can to some extent be viewed as surrogate markers for stages of illness progression.

The evolution of more formal staging models

Based on this kind of evidence, Berk et al. (2011) and Kapczinski et al. (2009) have proposed a classification of several stages of bipolar disorder progression. The simplest division of illness course into Early and Late already appears to have prognostic and treatment implications. Moreover, a number of neurobiological markers differ as a function of this early versus late distinction (Kauer-Sant'Anna et al. 2009).

This author has proposed a similar, but more detailed staging concept that would allow for consideration of the additional effects of comorbid substance and alcohol abuse, social stressors, loss of social support, multiple recurrences, and other illness complications that may further contribute prognosis (Post 2010; Post et al. 2012).

In this framework we have suggested eight stages, each with the possibility of multiple subcategories and classifications. These would include: Stage I, vulnerability; II, well interval; III, prodrome; IV, syndrome; V, recurrence; VI, progression; VII, treatment resistance; and VIII, late deterioration or end stage (Fig. 1.4). Stage I would include the degree of (a) genetic or (b) environmental predisposition, and further predisposing factors would be classified in II (the well interval) for a variety of childhood adversities, including different kinds of abuse neglect, parental loss, etc. Stages III (prodrome) and IV (syndrome) would be further subclassified for bipolar I, II, NOS subtypes, as well as other critical characteristics of prognostic significance, such as anxiety or substance abuse comorbidity.

One suggested schema is presented in Table 1.1 and is modelled after that used for staging progression in colon cancer. In that instance, subcategorizing the depth and degree of invasion of malignant cell and the spread of tumours in Stages IIa, IIb, or IIc has been shown to have very substantial prognostic implications for survival.

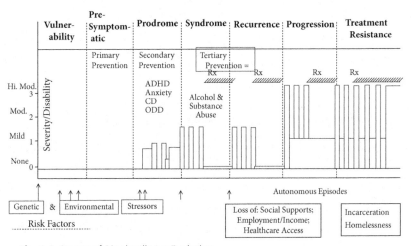

Fig. 1.4 Stages of Bipolar Illness Evolution

Table 1.1 Staging of bipolar illness

Early stages

Stage I VULNERABILITY	II WELL INTERVAL	III PRODROME	IV SYNDROME ONSET
A. Genetic 　1.Unilineal 　　a. S/SA 　　b. BP 　　c. UP 　2. Bilineal 　　a. S/SA 　　b. BP 　　c. UP 　3.Genetic markers 　　a. CACA 　　b. val66val 　　　proBDNF	A. Childhood 　adversity/abuse 　1. Verbal 　2. Physical 　3. Sexual 　4. Neglect	A. Antecedent Dx 　1. ADHD 　2. ODD 　3. Anxiety disorder 　　a. Separation 　　b. School 　　c. Phobia 　　d. Social p. 　　e. GAD 　　f. panic 　　g. OCD 　　h. PTSD 　4. Depression 　5. DMDD 　6. Substance abuse	A. BP-I 　At age 　Duration
B. Prenatal 　1. Low birth weight 　2. Preterm 　3. Viral infection 　4. Other	B. Parental loss 　1. Mother 　　a. Absent 　　b. Deceased 　2. Father 　　a. Absent 　　b. Deceased	B. Symptom 　emergence 　1. Brief euphoria 　2. Extended 　　euphoria 　3. Decreased sleep 　4. Grandiosity 　5. Hallucinations 　6. Hypersexual 　7. Extreme mood 　　lability 　8. Aggression 　9. Cyclothymia 　10. Suicidal threats 　11. Other	B. BP II 　At age 　Duration
C. Perinatal 　1. Low anger 　2. Anoxia 　3. Neonatal	C. Adolescent/adult 　adversity/abuse 　1. Verbal 　2. Physical 　3. Sexual 　4. Neglect 　5. Bullied		C. BP NOS 　At age 　Duration
D. Peripheral markers 　1. Homocysteine 　2. Antibodies	D. Low SES (family 　income) 　1. Below poverty 　　line 　2. Marginal/barely 　　adequate		D. Depression 　(followed by 　mania) 　At age: 　Duration

(*continued*)

Table 1.1 (continued) Staging of bipolar illness

Early stages

Stage I VULNERABILITY	II WELL INTERVAL	III PRODROME	IV SYNDROME ONSET

	E. Neuropsychology
	  1. Poor face
	    emotion
	    recognition		

	F. High achievement
	  1. All A's in high
	    school		

	G. Blood markers		

	H. Brain markers
	  1. MRI
	  2. fMRI
	  3. PET		

Later Stages

V RECURRENCE	VI PROGRESSION	VII TREATMENT RESISTANCE	VIII LATE STAGE

A. Manias
  1. #
  2. Rapid cycling
    (RC)
  3. Ultra RC
  4. Ultradian
    cycling
	A. Episodes (Ma, Dep,
	  Mix)
	  1. Faster
	  2. Increased
	    severity
	  3. Increased
	    chronicity
	  4. Continuous
	  5. Psychosis
	  6. Dysthymic or
	    hyperthymic
	    baseline persists
		A. Acute mania
		  Non-response to:
		  1. Lithium
		  2. A.C.
		  3. A.A.
		  4. Other
		  5. ECT
			A. Functionally
			  disabled

B. Depressions
  1. #
  2. –4
	B. Stressors
	  1. Separation
	  2. Divorce
	  3. Job loss
	  4. Home loss
	  5. Insurance loss
	  6. Legal
	  7. Jail
		B. Depression
		  Non-response to:
		  1–5 above
		  6. ADs
		  7. rTMS
		  8. Adjuncts: folate,
		    D3, T3, Li, NAC
			B. On disability

C. Mixed state
  1. #
  2–4.
D. D-M-I
 	
E. M-D-I
	C. Comorbidities
	New onset/
	progression
	  1. Substance use
	    a. Alcohol
	    b. Marijuana
		C. Prophylaxis
		  Non-response to:
		  1–8 above
		D. Dual agents
		
		  Non-response to:
			C. Homeless
			
			D. Halfway home
			
			E. Chronic hospital
			  or jail

Table 1.1 (continued) Staging of bipolar illness

Later Stages

V RECURRENCE	VI PROGRESSION	VII TREATMENT RESISTANCE	VIII LATE STAGE
	c. Stimulant d. Opiates e. Hallucinogenic f. Other 2. Anxiety disorder a–h (see stage III) 3. Cognitive dysfunction 4. Medical syndrome	E. Complex combination Rx	F. Medical disability
			G. Dementia
			H. Early death by: 1. Suicide 2. Medical illness 3. Accident 4. Other

CACNA1C, alpha subunit of the dihydropyridine calcium channel; Onset at age____(age to be filled in). Duration____(duration of episode to be filled in); S/SA: schizophrenia/schizoaffective; CRP, C-reactive protein; ODD = oppositional defiant disorder; DMDD = dysphoric mood dysregulation disorde; BP, bipolar; UP, unipolar; LowSES: low socieconomic status; BP-type I: type I bipolar disorder; BP NOS: Bipolar disorder not otherwise specified.

The case for multiple stages and subcategories

As in the case of tumour progression, we suggest the utility of starting with more comprehensive and multiply staged and subdivided models for affective illness progression. This would have multiple advantages over more truncated staging models even though the later would initially be easier to validate. Having more stages from the outset would allow multiple investigative groups to speak a common language in their future investigations and provisional categories could later be combined or simplified if the data warranted. Having more stages and subcategories would also speak to the complexity of bipolar disorder itself, which perhaps has more psychiatric and medical comorbidities, patterns and subtypes of episodes, and frequencies of recurrence, than any other psychiatric disorder.

If one starts with only a few discrete stages or simply the early–late dichotomy, as the field matures, more distinctions will have to be created and this will lead to the creation of multiple different staging models. This would particularly be the case as staging models would have many different uses and implications.

As implicit in the early staging ideas and explicit in the more recent proposals, the idea of stages is most cogent for considering differential treatment interventions as a function of stage of illness, with the assumption that earlier treatment would be more effective than later and perhaps also less complex (Berk et al. 2010). Having pre-illness risk status well characterized in the I (vulnerability) and II (well interval) stages from the outset will allow the integration of genetic and other neurobiological markers into the staging process, and ultimately will facilitate the development of early intervention and even primary prophylaxis for those at ultra-high risk (Post et al. 2013).

Similarly, including subcategories, for example involving the presence or absence of current or lifetime anxiety and substance disorders, will allow delineation of their effects on course of illness, treatment response, and ultimately more specific clinical trials to assess optimal treatments for these comorbidities, which complicate treatment and portend a poor outcome. The development of treatment algorithms and the application of personalized medicine will likely depend on a combination of clinical attributes and stages and ultimately their neurobiological correlates.

Examining neurobiological correlates of illness stage and attempting to validate stages as a function of degree of neurobiological abnormality will also vary greatly. In some instances, only gross distinctions such as early versus late may be adequate (Kauer-Sant'Anna et al. 2009), but more refined biological measures with continuous variables may be more suitable for allocation to multiple stages or numbers, type, or complexity of episodes. Having these multiple, detailed stage categories defined at the outset will facilitate collection of these data and comparison across investigative groups, with the view that the stages could then be further subcategorized as needed, or easily be collapsed and truncated if required by the data.

As noted earlier, a number of variables, including cognitive dysfunction, treatment response, and neurobiological abnormalities, have already been linked to the number of previous episodes, so only dealing a first versus a recurrent episode, for example, would not allow the analyses of more detailed relationships that might be possible with the full delineation of number of episodes. Moreover, the ability to use continuous rather than dichotomous variables will enhance the likelihood of finding statistically significant relationships.

In the staging of colon cancer, subtle differences in the degree of invasion of the basement membrane or distance of spread to other organs have been found to have notable prognostic implications. While not as well worked out, colon cancer stages also have pathophysiological implications in terms of the progressive development of somatic mutations involving both successive loss of tumour suppressor factors and gain of function mutations in oncogenic and cell proliferative processes (Vogelstein et al. 2013). We would surmise that a similar progression of successive alterations in gene expression would occur on an epigenetic basis in bipolar disorder and analogously involve both suppression of positive adaptive neurobiological alterations and enhancement of the primary pathological ones (Post 2007). The increasing ratio of pathological to adaptive alterations would hypothetically drive ill versus well phases, cycle acceleration, inability to achieve a well interval, and ultimately, treatment non-responsiveness.

The potential pathophysiological mechanisms in bipolar disorder have been examined in the last 50 years at many, and sequentially, deeper levels of analysis in multiple domains. Studies have evolved: in signal transduction pathways from neurotransmitters, to receptors, second messengers, kinases, transcription factors, immediate early genes, and epigenetic modifications; in type of tissue examined from blood, to cerebrospinal fluid and brain measures of endocrine, cytokine, and oxidative stress; and in static to functional brain imaging of multiple types. Therefore, having clinically defined, very detailed stages from the outset would facilitate the analysis of so many of these diverse measures, which will only grow in number with time. Once the neurobiological findings become replicable and consistent, they themselves could be added to the clinical stage definitions and (as in colon cancer Stages II a, b, and c) be examined for treatment implications and prognostic relationships.

Similarly, in the relatively late stage of VII (treatment resistance), having precise subcategories of the degree of treatment resistance to lithium, mood stabilizing anticonvulsants, atypical antipsychotics, repeated transcranial magnetic stimulation (rTMS), and electroconvulsive therapy, or their combinations, will allow analysis of these gradations in treatment resistance in relationship to functional outcome, cognition, and neurobiology.

Describing and defining stages in bipolar disorder would have other benefits as well. It would help in the public perception of the illness as potentially progressive and in need for concerted efforts at treatment and prevention. As neurobiological correlates of illness stage progression are better defined, this should also help greatly with destigmatization. Efforts at early intervention in an attempt to prevent or delay the development of the full-blown syndrome are more than a decade more advanced in schizophrenia compared to bipolar disorder, in part because of careful definition of the at-risk or prodromal stage (McGorry et al. 2006).

The recognition that about ¼ of adults in the United States had onset of their bipolar illness prior to age 13 and about 2/3 prior to age 19 (Perlis et al. 2004; Post et al. 2013) and that these early onsets are a poor prognostic factor, which emphasizes the importance of staging definitions pertinent to children. This might further help to shorten the long delays to first treatment which are themselves an independent contributor to a poor outcome in adulthood (Post et al. 2010), and encourage more robust study of early intervention with the goal of developing effective and well-tolerated preventive strategies (Post et al. 2013).

It would appear prudent and useful to view the staging of bipolar disorder in its historical context so that staging exercise itself can be seen as an iterative and progressively evolving process. Constructing a comprehensive framework for staging in bipolar disorder that will allow maximum flexibility for incorporating future data and concepts might be an optimal way to proceed.

References

Antelman SM, Eichler AJ, Black CA, et al. (1980) Interchangeability of stress and amphetamine in sensitization. Science 207(4428):329–331.

Ballenger JC and Post RM (1978) Kindling as a model for alcohol withdrawal syndromes. Brit J Psychiat 133:1–14.

Berk M, Brnabic A, Dodd S, et al. (2011) Does stage of illness impact treatment response in bipolar disorder? Empirical treatment data and their implication for the staging model and early intervention. Bipolar Disord 13(1):87–98. doi: 10.1111/j.1399–5618.2011.00889.x

Berk M, Hallam K, Malhi GS, et al. (2010) Evidence and implications for early intervention in bipolar disorder. J Ment Health 19(2):113–126.

Birmaher B, Axelson D, Goldstein B, et al. (2009) Four-year longitudinal course of children and adolescents with bipolar spectrum disorders: the Course and Outcome of Bipolar Youth (COBY) study. Am J Psychiat 166(7):795–804.

Davanzo PA, Krah N, Kleiner J, et al. (1999) Nimodipine treatment of an adolescent with ultradian cycling bipolar affective illness. J Child Adoles Psychopharmacol 9(1):51–61.

Dienes KA, Hammen C, Henry RM, et al. (2006) The stress sensitization hypothesis: understanding the course of bipolar disorder. J Affect Disorders 95(1–3):43–49.

Dunner DL, Murphy D, Stallone F, et al. (1979) Episode frequency prior to lithium treatment in bipolar manic-depressive patients. Compr Psychiat 20(6):511–515.

Geller B, Williams M, Zimerman B, et al. (1998) Prepubertal and early adolescent bipolarity differentiate from ADHD by manic symptoms, grandiose delusions, ultra-rapid or ultradian cycling. J Affect Disorders 51(2):81–91.

Kalivas PW and Stewart J (1991) Dopamine transmission in the initiation and expression of drug- and stress-induced sensitization of motor activity. Brain Res Rev 16(3):223–244.

Kapczinski F, Dias VV, Kauer-Sant'Anna M, et al. (2009) Clinical implications of a staging model for bipolar disorders. Expert Rev Neurother 9(7):957–966. doi: 10.1586/ern.09.31

Kauer-Sant'Anna M, Kapczinski F, Andreazza AC, et al. (2009) Brain-derived neurotrophic factor and inflammatory markers in patients with early- vs. late-stage bipolar disorder. Int J Neuropsychoph 12(4):447–458. doi: 10.1017/S1461145708009310

Kendler KS, Thornton LM, and Gardner CO (2000) Stressful life events and previous episodes in the etiology of major depression in women: an evaluation of the 'kindling' hypothesis. Am J Psychiat 157(8):1243–1251.

Kendler KS, Thornton LM, and Gardner CO (2001) Genetic risk, number of previous depressive episodes, and stressful life events in predicting onset of major depression. Am J Psychiat 158(4):582–586.

Kessing LV, Andersen PK, and Mortensen PB (1998) Predictors of recurrence in affective disorder. A case register study. J Affect Disorders 49(2):101–108.

Kraepelin E (1921) Manic-depressive Illness and Paranoia. Edinburgh: ES Livingstone.

Kramlinger KG and Post RM (1996) Ultra-rapid and ultradian cycling in bipolar affective illness. Brit J Psychiat 168(3):314–323.

Kupka RW, Luckenbaugh DA, Post RM, et al. (2005) Comparison of rapid-cycling and non-rapid-cycling bipolar disorder based on prospective mood ratings in 539 outpatients. Am J Psychiat 162(7):1273–1280.

McGorry PD, Hickie IB, Yung AR, et al. (2006) Clinical staging of psychiatric disorders: a heuristic framework for choosing earlier, safer and more effective interventions. Aust NZ J Psychiat 40(8):616–622.

Pazzaglia PJ, Post RM, Ketter TA, et al. (1993) Preliminary controlled trial of nimodipine in ultra-rapid cycling affective dysregulation. Psychiat Res 49(3):257–272.

Perlis RH, Miyahara S, Marangell LB, et al. (2004) Long-term implications of early onset in bipolar disorder: data from the first 1000 participants in the systematic treatment enhancement program for bipolar disorder (STEP-BD). Biol Psychiat 55(9):875–881.

Post RM (1992) Transduction of psychosocial stress into the neurobiology of recurrent affective disorder. Am J Psychiat 149(8):999–1010.

Post RM (2007) Kindling and sensitization as models for affective episode recurrence, cyclicity, and tolerance phenomena. Neurosci Biobehav R 31(6):858–873. doi: 10.1016/j.neubiorev.2007.04.003

Post RM (2010) Mechanisms of illness progression in the recurrent affective disorders. Neurotoxicol Res 18(3–4):256–271.

Post RM, Chang K, and Frye MA (2013) Paradigm shift: preliminary clinical categorization of ultrahigh risk for childhood bipolar disorder to facilitate studies on prevention. J Clin Psychiat 74(2):167–169.

Post RM, Fleming J, and Kapczinski F (2012) Neurobiological correlates of illness progression in the recurrent affective disorders. J Psychiatr Res 46(5):561–573.

Post RM and Leverich GS (2008) Treatment of Bipolar Illness: A Casebook for Clinicians and Patients. New York: W.W. Norton and Company.

Post RM, Leverich GS, Kupka RW, et al. (2010) Early-onset bipolar disorder and treatment delay are risk factors for poor outcome in adulthood. J Clin Psychiat 71(7):864–872.

Post RM and Miklowitz D (2010) The role of stress in the onset, course, and progression of bipolar illness and its comorbidities: implications for therapeutics. In: Miklowitz D and Cicchetti D, eds. Bipolar Disorder: A Developmental Psychopathology Approach. New York: Guilford Press, pp. 370–416.

Post RM, Weiss SR, and Pert A (1987) The role of context and conditioning in behavioral sensitization to cocaine. Psychopharmacol Bull 23(3):425–429.

Scott J, Leboyer M, Hickie I, et al. (2013) Clinical staging in psychiatry: a crosscutting model of diagnosis with heuristic and practical value. Br J Psychiatry 202(4):243–245.

Slavich GM, Monroe SM, and Gotlib IH (2011) Early parental loss and depression history: associations with recent life stress in major depressive disorder. J Psychiatr Res 45(9):1146–1152.

Vogelstein B, Papadopoulos N, Velculescu VE, et al. (2013) Cancer genome landscapes. Science 339(6127):1546–1558.

Chapter 2

Staging systems in bipolar disorder

Ralph W. Kupka, Manon H. J. Hillegers, and Jan Scott

Introduction

In this chapter we review some of the staging systems employed in medicine and highlight how these models are gradually being introduced in psychiatry in general. We then focus on the staging systems that have been described specifically for use in bipolar disorder and summarize some of the basic assumptions of the staging model. To set the scene, we provide a brief overview of the basic characteristics and current classification systems employed for bipolar disorders.

Bipolar disorder is a severe, chronic mood disorder characterized by recurrent episodes of mania, hypomania, and depression, separated by euthymic intervals of shorter (days to weeks) or longer (months to years) duration (Fig. 2.1). The lifetime prevalence of bipolar disorder is estimated at 2.4% of the world's population (Merikangas et al. 2011) and it is ranked among the top ten most burdensome diseases worldwide (WHO 2001).

In the *Diagnostic and Statistical Manual of Mental Disorders*, 5th edition (DSM-5) (APA 2013), bipolar and related disorders are deliberately placed between schizophrenia spectrum disorders and depressive disorders in recognition of their place as a bridge between these diagnostic classes in terms of shared symptomatology, family history, and genetic liability. In the DSM system, bipolar I disorder corresponds to classic descriptions of manic–depressive illness with the lifetime occurrence of manic and depressive episodes meeting full syndromal criteria, with or without psychotic features. Bipolar II disorder requires the lifetime occurrence of at least one major depressive episode and at least one

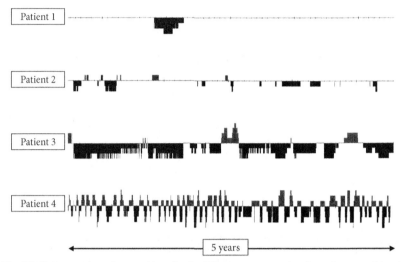

Fig. 2.1 Heterogenic patterns of longitudinal illness course and various degrees of treatment resistance in four treated outpatients with bipolar I disorder; manic/hypomanic episodes shown above baseline, depressive episodes below baseline (examples of daily rated prospective Life Charts from the Stanley Foundation Bipolar Network, data from Post et al. 2003; Kupka et al. 2005).

hypomanic episode, but no syndromal episodes of mania. In cyclothymic disorder, there are numerous subsyndromal episodes of mania and depression, none of which fulfil the formal criteria for a manic, hypomanic, or depressive episode. In addition to these more specifically described syndromes, several other subcategories are defined; taken together all these presentations are referred to as the bipolar spectrum (Table 2.1).

Bipolar disorder typically becomes manifest in adolescence and early adulthood (Goodwin and Jamison 2007). Whilst the diagnostic criteria in DSM-5 are applicable for adolescents and adults, in some countries these criteria are applied to children. However, debate on the validity of the diagnosis of mania in children spans more than half a century (Carlson and Glovinsky 2009). Between 1994 and 2003 in the United States the prevalence of the paediatric bipolar disorder diagnosis in outpatient clinics increased 40-fold (Moreno et al. 2007). Possible explanations for this increase included sampling bias (e.g. more offspring of bipolar parents being taken for clinical assessments), changes in conceptualization

Table 2.1 DSM-5 classification of bipolar and related disorders (Data from APA 2013)

Code	Definition	Episode	Specifier (with . . .)
296.xx	Bipolar I disorder	Manic	Anxious distress
		Hypomanic	Mixed features
		Depressed	Rapid cycling
		Unspecified	Melancholic features
			Atypical features
			Psychotic features
			Catatonia
			Peripartum onset
			Seasonal pattern
296.89	Bipolar II disorder	Hypomanic	As in bipolar I disorder
		Depressed	
301.13	Cyclothymic disorder	n/a	Anxious distress
296.89	Other specified bipolar and related disorder	n/a	n/a
296.80	Other unspecified bipolar and related disorder	n/a	n/a
293.83	Bipolar and related disorder due to another medical condition	n/a	Manic features
			Manic- or hypomanic-like episode
			mixed features
___.__	Substance/medication-induced bipolar and related disorders		Onset during intoxication
			Onset during withdrawal

of the disorder (e.g. the introduction of 'juvenile' or 'paediatric' bipolar disorder), and the inappropriate application of the bipolar disorder diagnosis (e.g. to young children with brief periods of hyperactivity and expressing grandiose ideas or chronic irritability). A major question was whether children and adolescents with severe, non-episodic irritability and symptoms of attention deficit hyperactivity disorder (ADHD) should be considered to have a diagnosis of bipolar disorder. Longitudinal studies showed that these children and adolescents with severe, non-episodic irritability differ from those with bipolar disorder in course, family history, and performance tasks linked to pathophysiology and are not significantly more likely than 'control group' cases to manifest bipolar disorders in adulthood (Brotman et al. 2006; Birmaher et al. 2006; Rich et al. 2007; Baroni et al. 2009; Margulies et al. 2012; Skirrow et al. 2012). Consequently, the diagnosis of bipolar disorder should be reserved for those children and adolescents who have a history of one or more distinct episodes of mania or hypomania meeting full DSM-5 criteria—that is, the diagnosis should be made on the basis of longitudinal rather than cross-sectional assessment. This is important, as an early putative phenotype for bipolar disorder (severe mood dysregulation) was shown to prospectively predict unipolar depression but not bipolar disorder. To reduce the confusion between severe mood dysregulation and non-episodic irritability with bipolar disorder not otherwise specified (NOS) or bipolar spectrum, a new diagnostic category has been added in DSM-5: disruptive mood dysregulation disorder. However, such approaches demonstrate the difficulties with the current classification system—namely that it overemphasizes reliability. Presently, this 'new' diagnosis is not supported by any empirical studies on this DSM-5 proposed disorder, and the diagnostic utility in clinical populations is still unclear (Axelson et al. 2012; Copeland et al. 2013).

Among the group of patients diagnosed with bipolar disorder there is a vast variety of clinical presentations, previous illness and treatment histories, treatment responses, and degrees of residual symptoms with cognitive or functional impairment. Moreover, patients may or may not have a family history of mood disorders, a personal biography complicated by traumatic life events, or a comorbid anxiety disorder, substance abuse disorder, or personality disorder. Still, treatment practice, treatment guidelines, and clinical trials tend to disregard this heterogeneity and lump patients together under the shared diagnosis of bipolar disorder, only to be differentiated into large subcategories such as bipolar I, bipolar II, or bipolar NOS. Although the cross-sectional clinical syndromes of mania, hypomania, and depression may have many similarities among patients, it is in the longitudinal illness progression where the individual differences become apparent. It is therefore not surprising that treatment response and outcome may differ considerably within a group of bipolar patients, be it in an outpatients treatment programme or in a formal clinical trial. In an era where early intervention and personalized treatment become issues of growing interest, clinical staging of psychiatric disorders is one approach to deal with individual differences in illness progression, complementing traditional classification.

Staging in medicine and psychiatry

The prototypical example of staging systems in medicine is the TNM system in oncology. This classification scheme that was intended to encompass all aspects of cancer in terms of primary tumour (T), regional lymph nodes (N), and distant metastasis (M) was first introduced by the International Union Against Cancer (UICC) in 1958 for worldwide use. Numbers are added to denote tumour size and degree of involvement; for example, 0 indicates undetectable, and 1, 2, 3, and 4 a progressive increase in size or involvement. Thus, a tumour may be described as T1, N2, M0. The TNM staging system is a 'bin model'; the TNM prognostic factors are used to create a mutually exclusive and exhaustive partitioning of patients, so that every patient is in one particular bin, and the bins are grouped together into larger bins called stages (Burke and Henson 1993). Stages range from 0 (carcinoma in situ) via stage I, II, and III (indicating progressively extensive disease with larger tumour size and/or spread of the cancer beyond the organ in which it first developed to nearby lymph nodes and/or tissues or organs adjacent to the location of the primary tumour) to stage IV (indicating that the cancer has spread to distant tissues or organs). The utility of the system arises from its ability to order patients by a decreasing probability of survival. It can be used for selecting patients for therapy and for providing patients with an estimate of their prognosis. The TNM system is adapted for various sorts of solid tumours but is not applicable to every form of cancer.

In the field of cardiology, a staging system used by the American College of Cardiology/American Heart Association for grading heart failure is defined by the following four stages (Hunt et al. 2009): stage A (high risk of heart failure but no structural heart disease or symptoms of heart failure), stage B (structural heart disease but no symptoms of heart failure), stage C (structural heart disease and symptoms of heart failure), and stage D (refractory heart failure requiring specialized interventions). Staging systems are used in many other areas of medicine, like rheumatology, neurology, endocrinology, and nephrology.

Staging systems in psychiatry are hampered by the fact that the pathophysiology of psychiatric illness is still largely unknown, and recognition of structural or neurobiological markers is currently in its infancy. Disorders are defined by their clinical symptomatology and, to a lesser extent, by their longitudinal clinical course. Moreover, there is a considerable overlap between the phenomenology of many diagnostic categories. Nevertheless there is a need for timely recognition, applying effective treatments, and making a reasonably reliable prognosis. In this chapter we discuss how staging complements traditional diagnostic approaches to bipolar disorders. Fava and Kellner (1993) are credited with the first attempts to construct staging models for psychiatry. Their first proposals included outlines for schizophrenia, depression, bipolar disorder, and panic disorder. In that original article, they described a staging model of mania with four phases: (1) prodromal, that is, increased self-confidence, energy, and elated mood; (2) hypomania; (3) manic episode without psychotic features; and (4) manic episode with psychotic features. Their model of mania was restricted to a single manic episode, and thus did not refer to bipolar disorder, let alone its longitudinal course. Recently, Cosci and Fava (2013) reviewed the literature on staging of a range of mental disorders, and derived a general template with the following stages: (1) prodromal phase, (2) acute manifestations, (3) residual phase, and (4) recurrent or chronic disorder. Critics of this approach highlight that the model does not incorporate the 'at risk' phase that is typical of medical models (Hickie et al. 2013; Scott et al. 2013). As summarized in Table 2.2, other researchers, especially McGorry et al. (2006, 2010), have proposed a model for psychosis and severe mood disorders that extends from an asymptomatic at-risk stage (stage 0) to a severe, persistent illness (stage 4). These authors have a more transdiagnostic approach to staging, in contrast to the disorder-specific approach taken in this chapter.

Table 2.2 Proposed 'combined' or trans-diagnostic staging model for psychotic and severe mood disorders (data from Scott et al. (2013) and McGorry et al. (2006, 2010))

Stage	Definition of stage (psychosis or severe mood disorder)
0	Increased risk of psychotic or severe mood disorder. No symptoms currently
Ia	Mild or non-specific symptoms (including subtle neurocognitive deficits) of psychosis or severe mood disorder. Mild functional change or decline
Ib	Ultra-high risk: moderate but subthreshold symptoms, with neurocognitive changes and functional decline to caseness (GAF < 70)
II	First episode of psychotic or severe mood disorder. Full threshold disorder with moderate to severe symptoms, neurocognitive deficits and functional decline (GAF 30–50)
IIIa	Incomplete remission from first episode of care (patient's management could be linked or fast-tracked to stage IV)
IIIb	Recurrence with relapse of psychotic or mood disorder which stabilizes with treatment at a GAF level ≤ 30, or with residual symptoms or neurocognition below the best level achieved after remission from the first episode
IIIc	Multiple relapses with worsening in clinical extent and impact of illness objectively present
IV	Severe, persistent or unremitting illness as judged by symptoms, neurocognition and disability criteria

GAF, Global Assessment of Functioning Scale.

Staging in bipolar disorder

As outlined by Post in Chapter 1, systematic longitudinal observations of manic–depressive illness initiated by Kraepelin and others in the late nineteenth century have delineated various patterns of illness progression, and given rise to several theories about the underlying mechanisms. There is a general tendency of recurrence, with increasing frequency of episodes, and decreasing levels of cognitive and psychosocial functioning, although not all patients progress to such a poor prognosis. As bipolar disorder has its peak age at onset in adolescence or early adulthood, the illness process may interfere significantly with educational, vocational, and interpersonal development. There is evidence that repeated episodes of mania (especially when accompanied by psychotic features) may lead to neurocognitive decline, and alongside the debilitating effects of interepisode subsyndromal symptoms it is hypothesized that individuals develop both a neurobiological scar and an emotional/psychosocial scar.

This evidence of decline in psychobiosocial functioning underlines the need for (as) early (as possible) intervention, and thus the identification of risk factors, prodromal symptoms, and effective diagnosis of initial illness episodes. Staging models therefore typically start before the illness becomes manifest. Currently, two complementary 'bipolar-specific' staging models have been described: the one mainly focused on illness episodes (Berk et al. 2007), the other mainly on inter-episode functioning (Kapczinski et al. 2009a) (Table 2.3). Other researchers (e.g. McNamara et al. 2010) have proposed similar models, but we focus in this chapter on the two original published systems.

The staging model by Berk et al.

The staging model of bipolar disorder as proposed by Berk et al. (2007) is based on the McGorry model described previously (Table 2.3 and Fig. 2.2). Illness progression is mainly defined by the occurrence, remission, and recurrence of mood episodes.

Table 2.3 Comparison of the complementary staging models of bipolar disorder as data from Berk et al. (2007) with emphasis on episode recurrence, and Kapczinski et al. (2009a) with emphasis on interepisode functioning; the respective timing and numbering of stages do not fully correspond due to different focus.

Stage	Berk et al. staging model	Stage	Kapczinski et al. staging model
0	Increased risk of bipolar disorder	Latent	Increased risk of bipolar disorder
1a	Mild or non-specific symptoms of mood disorder		Mood or anxiety symptoms without criteria for threshold BD
1b	Prodromal features: ultra-high risk		
2	First threshold mood episode	1	Well-defined periods of euthymia without overt psychiatric symptoms
3a	Recurrence of sub-threshold mood symptoms		
3b	First threshold relapse	2	Symptoms in interepisode periods related to comorbidities
3c	Multiple relapses	3	Marked impairment in cognition and functioning
4	Persistent unremitting illness	4	Unable to live autonomously owing to cognitive and functional impairment

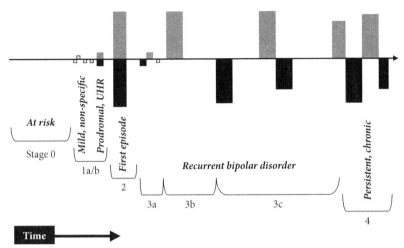

Fig. 2.2 Graphic representation of the staging model of bipolar disorder as proposed by Berk et al. (2007). Mania/hypomania above baseline, depression below baseline. First episode may be depression or (hypo)mania, or biphasic, but bipolar disorder can only be diagnosed after a first (hypo)manic episode (see text).

Reprinted from Bipolar Disorders, 9:, Berk M, Conus P, Lucas N, et al., Setting the stage: from prodrome to treatment resistance in bipolar disorder, pp. 671–8, Copyright (2007), with permission from John Wiley & Sons Ltd.

Persons at risk (stage 0) are mainly those with a family history of bipolar disorder. However, in practice, clinicians also recognize the role of additional psychosocial risk factors, including childhood physical or sexual abuse, death of a close relative, and substance abuse. During the prodromal stages(1a and 1b) mild and non-specific symptoms occur, such as mood lability, anxiety, sleep disturbances, irritability, aggressiveness, and hyperactivity (Reichart et al. 2004; Skjelstad et al. 2010). Non-specific symptoms may evolve to subsyndromal mood disorder (dysthymia or cyclothymia) as a sign of ultra-high risk, or may resolve with no further progression (Hickie et al. 2013). Stage 2 is defined by the occurrence of the first mood episode that meets traditional diagnostic criteria. If this is a clear-cut manic episode, then the formal diagnosis of bipolar disorder is established. However, first-episode mania can present with significant psychotic features, in which case the differential diagnosis between affective or non-affective psychosis can be difficult. In the case of a hypomanic first episode, this may not be recognized as a pathological state. In the majority of individuals, bipolar disorder starts

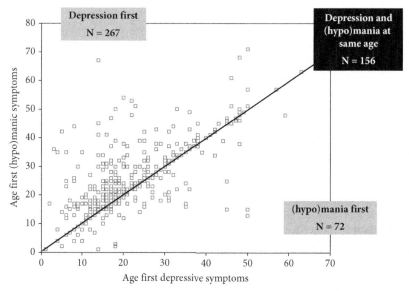

Fig. 2.3 Age at onset in 495 patients with bipolar I or II disorder, as retrospectively assessed in the Stanley Foundation Bipolar Network. In patients with depression as first episode a definite diagnoses of bipolar disorder will be delayed (data from Kupka et al. 2005).

with a depressive episode. Retrospective assessment of first mood episode in 495 patients with bipolar I or II disorder revealed that in more than half of the patients depression preceded (hypo)mania, often by many years (Kupka et al. 2005) (Fig. 2.3).

Prospective assessments of offspring of bipolar parents have shown that in virtually all patients a depressive episode precedes the occurrence of the first hypomanic or manic episode by years (Hillegers et al. 2005; Duffy et al. 2010; Mesman et al. 2013). In all these cases a diagnosis of depressive disorder will be made, which may or may not evolve to bipolar disorder depending on the later incidence of (hypo)mania. If so, then the age at onset of bipolar disorder is technically the age of the first depressive episode. Patients frequently have two to four depressions before a (hypo)manic episode. Such a clinical course demonstrates the inadequacies of the current systems, as the individual will initially be diagnosed with recurrent depression rather than bipolar disorder. Also it shows that the 'staging' system is imperfect, as in a staging system for depression the patient will be viewed as stage 3, whilst in a bipolar disorder system, they would be viewed as stage 2 (this issue is discussed elsewhere in the book).

Thus, from a prospective point of view, there are limitations to the Berk et al. model, especially when early recognition and intervention is aimed at bipolar disorder, and not at mood disorders in general. The occurrence of one or more depressive episodes in a young person at risk for bipolar disorder (i.e. those in stage 0 or 1a/b) should therefore be viewed with extra caution. If bipolar disorder is a potential long-term outcome, one of the clinical dilemmas may be when to start long-term prophylactic treatment.

When mood symptoms or mood episodes recur, the patient enters stage 3. Longitudinal studies give strong evidence that bipolar disorder has a recurrent course in most cases (Goodwin and Jamison 2007). Outpatients with bipolar disorder who were prospectively followed in naturalistic studies were, on average, half of the time symptomatic, despite treatment (Judd et al. 2002, 2003; Kupka et al. 2007). Subsyndromal depression prevails, and is a risk factor for recurrence of any type of episode of bipolar disorder. Residual depressive symptoms also may account for the considerable degree of functional impairment in patients in stages 3 and 4.

At stage 4 symptoms have become chronic, often manifested as either persistent depression or rapid cycling (Fig. 2.1). Post et al. (2003) reported that about a quarter of bipolar patients in a naturalistic cohort had a chronic course. Rapid cycling is prevalent in about 16% of bipolar patients in clinical research samples, and can be temporary or occur continuously over longer periods, and is in general a predictor of poor outcome (Kupka et al. 2003). The patients classified as being in stage 4 bipolar disorders are often middle-aged adults with established bipolar disorder who also may be unresponsive to multiple treatment modalities, although treatment resistance may also be caused by inadequate treatment trials or non-adherence. Risk-factors that play a role in early onset of bipolar disorder (e.g. a family history of bipolar disorder, a history of childhood abuse, a history of anxiety disorder or substance abuse) are also associated with subsequent progression to stage 4 (Kupka et al. 2005). As can be seen from this description, cases presenting in this stage resemble those typically seen in psychiatric settings. However, a clear goal of employing staging models is to 'shift' the interventions towards the initial phases of illness in order to target treatment preferably at stages 2 and 3 (and ultimately at even earlier stages), in order to try to minimize the number of individuals who progress to stage 4.

The staging model by Kapczinski et al.

Whereas the staging model of Berk et al. fundamentally uses mood symptomatology and the pattern of episode recurrence as the main determinant of illness progression, Kapczinski et al. (2009a, b) and Fries et al. (2012) proposed a staging model that emphasizes the assessment of patients in the interepisode period, focusing on the level of cognitive and psychosocial functioning rather than on the number, recurrence, and severity of mood episodes per se. The basic assumption in this model is that functional disability and cognitive decline are more direct measures of underlying neuroprogression, and as such would be able to more accurately predict long-term treatment needs. The latent stage in this model allows the presence of subsyndromal mood and anxiety symptoms in persons at risk for bipolar disorder based on a positive family history, but without cognitive impairment. In stage 1 the patient fully recovers from mood episodes (regardless of their number and severity) without psychiatric morbidity or cognitive impairment in the interepisode period. It is important to notice however that incomplete functional recovery is common, even after a first major mood episode, especially psychotic mania (Conus et al. 2006). In stage 2 psychiatric symptoms persist, either from rapid cycling bipolar disorder or psychiatric comorbidities like substance abuse, anxiety disorders, or personality disorders, but there is only transient cognitive impairment. Stage 3 is characterized by subsyndromal symptoms of bipolar disorder and/or marked cognitive impairment associated with functional impairment, leading to inability to work or the ability to work only with very impaired performance. In stage 4, the patient is unable to live autonomously due to severe cognitive and functional disability.

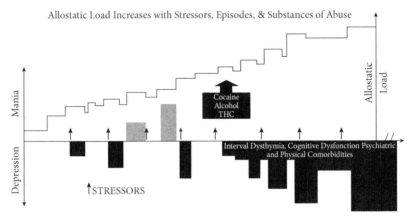

Fig. 2.4 Graphic representation of allostatic load in the staging model of bipolar disorder as proposed by Kapczinski et al. (2008). Allostatic load can be defined as 'the wear and tear on the body' which grows over time when the individual is exposed to repeated or chronic stress.

Reprinted from Neurosci Biobehav Rev, 32, Kapczinski F, Vieta E, Andreazza AC, Frey BN, Gomes FA, Tramontina J, Kauer-Sant'anna M, Grassi-Oliveira R, Post RM., Allostatic load in bipolar disorder: implications for pathophysiology and treatment, 675–92, Copyright (2008), with permission from Elsevier.

Critics of this model suggest that it is overly focused on the post-illness onset bipolar disorder subtypes, but Kapczinski and his group highlight that the clinical stages they describe are compatible with the biological concept of allostatic load, defined as the 'wear and tear' of the body and the brain resulting from chronic overactivity or inactivity of physiological systems that are involved in the adaptation to environmental challenges (McEwen and Wingfield 2003; Kapczinski et al. 2008). They propose that allostatic load progressively increases with repeated episodes as a function of cumulative stressors, mood changes and exposure to other factors such as drugs of abuse. Increased allostatic load then leads to cognitive impairment, intermittent dysthymia and increased rates of physical and psychiatric comorbidities (Fig. 2.4).

The prodromal and early stages of bipolar disorder

Due to the non-specific nature of early psychiatric symptoms, with even (hypo)manic symptoms being transient in the majority of adolescents in the general population (Tijssen et al. 2010), and the difficulty in predicting whether early onset depression will evolve into a unipolar or bipolar disorder, the reliable and valid identification of a 'bipolar prodrome' is difficult. Further, in an ideal situation, we would not rely on prodromes (which by definition can only be fully described *after* a disease onset), but would have prospectively defined precursor syndromes to allow us to estimate future risk of bipolar disorder onset. These precursor syndromes consist of signs and symptoms from a diagnostic cluster that precede disorder, but do not predict the onset of a specific disorder with certainty (Eaton et al. 1995). Given the widespread prevalence of individual signs and symptoms of mental disorders in the general population, it is likely that not many individuals will go on to develop the full-blown disorder, or individuals who present with similar problems in early childhood may grow up to develop different adult mental disorders. Combining risk factors (i.e. individual characteristics associated with increased probability of later onset of disorder) and prodromal symptoms could facilitate the identification of target population for prevention. However, until such data are available, it is helpful to examine prodromal features.

The initial prodrome may be defined as the time interval from the onset of the first noticeable signs and symptoms to the onset of a fully developed and diagnosable disorder. A distinction between a distal and a proximal prodrome has been proposed which respectively denominate the early and late stages of the initial prodrome. In a review on the prodrome of bipolar disorder irritability and aggressiveness, sleep disturbances, affective dysregulation, hyperactivity, and anxiety are clusters representing common symptoms and signs of the distal prodrome of bipolar disorder (Skjelstad et al. 2013). As the individual progresses through stage 1 towards stage 2, symptoms of mania and depression seem to increase gradually in severity and prevalence, referring to the proximal prodrome (Zeschel et al. 2013). However, the specificity of prodromal symptoms and signs appears to be low (Skjelstad et al. 2013).

One way to understand the early stages of bipolar disorder is to examine groups that are known to be at high risk such as the offspring of parents with bipolar disorder. Although non-affective childhood psychiatric symptoms and diagnoses (e.g. anxiety, sleep, and behavioural problems) may have different significance in the offspring of bipolar disorder parents than in controls or unselected clinical paediatric samples, these prospective studies are proving invaluable in the exploration of the earliest manifestations of future bipolar disorder (Birmaher et al. 2006; Duffy et al. 2010, 2013). The findings in bipolar offspring also reinforce the importance of family history in evaluating the meaning of behavioural problems and diagnoses in children and adolescents, and support a different monitoring and management strategy for children and adolescents with a positive family history of bipolar disorder.

Implications of clinical staging systems

Neuroprogression, neuroprotection, and stage-specific biomarkers

Several biological hypotheses have tried to address the progressive nature of mood disorders, and these clearly link with the clinical notion of disease progression that is at the core of staging models. For example, the concepts of kindling, stress, and episode sensitization, and allostatic load all offer putative mechanisms to explain the phenomena of neuroprogression. This can be defined as the pathological rewiring of the brain that takes place when a clinical and cognitive deterioration occurs in the context of the progression of psychiatric disorders (Berk 2009; Berk et al. 2010; Fries et al. 2012). Neuroprogression can be viewed as a multifactorial and interactive process leading to a loss of cellular resilience and may include alterations in the dopaminergic system, inflammatory cytokines, oxidative stress, mitochondrial and endoplasmatic reticulum stress, as well as changes in neurotrophins such as brain-derived neurotrophic factor (BDNF) (Berk et al. 2011). It is hypothesized that every progressive stage of the illness has a particular set of putative genetic, structural, and biochemical biomarkers (Kapczinski et al. 2009b; Fries et al. 2012).

Given the emphasis on neuroprogressive changes, it is logical that the concept of neuroprotection is also part of the dialogue about staging. Neuroprotection refers to the putative mechanisms and pathways by which mood stabilizers such as lithium and sodium valproate counteract the process of neuroprogression, providing a further rationale for early intervention in established cases (those at stage 2 or more), although it is less clear whether these treatments are also the preferred interventions for stages 0 or 1 (Scott et al. 2013).

Clinical staging and intervention

An important goal of applying staging models is that it enhances the clinical treatment process by means of a more precise definition of stage-appropriate treatment interventions for individual patients (Scott et al. 2013; Berk et al. 2013). However, research on appropriate clinical interventions for stages 0 to 1 are in their infancy, so most attempts to link interventions to staging are based on clinical common sense (i.e. on what we know in general about the efficacy of treatments in bipolar disorder). For example, there is indirect support for the idea that introducing treatments at an earlier stage in the illness may produce more benefit than if these treatments are delayed until stage 4. Clinical trials demonstrated that both lithium and cognitive behavioural therapy were less effective in individuals with bipolar disorder who had experienced more than 12 prior mood episodes (Scott et al. 2006).

Berk et al. (2007) suggest potential interventions targeted to each stage of bipolar disorder. In their model, they suggest that in the early stages (stages 0 and 1a), interventions should include mental health literacy, self-help, family psychoeducation, cognitive therapy, and 'harm reduction' (reducing use or misuse of alcohol and other substances). In the first symptomatic stages (stages 1b and 2), phase specific or mood stabilizing pharmacotherapy is added, and attention is given to vocational rehabilitation. In the later stages (stage 3a–c), the emphasis lies on maintenance medications, often involving the use of combinations of mood stabilizers, and relapse prevention techniques such as psychosocial therapies. In stage 4, treatment is more focused on rehabilitation, and symptomatic treatments, plus efforts to retain or enhance social participation, despite disability.

Kapczinski et al. (2009a, b) also delineate treatments to prevent disease progression, but discuss more explicitly the notion of reducing the exposure to pathogenic risk factors (e.g. substance abuse) in the latent stage. The other interventions mirror those suggested by Berk and colleagues, including mood stabilizer monotherapy, psychoeducation, and cognitive-behavioural therapy at stage 1; combined pharmacotherapy plus psychotherapy, vocational rehabilitation, and a focus on the treatment of comorbidities at stage 2; the use of complex combination pharmacotherapy regiments and treatment in specialized centres at stage 3; and then a 'palliative care' approach to stage 4 illness.

Conclusion

Several staging models of bipolar disorder have been proposed, each approaching illness progression from a different perspective. The two main 'disorder-specific' models used in bipolar disorder research are based on an increasing episode recurrence (Berk's model) and a decreasing interepisode functioning (Kapczinski's model), and thus these approaches can be viewed as complementing each other. In contrast to classification systems such as DSM-5, these staging models do not take illness subtypes, risk factors, and specifiers into account. Combining both approaches might be a further step towards a more refined, personalized diagnosis. Both staging models assume an underlying pathophysiological process of neuroprogression, associated with neuroanatomical changes, loss of cellular resilience, and cognitive decline. However, not every patient will proceed through all stages. Much current research in bipolar disorder has been performed in samples of relatively late stage bipolar disorder, and might give an overly pessimistic view of illness progression and prognosis. Both staging models promote the notion of timely diagnosis and early intervention to prevent future decline. Early detection is, however, hampered by the lack of specificity of the earliest stages of bipolar disorder and the lack of transdiagnostic data to allow better characterization of any specific precursors of bipolar disorder. This makes a distinction between the early stages of psychotic, depressive, and bipolar disorders difficult, but also means it is not straightforward to differentiate normal temperament and transient behavioural changes in young adults from psychopathology indicative of an emerging severe mental disorder. At the other end of the disease timeline, late stages of severe mental disorders may also be difficult to differentiate, since disorder-specific symptomatic episodes may be overshadowed by a more generic disability resulting from cognitive and functional decline (Scott et al. 2013). Thus, attracting more support for clinical staging models will be partly dictated by our ability to identify stage-specific and potentially disorder-specific biomarkers that help to choose the most effective acute and prophylactic treatment.

Overall, this chapter offers an introduction to staging models, but it is important to emphasize that this is a rapidly expanding field of research in psychiatry. So, although staging models in psychiatry are still in their early stages, we anticipate that there will be further discussion about both disease-specific and trans-diagnostic staging models. The evidence for these will evolve when they are formally tested in longitudinal designs combining clinical and neurobiological studies.

References

American Psychiatric Association (2013) Diagnostic and Statistical Manual of Mental Disorders, fifth edition. Washington: American Psychiatric Publishing.

Axelson D, Findling RL, Fristad MA, et al. (2012) Examining the proposed disruptive mood dysregulation disorder diagnosis in children in the Longitudinal Assessment of Manic Symptoms study. J Clin Psychiat 73:1342–1350.

Baroni A, Lunsford JR, Luckenbaugh DA, et al. (2009) Practitioner review: the assessment of bipolar disorder in children and adolescents. J Child Psychol Psyc 50:203–215.

Berk M (2009) Neuroprogression: pathways to progressive brain changes in bipolar disorder. Int J Neuropsychoph 12:441–445.

Berk M, Berk L, Dodd S, et al. (2014) Stage managing bipolar disorder. Bipolar Disord 16:471–477.

Berk M, Conus P, Kapczinski F, et al. (2010) From neuroprogression to neuroprotection: implications for clinical care. Med J Aust 193(4 Suppl):S36–40.

Berk M, Conus P, Lucas N, et al. (2007) Setting the stage: from prodrome to treatment resistance in bipolar disorder. Bipolar Disord 9:671–678.

Berk M, Kapczinski F, Andreazza AC, et al. (2011) Pathways underlying neuroprogression in bipolar disorder: focus on inflammation, oxidative stress and neurotrophic factors. Neurosci Biobehav R 35:804–817.

Birmaher B, Axelson D, Strober M, et al. (2006) Clinical course of children and adolescents with bipolar spectrum disorders. Arch Gen Psychiat 63:175–183.

Brotman MA, Schmajuk M, Rich BA, et al. (2006) Prevalence, clinical correlates, and longitudinal course of severe mood dysregulation in children. Biol Psychiat 60:991–997.

Burke HB and Henson DE (1993) Criteria for prognostic factors and for an enhanced prognostic system. Cancer 72:3131–3135.

Carlson GA and Glovinsky I (2009). The concept of bipolar disorder in children: a history of the bipolar controversy. Child Adolesc Psychiatr Clin N Am **18**:257–271.

Conus P, Cotton S, Abdel-Baki A, et al. (2006) Symptomatic and functional outcome 12 months after a first episode of psychotic mania: barriers to recovery in a catchment area sample. Bipolar Disord **8**:221–231.

Copeland WE, Angold A, Costello EJ, et al. (2013) Prevalence, comorbidity, and correlates of DSM-5 proposed disruptive mood dysregulation disorder. Am J Psychiat **170**:173–179.

Cosci F and Fava GA (2013) Staging of mental disorders: systematic review. Psychother Psychosom **82**:20–34.

Duffy A, Alda M, Hajek T, et al. (2010) Early stages in the development of bipolar disorder. J Affect Disorders **121**:127–135.

Duffy A, Horrocks J, Doucette S, et al. (2013) Childhood anxiety: an early predictor of mood disorders in offspring of bipolar parents. J Affect Disorders **150**:363–369.

Eaton WW, Badawi M, and Melton B (1995) Prodromes and precursors: epidemiologic data for primary prevention of disorders with slow onset. Am J Psychiat **152**:967–972.

Fava GA and Kellner R (1993) Staging—a neglected dimension in psychiatric classification. Acta Psychiat Scand **87**:225–230.

Fries GR, Pfaffenseller B, Stertz L, et al. (2012) Staging and neuroprogression in bipolar disorder. Curr Psychiat Rep **14**:667–675.

Goodwin FK and Jamison KR (2007) Manic-depressive Illness, 2nd edition. New York: Oxford University Press.

Hickie IB, Scott J, Hermens DF, et al. (2013) Clinical classification in mental health at the cross-roads: which direction next? BMC Med **11**:125.

Hillegers MH, Reichart CG, Wals M, et al. (2005) Five-year prospective outcome of psychopathology in the adolescent offspring of bipolar parents. Bipolar Disord **7**:344–350.

Hunt SA, Abraham WT, Chin MH, et al., and the American College of Cardiology Foundation; American Heart Association (2009) Focused update incorporated into the ACC/AHA 2005 guidelines for the diagnosis and management of heart failure in adults: a report of the American College of Cardiology Foundation/ American Heart Association Task Force on practice guidelines developed in collaboration with the International Society for Heart and Lung Transplantation. J Am Coll Cardiol **53**(15):e1–e90.

Judd LJ, Akiskal HS, Schettler PJ, et al. (2002) The long-term natural history of the weekly symptomatic status of bipolar I disorder. Arch Gen Psychiat **59**:530–537.

Judd LJ, Akiskal HS, Schettler PJ, et al. (2003) A prospective investigation of the natural history of the long-term weekly symptomatic status of bipolar II disorder. Arch Gen Psychiat **60**:261–269.

Kapczinski F, Dias VV, Kauer-Sant'Anna M, et al. (2009a) Clinical implications of a staging model for bipolar disorders. Expert Rev Neurother **9**:957–966.

Kapczinski F, Dias VV, Kauer-Sant'Anna M, et al. (2009b) The potential use of bio-markers as an adjunctive tool for staging bipolar disorder. Prog Neuropsychopha **33**:1366–1371.

Kapczinski F, Vieta E, Andreazza AC, et al. (2008) Allostatic load in bipolar disorder: implications for pathophysiology and treatment. Neurosci Biobehav R **32**:675–692.

Kupka RW, Altshuler LL, Nolen WA, et al. (2007) Three times more depression than mania in both bipolar I and bipolar II disorder. Bipolar Disord **9**:531–535.

Kupka RW, Luckenbaugh DA, Post RM, et al. (2003) Rapid and non-rapid cycling bipolar disorder: a meta-analysis of clinical studies. J Clin Psychiat **64**:1483–1494.

Kupka RW, Luckenbaugh DA, Post RM, et al. (2005) Comparison of rapid-cycling and non-rapid-cycling bipolar disorder based on prospective mood ratings in 539 outpatients. Am J Psychiat **162**:1273–1280.

Leibenluft E, Cohen P, Gorrindo T, et al. (2006) Chronic versus episodic irritability in youth: a community-based, longitudinal study of clinical and diagnostic associations. J Child Adol Psychop **16**:456–466.

Margulies DM, Weintraub S, Basile J, et al. (2012) Will disruptive mood dysregulation disorder reduce false diagnosis of bipolar disorder in children? Bipolar Disord **14**:488–496.

McEwen BS and Wingfield JC (2003) The concept of allostasis in biology and biomedicine. Horm Behav **43**:2–15.

McGorry PD, Hickie IB, Yung AR, et al. (2006) Clinical staging of psychiatric disorders: a heuristic framework for choosing earlier, safer and more effective interventions. Aust NZ J Psychiat **40**:616–622.

McGorry PD, Nelson B, Goldstone S, et al. (2010) Clinical staging: a heuristic and practical strategy for new research and better health and social outcomes for psychotic and related mood disorders. Can J Psychiat **55**:486–497.

McNamara RK, Nandagopal JJ, Strakowski SM, et al. (2010) Preventative strategies for early-onset bipolar disorder: towards a clinical staging model. CNS Drugs **24**:983–996.

Merikangas KR, Jin R, He JP, et al. (2011) Prevalence and correlates of bipolar spectrum disorder in the world mental health survey initiative. Arch Gen Psychiat **68**:241–251.

Mesman E, Nolen WA, Reichart CG, et al. (2013) The Dutch bipolar offspring study: 12-year follow-up. Am J Psychiat **170**:542–549.

Moreno C, Laje G, Blanco C, et al. (2007) National trends in the outpatient diagnosis and treatment of bipolar disorder in youth. Arch Gen Psychiat **64**:1032–1039.

Post RM, Denicoff KD, Leverich GS, et al. (2003) Morbidity in 258 bipolar outpatients followed for 1 year with daily prospective ratings on the NIMH Life Chart Method. J Clin Psychiat **64**:680–690.

Reichart CG, Wals M, Hillegers MH, et al. (2004) Psychopathology in the adolescent offspring of bipolar parents. J Affect Disorders **78**:67–71.

Rich BA, Schmajuk M, Perez-Edgar KE, et al. (2007) Different psychophysiological and behavioral responses elicited by frustration in pediatric bipolar disorder and severe mood dysregulation. Am J Psychiat 164:309–317.

Scott J, Leboyer M, Hickie I, et al. (2013) Clinical staging in psychiatry: a cross-cutting model of diagnosis with heuristic and practical value. Brit J Psychiat 202:243–245.

Scott J, Paykel E, Morriss R, et al. (2006) Cognitive-behavioural therapy for severe and recurrent bipolar disorders: randomised controlled trial. Brit J Psychiat 188:313–320.

Skirrow C, Hosang GM, Farmer AE, et al. (2012) An update on the debated association between ADHD and bipolar disorder across the lifespan. J Affect Disorders 141:143–159.

Skjelstad DV, Malt UF, and Holte A (2010) Symptoms and signs of the initial prodrome of bipolar disorder: a systematic review. J Affect Disorders 126:1–13.

Tijssen MJ, van Os J, Wittchen HU, et al. (2010) Evidence that bipolar disorder is the poor outcome fraction of a common developmental phenotype: an 8-year cohort study in young people. Psychol Med 40:289–299.

World Health Organization (2001) The World Health Report 2001, Mental Health: New Understanding, New Hope. Geneva: World Health Organization.

Zeschel E, Correll CU, Haussleiter IS, et al. (2013) The bipolar disorder prodrome revisited: Is there a symptomatic pattern? J Affect Disorders 151:551–560.

Chapter 3

Allostatic load and accelerated ageing in bipolar disorder

Iria Grande and Flavio Kapczinski

Introduction

Bipolar disorder (BD) is among the world's 10 most disabling conditions regarding burden of disability (Kupfer 2005). This global load encompasses not only the inner chronicity of the affective disorder with mood swings but a wide range of comorbid medical and psychiatric conditions as well as neurocognitive deterioration that have been reported to be more prevalent in patients with BD compared to the healthy population.

Regarding comorbidities, patients with BD mostly develop cardiovascular morbidity and mortality (Angst et al. 2002; Birkenaes et al. 2007). It could be advocated that this is a consequence of psychiatric treatment, and is certainly so to some extent—concerning atypical antipsychotic treatment. Nevertheless, many reports support the independent link between cardiovascular disorders and BD (Garcia-Portilla et al. 2009). Moreover, the prevalence of psychiatric comorbidity is high in BD, substance use and anxiety disorders being the most frequent (Merikangas et al. 2007; Mantere et al. 2010). BD has also been associated with significant neurocognitive deficits across all mood states, as well as in euthymia (Martínez-Arán et al. 2004b). Such dysfunction seems to be related to the severity of disease as well as the presence of psychotic symptoms, longer duration of the illness, and higher number of manic episodes (Robinson and Ferrier 2006).

The aforementioned systemic consequences of BD, which embrace comorbidities and neurocognitive deficits, can be studied in the light of the concept of allostatic load (Kapczinski et al. 2008; Grande et al. 2012). Sterling and Eyer (1988) first employed the term of *allostasis* and in the following years, McEwen and Stellar (1993) used it to define a wider concept of stress and its consequences. Allostasis is the ability to achieve stability through change produced by adaptive mechanisms that help us to deal with daily life situations. The term to define the systemic consequences of these adaptive mechanisms is *allostatic load* (AL).

In this chapter, we will portray the concept of allostasis, AL, and allostatic overload (AO), and their application to neuropsychiatric illnesses, especially BD, to explain the dimensional impact of mental disorders on the organism.

Coping with life events: allostasis and allostatic load

The brain is the key organ in the orchestration of stress response. It determines which events are threatening, and therefore potentially stressful, and also controls the behavioural and physiological responses, which are as important as the stressful experiences themselves to develop AL (McEwen 2008) (Fig. 3.1).

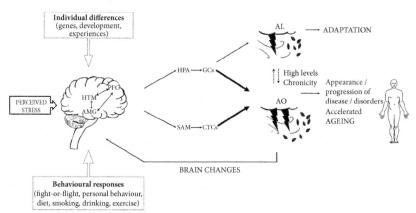

Fig. 3.1 Stress response and allostasis: the perception of stress is influenced by individual differences in constitution (genetic, development, experience) and behaviour (coping and health habits) that ultimately modulate individual resiliency to stress. When the brain perceives an event as stressful, physiologic responses are initiated mainly by the release of glucocorticoids and catecholamines by the hypothalamic-pituitary-adrenal (HPA) axis and the sympathetic-adrenal-medullary (SAM) axis, respectively, leading to the process of adaptive allostasis. If the allostatic load (AL) increases dramatically or becomes chronic and resiliency is not sufficient, AL will become AO, which serves no useful purpose, but rather conversely predisposes the individual to accelerated ageing and diseases.

HTM, hypothalamus; AMG, amygdala; PFC, prefrontal cortex; HPA, hypothalamic-pituitary-adrenal axis; GCs, glucocorticoids; SAM, sympathetic-adrenal-medullary axis; CTCs, catecholamines; AL, allostatic load; AO, allostatic overload.

Furthermore, individual differences also play a paramount role in the response to stress (Korte et al. 2005), based upon the experiences of the individual throughout life. For instance, positive or negative experiences in school, at work, or in interpersonal relationships can bias an individual towards either a positive or negative response in a new situation (McEwen 2008); this can be low familiar affection, which is known to produce long-lasting emotional problems in children (Repetti et al. 2002). Animal models have been useful in providing insight into behavioural and physiological mechanisms. For instance, early-life maternal care in rodents is a powerful determinant of stress hormone reactivity, and therefore life-long emotional reactivity in the offspring, as well as in future generations (Francis et al. 1999; Cavigelli and McClintock 2003). All these events may produce detained effects on brain structure and function, which may be observed later in life, and can increase the risk for developing psychiatric disorders (Kaufman et al. 2000; Vermetten et al. 2006). In particular, early-life experiences may carry even greater weight in terms of how an individual reacts to new situations, as early-life physical and sexual abuse are known to lead to a life-long burden of behavioural and pathophysiological problems (Garno et al. 2005; Leverich and Post 2006).

The brain assesses the threat and the execution of action by the hippocampal, amygdala, and prefrontal cortical regulation (McEwen 2007; Jankord and Herman 2008). Chronic stress is known to induce hyperactivation of the amygdala, enhancing amygdala-dependent unlearned fear, fear conditioning, and aggression (McEwen 2004). In BD, abnormalities in emotional processing involving this circuitry have been described, and an enlargement of the amygdala has been portrayed as the most prominent neurostructural abnormality in BD (Phillips and Vieta 2007; Strakowski et al. 2012; Townsend and Altshuler 2012). Similar results have also been found in functional neuroimaging, indicating increased activity in the amygdala during acute mood episodes and dysfunctional connectivity between the ventral prefrontal cortex and amygdala in the resting state (Versace et al. 2010; Pomarol-Clotet et al. 2012). Using amygdala-dependent tasks, manic and depressed subjects have also displayed alterations in facial recognition tests, identifying facial expressions less accurately than euthymic bipolar or healthy subjects (Chen et al. 2006). It has been also shown that patients with bipolar depression or mania may present increased subcortical and ventral prefrontal cortical responses to both positive and negative emotional facial expressions compared with healthy controls and major depression patients. Regarding episodic emotional memory, BD patients reportedly had no memorial enhancement for the emotional content of a story, and mislabelled the neutral information as emotional, contrary to the control subjects (Kauer-Sant'anna et al. 2008). These findings suggest that the amygdala and its related circuits seem to be overactive, but dysfunctional, in patients with BD. Therefore, it is likely that the gate system coding experiences as stressful is overactive but defective in patients with BD. Such dysfunction would render bipolar patients more vulnerable to stress and its neurobiological consequences.

Because the brain is the major regulator of the neuroendocrine, autonomic, and immune systems, as well as behaviour, alterations in brain function due to chronic stress can, therefore, have direct and indirect effects on the cumulative AL. These changes may induce synaptic and dendritic remodelling and structural atrophy or hypertrophy (Radley et al. 2006; Sotiropoulos et al. 2008; Bessa et al. 2009; Dias-Ferreira et al. 2009; Yu et al. 2010), which further diminish the body's ability to cognitively process and physiologically respond to stresssors (McEwen 2000; Liston et al. 2006). Real or interpreted threats in the brain initiate the hypothalamic-pituitary-adrenal (HPA) axis secretion of glucocorticoids and the sympathetic-adrenal-medullary (SAM) axis release of catecholamines that mobilize the energy necessary for fight-or-flight responses, increasing the AL so as to achieve allostatic equilibrium (Sapolsky et al. 2000) (Fig. 3.1).

On the one hand, mechanisms of adjustment are protective to obtain allostasis but on the other hand, adaptation is the price to pay for this forced re-setting of parameters while the body is forced to cope with adverse psychosocial or physical situations. AL represents either the presence of too much stress or the inefficiency of the stress hormone response system for instance, when mediators of allostasis are not turned off once stress is over, when they are not turned on adequately during stress, or when they are overused by many stressors (McEwen 1998). As mentioned previously, the HPA and SAM axes play a main role in allostasis. While they are acutely adaptive, their chronic overactivation induces a 'domino-effect' on interconnected biological systems that overcompensate and eventually collapse, leaving the organism susceptible to future stress-related diseases (McEwen 1998; Juster et al. 2010). Within limits, mechanisms related to allostasis are an adaptive response to internal and external demands (McEwen 2000). However, when there are extra loads, AL can increase. When the additional load grows dramatically, most often due to unpredictable events, AL becomes AO, which, contrary to AL, no longer holds a useful purpose and predisposes the individual to disease (Fig. 3.1). For instance, acute physiological increase of glucocorticoids promotes allostasis by regulation of the availability of energetic compounds, as previously mentioned. However, chronic elevated levels of adrenal steroids that result from overactivation of the HPA axis may induce insulin resistance, diabetes, obesity, atherosclerosis, and hypertension. In fact, patients with high AL have been described to have increased risk for incident cardiovascular disease, physical and cognitive decline, and all-cause mortality in cross-sectional and follow-up studies (Seeman et al. 1997, 2001, 2004; Karlamangla et al. 2002, 2005, 2006; Juster et al. 2010). As McEwen pointed out, there are differences between 'being stressed or stressed-out' (McEwen 2005).

Allostatic states are engendered by several factors such as catecholamines, glucocorticoids, inflammatory cytokines, and oxidative stress mediators which interact in a nonlinear manner (McEwen 1998; Juster et al. 2010). These represent the *primary mediators* (McEwen 2003a), and can be classified as *biomarkers*. Synergic effects of these molecules exert *primary effects* on cellular activities of enzymes, receptors, ion channels, or even genomics that compromise the physiological integrity of allostatic mechanisms. Over time, subsidiary biological systems compensate for over- and/or under-production of primary mediators and, in turn, shift their own operating ranges to maintain abated chemical, tissue, and organ functions. This state is characterized by the *secondary outcomes* whereby metabolic, cardiovascular, and immune parameters reach sub-clinical levels and define a prodromal condition. At a final stage, the culmination of physiological dysregulation leads to the *tertiary outcomes*, defined by disorders and diseases that result from AO (Juster et al. 2010). This interaction can be illustrated by the prolonged secretion of the stress hormones epinephrine (adrenaline), norepinephrine (noradrenaline), and cortisol that can falter in their ability to protect the distressed individual and instead begin to damage the brain and body (McEwen 2007). Stress hormones and their antagonists, in this case dehydroepiandrosterone, in conjunction with pro- and anti-inflammatory cytokines, such as interleukin-6 and tumour necrosis factor-alpha, represent the AL biomarkers. Synergistic effects of these molecules induce primary effects, which can lead to premorbid conditions such as alterations in parameters like levels of insulin, glucose, visceral fat deposits, and systolic and diastolic blood pressure. If this situation is maintained, the individual may develop diabetes, lipid disorders, or hypertension.

In nature, allostasis and AL are widespread concepts, which are not specific for humans and give an explanation to animal adaptive responses. For instance, bears eating large quantities of food and putting on body fat act as an energy source during hibernation in winter (Nelson 1980). This anticipatory accumulation of fat, which is useful for survival during winter, has an important adaptive value, albeit AL impact. The fat accumulation of bears that eat out of boredom while held captive in zoos could exemplify the pathophysiological state of AO. Along this same line, even adaptive situations such as the seasonal migration of salmon against the river current may lead to immune system alterations, accelerated ageing, and ultimately the death of individuals for the sake of the preservation of the species (Maule et al. 1989; McEwen and Wingfield 2003; Götz et al. 2005; Navarro and Boveris 2007). Increased levels of stress hormones (Vieta et al. 1997, 1999; Daban et al. 2006a), early ageing (Yatham et al. 2009), and dysfunction of the immune system (Brietzke et al. 2009) have also been reported among BD patients. In the successive section, we will describe the proposed relationship between AL and BD in depth.

Allostatic load in bipolar disorder

The concept of AL has been instrumental in the study of neuropsychiatric illnesses such as Alzheimer's disease (Swaab et al. 2005), post-traumatic stress disorder (Glover 2006), substance use disorder (Zimmermann et al. 2007), major depression (McEwen 2003b), and BD (Kapczinski et al. 2008) since it has provided a link between apparently separated dimensions such as cognitive dysfunction and bodily 'wear and tear' that have been reported among patients with chronic mental disorders. In the field of BD, our group and others have suggested that AL may provide a means to understand the consequences of the exposure to chronic stress such as accelerated ageing, deterioration, and diseases (Fig. 3.2).

Considering accelerated ageing, telomere length has been the focal point, as it is considered to be the 'molecular clock' of the cell. Telomeres shorten with time, and when they become critically short the risk of apoptosis increases and proliferation is arrested (Blasco 2007). In a preliminary study of accelerated ageing using a model of chronic stress, Simon et al. (2006) reported shortening of telomere length equivalent to 10 years in BD patients as compared to controls. Recently, Elvsåshagen et al. (2011) described an increased load of short telomeres in patients with bipolar type II disorder.

Regarding deterioration, significant neurocognitive deficits across all mood states have been reported as well as in euthymia (Martínez-Arán et al. 2004b). The more persistent cognitive deficits described in euthymia include attention, executive function, and verbal memory impairment (Martínez-Arán et al. 2004a; Mur et al. 2007; Bourne et al. 2013). These cognitive dysfunctions may reflect abnormal activation patterns in the brain, implicating the prefrontal cortex in the aetiopathogenesis of BD and indicating cortical-subcortical-limbic disruption as the underlying causes (Benabarre et al. 2005; Strakowski et al. 2012). Such deficits do not seem to be specific for BD and their pattern is quite similar to that described in patients with another chronic mental disorder such as schizophrenia (Martínez-Arán et al. 2002; Balanzá-Martínez et al. 2005; Daban et al. 2006b).

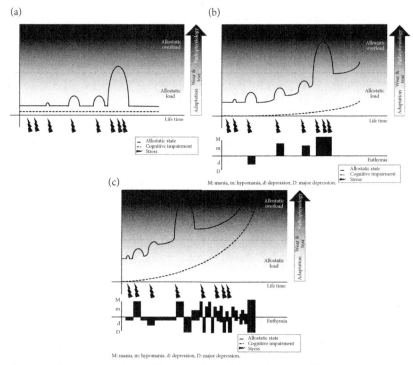

Fig. 3.2 Allostatic state during lifetime. Allostatic state is the equilibrium between stress and resilience. When stress is managed, the basal allostatic state is regained via mechanisms of resilience. An individual with a favourable genetic background, uneventful history, and personal abilities to handle problems will successfully cope with stressors during life and few dramatic allostatic state alterations will take place. (a) In the case of BD patients, basal resilience may not be as favourable and stress events can more easily facilitate AL or AO in the form of mood episodes. This can be exemplified by two possible scenes of BD evolution: (b) benign progression, in which resilience is able to deal with different stressors at the beginning, but as the AL increases, stressors result in mood episodes and cumulative AL and AO, (c) malignant evolution, in which resilience has difficulties in dealing with the load of stress from the very start. Cognitive impairment is also related to the allostatic state. In the benign progression, cognitive impairment would be expected to be rare but in the malignant forms it would be the rule rather than the exception.

M, mania; m, hypomania; d, depression; D, major depression.

BD carries a higher risk for medical comorbidity, including cardiovascular, metabolic, infectious, neurological, and respiratory disorders and has an earlier presentation (Kilbourne et al. 2004; Carney and Jones 2006). In addition, BD is associated with higher rates of the most frequent natural causes of death (Angst et al. 2002). This situation entails four times greater healthcare costs for patients with BD than costs for non-bipolar patients (Bryant-Comstock et al. 2002), being assigned a considerable part of the budget to medical illness (Gardner et al. 2006). Furthermore, several drugs used in the treatment of BD may account for higher medical comorbidity. For example, second-generation antipsychotics are associated with increased risk of weight gain and diabetes mellitus (McIntyre et al. 2001; Newcomer 2006; Torrent et al. 2008). It might be argued that the reasons for high medical comorbidity would be inadequate access to quality care, poor lifestyle choices, and adverse effects of treatment (McIntyre 2009). However, it is highly probable that the pathophysiology underlying BD fosters the development of a variety of medical disorders.

In addition to medical disorders, psychiatric comorbidities have been reported to occur among 50 and 70% in BD patients (Vieta et al. 2001). The presence of comorbidities is associated with worse prognosis, more severe subtypes, earlier onset, lower remission rates, suicidal behaviour, lower response to treatment, as well as worse functioning and quality of life (Vieta et al. 2001; McIntyre et al. 2008; Nery-Fernandes et al. 2009; Mantere et al. 2010). A growing body of evidence indicates that some of the neuroadaptive changes that occur in the 'brain stress systems' in patients with addiction disorders (Koob 2008) are comparable to those described as associated with AL in BD. That is to say, the incremental burden of AL translates into cognitive impairment, disability, disorders, and premature death (Soreca et al. 2009). In fact, the number of affective episodes boosts the vulnerability to subsequent episodes as well as a lowered response to pharmacological treatment such as lithium (Swann et al. 1999) or olanzapine (Ketter et al. 2006) or psychological treatment, such as psychoeducation or familiar psychoeducation (Scott et al. 2006; Reinares et al. 2010). In fact, the notion that cumulative episodes translate in more severe psychopathology can be tracked down to Griesinger (1867). Therefore, these new developments help to bridge historical clinical observations with emerging science in the field of pathophysiology. Overall, the concept of AL is instrumental in highlighting the importance of early intervention in order to prevent the malignant transformation of progressive disorders such as BD (Post 1992).

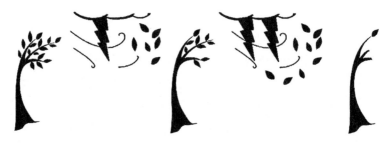

Allostasis   Allostatic load   Allostatic overload

Fig. 3.3 Allostasis, allostatic load (AL), and allostatic overload (AO): A graphic simile would be the state of a tree in a windy land. The tree would be bent as an adaptive state to the windy conditions (allostasis), even some branches would be damaged from time to time because of inclement weather (AL). However, a heavy storm would ruin the tree and it would take a long time to recover and not without injuries (AO).

Conclusions

There is evidence that a significant percentage of individuals with BD exhibits dysregulation of the HPA axis and altered stress hormones and catecholamines. Such changes can occur during euthymia but they are more pronounced during mood episodes. These variations are currently being studied and have been compiled in a systemic toxicity index (Kapczinski et al. 2010). These findings represent abnormalities in major indicators of AL, making BD more vulnerable to early ageing, medical and psychiatric comorbidities, as well as cognitive impairment. AL provides a means to understand the reaction to chronic toxicity, while acute toxicity may be better understood in the light of the concept of AO (Fig. 3.3).

References

Angst F, Stassen HH, Clayton PJ, et al. (2002) Mortality of patients with mood disorders: follow-up over 34–38 years. J Affect Disord **68**:167–181.

Balanzá-Martínez V, Tabarés-Seisdedos R, Selva-Vera G, et al. (2005). Persistent cognitive dysfunctions in bipolar I disorder and schizophrenic patients: a 3-year follow-up study. Psychother Psychosom **74**:113–119.

Benabarre A, Vieta E, Martínez-Arán A, et al. (2005) Neuropsychological disturbances and cerebral blood flow in bipolar disorder. Aust NZ J Psychiat **39**:227–234.

Bessa JM, Ferreira D, Melo I, et al. (2009) The mood-improving actions of antidepressants do not depend on neurogenesis but are associated with neuronal remodeling. Mol Psychiatr **14**:764–773, 739.

Birkenaes AB, Opjordsmoen S, Brunborg C, et al. (2007) The level of cardiovascular risk factors in bipolar disorder equals that of schizophrenia: a comparative study. J Clin Psychiat **68**:917–923.

Blasco MA (2007) Telomere length, stem cells and aging. Nat Chem Biol **3**:640–649.

Bourne C, Aydemir O, Balanzá-Martínez V, et al. (2013) Neuropsychological testing of cognitive impairment in euthymic bipolar disorder: an individual patient data meta-analysis. Acta Psychiat Scand **128**:149–162.

Brietzke E, Kauer-Sant'Anna M, Teixeira AL, et al. (2009) Abnormalities in serum chemokine levels in euthymic patients with bipolar disorder. Brain Behav Immun **23**:1079–1082.

Bryant-Comstock L, Stender M, and Devercelli G (2002) Health care utilization and costs among privately insured patients with bipolar I disorder. Bipolar Disord **4**:398–405.

Carney CP and Jones LE (2006) Medical comorbidity in women and men with bipolar disorders: a population-based controlled study. Psychosom Med **68**:684–691.

Cavigelli SA and McClintock MK (2003) Fear of novelty in infant rats predicts adult corticosterone dynamics and an early death. Proc Natl Acad Sci U S A **100**:16131–16136.

Chen C-H, Lennox B, Jacob R, et al. (2006) Explicit and implicit facial affect recognition in manic and depressed States of bipolar disorder: a functional magnetic resonance imaging study. Biol Psychiat **59**:31–39.

Daban C, Martínez-Arán A, Torrent C, et al. (2006a) Cognitive functioning in bipolar patients receiving lamotrigine: preliminary results. J Clin Psychopharm **26**:178–181.

Daban C, Martinez-Aran A, Torrent C, et al. (2006b) Specificity of cognitive deficits in bipolar disorder versus schizophrenia. A systematic review. Psychother Psychosom **75**:72–84.

Dias-Ferreira E, Sousa JC, Melo I, et al. (2009) Chronic stress causes frontostriatal reorganization and affects decision-making. Science (New York, NY) **325**:621–625.

Elvsåshagen T, Vera E, Bøen E, et al. (2011) The load of short telomeres is increased and associated with lifetime number of depressive episodes in bipolar II disorder. J Affect Disorders **135**:43–50.

Francis D, Diorio J, Liu D, et al. (1999) Nongenomic transmission across generations of maternal behavior and stress responses in the rat. Science (New York, NY) **286**:1155–1158.

Garcia-Portilla MP, Saiz PA, Bascaran MT, et al. (2009) Cardiovascular risk in patients with bipolar disorder. J Affect Disorders **115**:302–308.

Gardner HH, Kleinman NL, Brook RA, et al. (2006) The economic impact of bipolar disorder in an employed population from an employer perspective. J Clin Psychiat **67**:1209–1218.

Garno JL, Goldberg JF, Ramirez PM, et al. (2005) Impact of childhood abuse on the clinical course of bipolar disorder. Brit J Psychiat **186**:121–125.

Glover DA (2006) Allostatic load in women with and without PTSD symptoms. Ann N Y Acad Sci **1071**:442–447.

Götz ME, Malz CR, Dirr A, et al. (2005) Brain aging phenomena in migrating sockeye salmon *Oncorhynchus nerka nerka*. J Neural Transm (Vienna, Austria: 1996) **112**:1177–1199.

Grande I, Magalhães PV, Kunz M, et al. (2012) Mediators of allostasis and systemic toxicity in bipolar disorder. Physiol Behav **106**:46–50.

Griesinger W (1867) Mental Pathology and Therapeutics. London: The New Sydenham Society.

Jankord R and Herman JP (2008) Limbic regulation of hypothalamo-pituitary-adrenocortical function during acute and chronic stress. Ann N Y Acad Sci **1148**: 64–73.

Juster R-P, McEwen BS, and Lupien SJ (2010) Allostatic load biomarkers of chronic stress and impact on health and cognition. Neurosci Biobehav R **35**:2–16.

Kapczinski F, Dal-Pizzol F, Teixeira AL, et al. (2010) A systemic toxicity index developed to assess peripheral changes in mood episodes. Mol Psychiatr **15**:784–786.

Kapczinski F, Vieta E, Andreazza AC, et al. (2008) Allostatic load in bipolar disorder: implications for pathophysiology and treatment. Neurosci Biobehav R **32**:675–692.

Karlamangla AS, Singer BH, Greendale GA, et al. (2005) Increase in epinephrine excretion is associated with cognitive decline in elderly men: MacArthur studies of successful aging. Psychoneuroendocrinology **30**:453–460.

Karlamangla AS, Singer BH, McEwen BS, et al. (2002) Allostatic load as a predictor of functional decline. MacArthur studies of successful aging. J Clin Epidemiol **55**:696–710.

Karlamangla AS, Singer BH, and Seeman TE (2006) Reduction in allostatic load in older adults is associated with lower all-cause mortality risk: MacArthur studies of successful aging. Psychosom Med **68**:500–507.

Kauer-Sant'anna M, Yatham LN, Tramontina J, et al. (2008) Emotional memory in bipolar disorder. Brit J Psychiat **192**:458–463.

Kaufman J, Plotsky PM, Nemeroff CB, et al. (2000) Effects of early adverse experiences on brain structure and function: clinical implications. Biol Psychiat **48**:778–790.

Ketter TA, Houston JP, Adams DH, et al. (2006) Differential efficacy of olanzapine and lithium in preventing manic or mixed recurrence in patients with bipolar I disorder based on number of previous manic or mixed episodes. J Clin Psychiat **67**:95–101.

Kilbourne AM, Cornelius JR, Han X, et al. (2004) Burden of general medical conditions among individuals with bipolar disorder. Bipolar Disord **6**:368–373.

Koob GF (2008) A role for brain stress systems in addiction. Neuron **59**:11–34.

Korte SM, Koolhaas JM, Wingfield JC, et al. (2005) The Darwinian concept of stress: benefits of allostasis and costs of allostatic load and the trade-offs in health and disease. Neurosci Biobehav R **29**:3–38.

Kupfer DJ (2005) The increasing medical burden in bipolar disorder. JAMA **293**:2528-2530.

Leverich GS and Post RM (2006) Course of bipolar illness after history of childhood trauma. Lancet **367**:1040-1042.

Liston C, Miller MM, Goldwater DS, et al. (2006) Stress-induced alterations in prefrontal cortical dendritic morphology predict selective impairments in perceptual attentional set-shifting. J Neurosci **26**:7870-7874.

Mantere O, Isometsä E, Ketokivi M, et al. (2010) A prospective latent analyses study of psychiatric comorbidity of DSM-IV bipolar I and II disorders. Bipolar Disord **12**:271-284.

Martínez-Arán A, Penadés R, Vieta E, et al. (2002) Executive function in patients with remitted bipolar disorder and schizophrenia and its relationship with functional outcome. Psychother Psychosom **71**:39-46.

Martínez-Arán A, Vieta E, Colom F, et al. (2004a) Cognitive impairment in euthymic bipolar patients: implications for clinical and functional outcome. Bipolar Disord **6**:224-232.

Martínez-Arán A, Vieta E, Reinares M, et al. (2004b) Cognitive function across manic or hypomanic, depressed, and euthymic states in bipolar disorder. Am J Psychiat **161**:262-270.

Maule AG, Tripp RA, Kaattari SL, et al. (1989) Stress alters immune function and disease resistance in chinook salmon (*Oncorhynchus tshawytscha*). J Endocrinol **120**:135-142.

McEwen BS (1998) Stress, adaptation, and disease. Allostasis and allostatic load. Ann N Y Acad Sci **840**:33-44.

McEwen BS (2000) Allostasis and allostatic load: implications for neuropsychopharmacology. Neuropsychopharmacology **22**:108-124.

McEwen BS (2003a) Interacting mediators of allostasis and allostatic load: towards an understanding of resilience in aging. Metab Clin Exp **52**:10-16.

McEwen BS (2003b) Mood disorders and allostatic load. Biol Psychiat **54**:200-207.

McEwen BS (2004) Protection and damage from acute and chronic stress: allostasis and allostatic overload and relevance to the pathophysiology of psychiatric disorders. Ann N Y Acad Sci **1032**:1-7.

McEwen BS (2005) Stressed or stressed out: what is the difference? J Psychiatr Neurosci **30**:315-318.

McEwen BS (2007) Physiology and neurobiology of stress and adaptation: central role of the brain. Physiol Rev **87**:873-904.

McEwen BS (2008) Central effects of stress hormones in health and disease: understanding the protective and damaging effects of stress and stress mediators. Eur J Pharmacol **583**:174-185.

McEwen BS and Stellar E (1993) Stress and the individual. Mechanisms leading to disease. Arch Intern Med **153**:2093-2101.

McEwen BS and Wingfield JC (2003) The concept of allostasis in biology and biomedicine. Horm Behav **43**:2–15.

McIntyre RS (2009) Overview of managing medical comorbidities in patients with severe mental illness. J Clin Psychiat **70**:e17.

McIntyre RS, McCann SM, and Kennedy SH (2001) Antipsychotic metabolic effects: weight gain, diabetes mellitus, and lipid abnormalities. Can J Psychiat **46**:273–281.

McIntyre RS, Nguyen HT, Soczynska JK, et al. (2008) Medical and substance-related comorbidity in bipolar disorder: translational research and treatment opportunities. Dialogues Clin Neurosci **10**:203–213.

Merikangas KR, Akiskal HS, Angst J, et al. (2007) Lifetime and 12-month prevalence of bipolar spectrum disorder in the National Comorbidity Survey replication. Arch Gen Psychiat **64**:543–552.

Mur M, Portella MJ, Martínez-Arán A, et al. (2007) Persistent neuropsychological deficit in euthymic bipolar patients: executive function as a core deficit. J Clin Psychiat **68**:1078–1086.

Navarro A and Boveris A (2007) The mitochondrial energy transduction system and the aging process. Am J Physiol Cell PH **292**:C670–686.

Nelson RA (1980) Protein and fat metabolism in hibernating bears. Fed Proc **39**:2955–2958.

Nery-Fernandes F, Quarantini LC, Galvão-De-Almeida A, et al. (2009) Lower rates of comorbidities in euthymic bipolar patients. World J Biol Psychiat **10**:474–479.

Newcomer JW (2006) Medical risk in patients with bipolar disorder and schizophrenia. J Clin Psychiat **67**(Suppl 9):25–30; discussion 36–42.

Phillips ML and Vieta E (2007) Identifying functional neuroimaging biomarkers of bipolar disorder: toward DSM-V. Schizophrenia Bull **33**:893–904.

Pomarol-Clotet E, Moro N, Sarró S, et al. (2012) Failure of de-activation in the medial frontal cortex in mania: evidence for default mode network dysfunction in the disorder. World J Biol Psychiat **13**:616–626.

Post RM (1992) Transduction of psychosocial stress into the neurobiology of recurrent affective disorder. Am J Psychiat **149**:999–1010.

Radley JJ, Rocher AB, Miller M, et al. (2006) Repeated stress induces dendritic spine loss in the rat medial prefrontal cortex. Cereb Cortex **16**:313–320.

Reinares M, Colom F, Rosa AR, et al. (2010) The impact of staging bipolar disorder on treatment outcome of family psychoeducation. J Affect Disorders **123**:81–86.

Repetti RL, Taylor SE, and Seeman TE (2002) Risky families: family social environments and the mental and physical health of offspring. Psychol Bull **128**:330–366.

Robinson LJ and Ferrier IN (2006) Evolution of cognitive impairment in bipolar disorder: a systematic review of cross-sectional evidence. Bipolar Disord **8**:103–116.

Sapolsky RM, Romero LM, and Munck AU (2000) How do glucocorticoids influence stress responses? Integrating permissive, suppressive, stimulatory, and preparative actions. Endocr Rev **21**:55–89.

Scott J, Paykel E, Morriss R, et al. (2006) Cognitive-behavioural therapy for severe and recurrent bipolar disorders: randomised controlled trial. Brit J Psychiat **188**:313–320.

Seeman TE, Crimmins E, Huang M-H, et al. (2004) Cumulative biological risk and socio-economic differences in mortality: MacArthur studies of successful aging. Soc Sci Med (1982) **58**:1985–1997.

Seeman TE, McEwen BS, Rowe JW, et al. (2001) Allostatic load as a marker of cumulative biological risk: MacArthur studies of successful aging. Proc Natl Acad Sci U S A **98**:4770–4775.

Seeman TE, Singer BH, Rowe JW, et al. (1997) Price of adaptation—allostatic load and its health consequences. MacArthur studies of successful aging. Arch Intern Med **157**:2259–2268.

Simon NM, Smoller JW, McNamara KL, et al. (2006) Telomere shortening and mood disorders: preliminary support for a chronic stress model of accelerated aging. Biol Psychiat **60**:432–435.

Soreca I, Frank E, and Kupfer DJ (2009) The phenomenology of bipolar disorder: what drives the high rate of medical burden and determines long-term prognosis? Depress Anxiety **26**:73–82.

Sotiropoulos I, Cerqueira JJ, Catania C, et al. (2008) Stress and glucocorticoid footprints in the brain-the path from depression to Alzheimer's disease. Neurosci Biobehav R **32**:1161–1173.

Sterling P and Eyer J (1988) Allostasis: a new paradigm to explain arousal pathology. In: Fisher S and Reason J, eds. Handbook of Life Stress, Cognition and Health, John Wiley & Sons Ltd., New York, pp. 629–649.

Strakowski SM, Adler CM, Almeida J, et al. (2012) The functional neuroanatomy of bipolar disorder: a consensus model. Bipolar Disord **14**:313–325.

Swaab DF, Bao A-M, and Lucassen PJ (2005) The stress system in the human brain in depression and neurodegeneration. Ageing Res Rev **4**:141–194.

Swann AC, Bowden CL, Calabrese JR, et al. (1999) Differential effect of number of previous episodes of affective disorder on response to lithium or divalproex in acute mania. Am J Psychiat **156**:1264–1266.

Torrent C, Amann B, Sánchez-Moreno J, et al. (2008) Weight gain in bipolar disorder: pharmacological treatment as a contributing factor. Acta Psychiat Scand **118**:4–18.

Townsend J and Altshuler LL (2012) Emotion processing and regulation in bipolar disorder: a review. Bipolar Disord **14**:326–339.

Vermetten E, Schmahl C, Lindner S, et al. (2006) Hippocampal and amygdalar volumes in dissociative identity disorder. Am J Psychiat **163**:630–636.

Versace A, Thompson WK, Zhou D, et al. (2010) Abnormal left and right amygdala-orbitofrontal cortical functional connectivity to emotional faces: state versus trait vulnerability markers of depression in bipolar disorder. Biol Psychiat **67**:422–431.

Vieta E, Colom F, Corbella B, et al. (2001) Clinical correlates of psychiatric comorbidity in bipolar I patients. Bipolar Disord 3:253–258.

Vieta E, Gasto C, Martinez de Osaba MJ, et al. (1997) Prediction of depressive relapse in remitted bipolar patients using corticotrophin-releasing hormone challenge test. Acta Psychiat Scand 95:205–211.

Vieta E, Martínez-De-Osaba MJ, Colom F, et al. (1999) Enhanced corticotropin response to corticotropin-releasing hormone as a predictor of mania in euthymic bipolar patients. Psychol Med 29:971–978.

Yatham LN, Kapczinski F, Andreazza AC, et al. (2009) Accelerated age-related decrease in brain-derived neurotrophic factor levels in bipolar disorder. Int J Neuropsychoph 12:137–139.

Yu S, Patchev AV, Wu Y, et al. (2010) Depletion of the neural precursor cell pool by glucocorticoids. Ann Neurol 67:21–30.

Zimmermann US, Blomeyer D, Laucht M, et al. (2007) How gene-stress-behavior interactions can promote adolescent alcohol use: the roles of predrinking allostatic load and childhood behavior disorders. Pharmacol Biochem Behav 86:246–262.

Chapter 4

Neuroprogression and biological underpinnings of staging in bipolar disorder

Gabriel R. Fries, Pedro V. S. Magalhães,
Flavio Kapczinski, and Michael Berk

Introduction

Clinical evidence shows that if not all, a substantial proportion of patients with bipolar disorder (BD) present a progressive course (Kessing et al. 1998). This progression is commonly associated with several unfavourable clinical outcomes, such as reduced interepisode intervals, inferior responsiveness to treatment, especially with lithium and cognitive behavioural therapy, higher rates of comorbidity, functional impairments, augmented risk of suicide and hospitalization, as well as worse treatment outcome of family psychoeducation (Reinares et al. 2010; Berk et al. 2011a; Fries et al. 2012; Rosa et al. 2012). Moreover, cognitive impairment worsens with cumulative episodes, affecting executive functions and other cognitive tests, such as verbal memory, response inhibition, sustained attention, psychomotor speed, abstraction, and set-shifting (Torres et al. 2007; López-Jamarillo et al. 2010).

The term 'neuroprogression' will be used in this chapter as the pathological rewiring of the brain that takes place when clinical and cognitive deterioration occurs in the context of the progression of BD. Historically, we can track the origins of this concept in the writings of Griesinger (1867):

> It generally happens, that with patients who fall into insanity, (. . .) the attacks, as time advances, become longer and more serious, the lucid intervals shorter, and with each new attack the prognosis becomes more unfavorable.

More than 100 years later, Post (1992) explored different pathways related to the cross-sensitization between mood episodes, stress, and drug abuse. In that paper he postulated that changes in these clinical domains would translate into changes in neuroplasticity that in turn would provide the biological basis for the proclivity for recurrences and worse outcomes. In a more recent review (Post 2007), the same author acknowledged two mechanisms as potentially important for episode sensitization:

> In this fashion, there could be two different mechanisms of episode sensitization; one could relate to the passive process of general cellular endangerment occurring with BDNF decreases, potentially increasing with each episode, and the other could be an active or learned associative process (. . .). These and other data have led Kapczinski and associates to postulate that BDNF [brain derived neurotrophic factor] could be related to aspects of episode-induced illness progression, because periods of low BDNF may enhance the likelihood for neuronal atrophy and even the possibility of cell death via apoptosis. Consistent with this view are the findings by Kapczinski and associates that reactive oxygen species associated with DNA damage are also increased in patients' white cells during both manic and depressive episodes, but not euthymic periods. Therefore, there is the possibility that episode-related decreases in neuroprotective factors (such as BDNF) and increases in free radicals and other neurotoxic influences could place individuals at risk for additional cellular damage as a function of the occurrence of each new episode, yielding one potential mechanism for episode sensitization and illness progression. Reprinted from Neuroscience and Biobehavioral Reviews, 31(6), Post, R.M., Kindling and sensitization as models for affective episode recurrence, cyclicity, and tolerance phenomena, pp. 858–873., Copyright (2007), with permission from Elsevier.

In order to make sense of the process of cellular endangerment that seemed to take place in portion with mood episodes, Kapczinski et al. (2008) used the concept of allostatic load (McEwen and Stellar 1993). Accordingly, changes in pathways of inflammation, oxidative stress, and autonomic dysfunction shown in BD could lead into allostatic load, meaning the wear and tear of the bodily systems and brain tissue (Kapczinski et al. 2008). At this point in time, it became clear that in addition to the constitutive changes in neuroplasticity suggested earlier by Robert Post (1992), further allostatic changes were in place to induce the pathological brain rewiring suggested by Kapczinski et al. (2009a). This set of ideas was reorganized by Michael Berk (2009), who then coined the term 'neuroprogression'.

In a follow-up to his seminal article, Berk et al. (2010) suggested a balance between neuroprogression and neuroprotection as a key factor to be considered in the field of psychiatry. Subsequently, inflammation, oxidative stress, and the activity of growth factors were postulated as the canonic pathways of neuroprogression (Berk et al. 2011b). At this point in time, it was clear to this group of authors that neuroprogression would have a broader use in psychiatry, encompassing the biological underpinnings of the illness progression in differential domains of psychopathology. In fact, at the time that this chapter was written 60 papers on the topic of neuroprogression had already been published in areas such as schizophrenia, early intervention in affective disorders, geriatric BD, ageing, obesity, and nicotine dependence. We believe that the concept has proven to be useful in understanding the multidimensional changes described in the context of illness progression in psychiatry.

Accordingly, on the one hand, neuroprogression seems to take place from a *constitutive* perspective, meaning that patients that experience multiple episodes, stress, and drugs of abuse may develop specific changes in neuronal plasticity that lead into more complex and refractory clinical presentations (Post et al. 2012). These changes are likely to be related to synaptic tagging and metaplastic changes, particularly in dopaminergic neurons. On the other hand, neuroprogression has been suggested to take place from an *allostatic perspective*. Mechanisms of allostatic load may explain the cumulative medical burden associated with the recurrent mood episodes and characterize the disorder as a stress-related condition (Kapczinski et al. 2008).

The study of the biological basis of neuroprogression has the potential to aid in the identification of relevant targets for treatment and a better management of the disorder. In the following sections, we will review and discuss anatomical alterations that take place along with BD progression, as well as potential cellular and biochemical mechanisms associated with it.

Neuroanatomical evidences of progression

Several neuroanatomical alterations have been reported in patients with BD, some of which tend to become more pronounced after repeated episodes. Among such alterations, a greater number of episodes have been related to deficits in the volume of the prefrontal cortex, ventral prefrontal cortex, and anterior cingulate in patients (López-Larson et al. 2002; Sassi et al. 2004). Moreover, some studies have shown that illness progression is associated with a decrease in the volume of hippocampus and temporal lobe grey matter, as well as with an increase in the volume of lateral ventricles (Strakowski et al. 2002; Moorhead et al. 2007; Javadapour et al. 2010). In addition, a reduction of grey matter volume of the orbital and medial prefrontal cortex, ventral striatum, and mesotemporal cortex also tend to be more pronounced after multiple episodes (López-Larson et al. 2002; Bora et al. 2010).

This neuroanatomical progression can also be found in other brain structures, such as the cerebellum. It has been suggested that an increase in the number of episodes is associated with a decrease in the volume of the cerebellum, particularly of the vermis (Mills et al. 2005; Monkul et al. 2008). Furthermore, an increase in the volume of the amygdala has been reported in BD as a function of duration of illness and previous manic episodes (Altshuler et al. 2000; Bora et al. 2010). A meta-regression study has also shown that the size of amygdala trajectory increases with development or age in patients with BD (Usher et al. 2010). This particular neuroanatomical alteration may explain some particular clinical features of BD, such as an impaired emotional memory, aggressiveness, among others.

Altogether, total brain volume has been shown to be smaller in multiple-episode patients compared to those at a first episode and control subjects (Frey et al. 2008). However, it has been suggested that BD is not a neurodegenerative disorder, but is rather associated with neuroplasticity impairments (Grande et al. 2010; Jakobsson et al. 2013). In this sense, the shrinkage in brain structures may result from reduced connections between neuronal and glial cells rather than simply cell death. In fact, a postmortem study has reported decreased levels of synaptic markers in the hippocampus of BD patients as a function of duration of illness (Eastwood and Harrison 2001).

Further imaging and postmortem studies are warranted for a better understanding of the neuroanatomical alterations that take place along with illness progression in BD. Nonetheless, they already suggest that a series of biological mechanisms alter with the increase in the number of episodes, ultimately leading to these neuroanatomical changes (Fig. 4.1). These are then responsible for altering the patients' behaviour, possibly making them more vulnerable to stressors, as discussed in the next section.

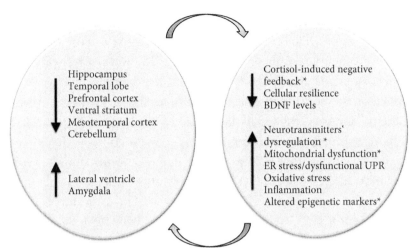

Fig. 4.1 Cross-talk between neuroanatomical and biochemical alterations taking place along with BD progression. The causal relationship between these mechanisms is still unknown. BDNF, brain-derived neurotrophic factor; ER, endoplasmic reticulum; UPR, unfolded protein response. * indicates proposed mechanisms that need to be confirmed in early vs. late-stage patients.

Biological mechanisms of neuroprogression

The role of stress and cortisol

Initial studies on BD describe a phenomenon of stress sensitization in patients, in which early episodes are often triggered by psychosocial stress, but end up occurring autonomously after a sufficient number of recurrences (Post et al. 2012). This sensitization, along with allostatic overload, indicates the relevance of stress and its modulation in the course of BD.

Cortisol is one of the main mediators of allostatic load, and its release is controlled by a hormonal physiological axis known as the 'stress hormone axis', or hypothalamus-pituitary-adrenal (HPA) axis. The HPA axis is clearly altered in mood disorders, and abnormalities in cortisol levels have been reported in patients with major depressive disorder (MDD) and BD (Daban et al. 2005). A high proportion of MDD and BD patients inefficiently suppresses cortisol release in response to the dexamethasone suppression test (DST) (Watson et al. 2004; Daban et al. 2005). In addition, they have been shown to present increased serum cortisol levels, independent of the phase of the illness. These observations indicate an impaired negative feedback of the HPA axis, which persists even after the remission of acute depression and can even present a prognostic value. For instance, patients presenting abnormalities in the HPA axis are more susceptible to depressive relapses during remission, either in unipolar or in bipolar depression (Varghese and Brown 2001).

Besides the already known HPA axis dysfunction in depression, evidences suggest that such a dysfunction also occurs during mania. Previous studies using the DST suggest an alteration in the function of glucocorticoids in manic episodes with mixes features (Evans and Nemeroff 1983; Krishnan et al. 1983; Godwin 1984; Swann et al. 1992). Patients with acute mania show an increased response to the test when compared to healthy controls, even after the remission of symptoms (Schmider et al. 1995). Likewise, another study was able to predict manic relapses based on the corticotropin-releasing hormone (CRH) stimulation test in BD patients on remission (Vieta et al. 1999). Studies with cortisol secreting profiles have also reported changes in HPA axis during mania (Linkowski et al. 1994; Cervantes et al. 2001). In this same vein, plasma cortisol levels have been shown to be significantly elevated during the night in manic patients when compared to healthy controls (Linkowski et al. 1994).

This deficiency of the HPA axis to regulate circulating cortisol results in a feed-forward mechanism of increased cortisol levels during stress and a decreased ability to return to resting conditions (Galigniana et al. 2012). In fact, such a dysfunction of the HPA axis has also been reported to take place along with illness progression (Fries et al. 2014). These increased cortisol levels may have important long-term consequences in BD patients, which will be further discussed in subsequent sections. Besides alterations in neuroplasticity, a dysfunctional HPA axis can alter various aspects of the circadian rhythm, including sleep regulation. Most of these parameters have been associated with BD pathophysiology and neuroprogression, and thus warrant more intricate studies. So far, no study has assessed HPA axis functioning in regard to the progression of BD. However, considering the reduction of resilience that takes place with the recurrence of episodes, it is plausible to assume that the

HPA axis may play a significant role in BD neuroprogression. In fact, a dysfunctional HPA axis might be an explanatory mechanism by which patients present reduced coping and increased stress reactivity along with BD progression. It may also be one of the mechanisms by which patients of the same age tend to progress more quickly than others, playing a key role on the susceptibility of ultra-high-risk subjects and their mechanisms of handling with stress.

Neurotransmitter alterations

Along with cortisol, there is now substantial evidence that other systems play key roles in BD pathophysiology, including in neurotransmitter levels and functions. Very few studies have focused on alterations of these systems over the course of illness in BD, but have rather examined their relevance on acute episodes and in remission. Nonetheless, by presenting specific changes in acute episodes, these neurotransmitter systems may lead to impairments in cell signalling pathways and oxidative stress commonly associated with BD neuroprogression, most of which will be discussed in the following sections.

It has been suggested that excessive dopamine is involved in the development of manic symptoms, and dopamine-inducing agents, such as amphetamine, have been used to induce animal models of mania in rodents (Joyce et al. 1995; Anand et al. 2000; Frey et al. 2006; Cousins et al. 2009). Meanwhile, dopamine antagonists typically present antimanic effects, whereas mood-stabilizing drugs such as lithium and valproate are known to share actions on dopamine transmission (Yatham et al. 2002). As a consequence, excessive dopamine can be oxidized and induce the formation of toxic oxidant molecules, thus causing cellular dysfunctions. This can be one of the mechanisms by which patients present increased oxidative stress during mood episodes.

Glutamate has been also implicated in BD, mainly due to the fact that mood stabilizers can modulate its functions (Zarate et al. 2010). Some studies show that glutamate levels reduce after treatment of acute episodes, being correlated with symptom severity, as well (Frye et al. 2007; Yoon et al. 2009). Moreover, excessive glutamate can lead to excitotoxicity and calcium influx, ultimately resulting in some of the features of

BD pathophysiology. For instance, patients with BD present increased markers of excitotoxicity in postmortem frontal cortex (Rao et al. 2010), some of which can be alleviated by mood stabilizers in vitro. This has been described in studies showing that lithium and valproate are able to protect rat cerebral cortical neurons against glutamate excitotoxicity (Hashimoto et al. 2002; Shao et al. 2005). Of note, a recent study found no differences in hippocampal glutamine + glutamate levels in patients after the first manic episode (Gigante et al. 2014). This suggests that glutamate alterations are not a feature of BD at its beginning, and may only take place along with the illness progression.

Cellular resilience mechanisms

Considering cellular resilience as the ability of cells to adapt to different insults or stress episodes, impaired cellular resilience may be one of the possible mechanisms leading to increased vulnerability of patients to stressful events. In fact, several studies have shown that patients with BD present alterations in cell signalling pathways, including neurotransmitters, trophic cascades, antiapoptotic factors, cell survival pathways, and calcium signalling, among others (Hunsberger et al. 2009; Fries et al. 2012; Pfaffenseller et al. 2013). These alterations may reduce the ability of cells to deal with extracellular stimuli and ultimately influence the way patients respond to environmental events.

Among several alterations, hyperactive intracellular calcium dynamics have been found in peripheral blood cells from patients with BD (Perova et al. 2008). Neuroimaging studies also report decreased levels of N-acetylaspartate in the living brain from patients (Stork and Renshaw 2005), which support the hypothesis that patients with BD present impaired neuronal viability and function. Moreover, cells of the olfactory neuroepithelium from patients showed an increased vulnerability to cell death when compared to healthy controls (McCurdy et al. 2006). This may be possibly linked to the activation of glycogen synthase kinase-3β (GSK-3β) by protein kinase C (PKC), which leads to the phosphorylation of β-catenin and increases the cells' susceptibility to apoptosis. Lithium, which is the most commonly used mood stabilizer for the treatment of BD, can inhibit GSK-3β and increase the expression of antiapoptotic proteins, thereby hindering this process (Brown and Tracy 2013). In fact, several apoptotic markers have been found to be increased in patients with BD, including increased DNA damage in peripheral blood of patients (Andreazza et al. 2007a), apoptotic serum activity (Politi et al. 2008), expression of molecules involved in cell death/survival (Benes et al. 2006; Herberth et al. 2011), and mitochondrial dysfunction (Shao et al. 2008). In addition, peripheral blood mononuclear cells from patients with BD have been shown to present an increased percentage of early apoptotic cells when compared to controls (Fries et al. 2014).

It is likely that this increased cell death and reduced cellular resilience may be a consequence to chronic stress. In vitro and animal studies have shown that chronic stress and chronic exposure to high levels of glucocorticoids can lead to mitochondrial dysfunctions, including reductions in oxygen consumption, mitochondrial membrane potential, and calcium holding capacity (Du et al. 2009; Gong et al. 2011). Impaired mitochondria can induce the opening of mitochondrial permeability transition pore, thus releasing cytochrome c from the intermembrane space and inducing apoptotic cascades. Up to date, no study has ever assessed the direct effect of illness progression on mitochondrial functions in BD, which will likely be clarified by the analysis of mitochondrial parameters in early- and late-stage patients. Nonetheless, the evidence of impaired mitochondrial functioning strongly supports a key role of this organelle in synaptic functioning, thus contributing to the atrophic changes underlying BD neuroprogression.

Even though only a few studies have examined cellular resilience in BD regarding the stage of illness, there is consistent evidence that the levels of synaptic subcellular markers of neuroplasticity are not only reduced in the anterior cingulate cortex of patients but also correlate with illness duration (Eastwood and Harrison 2001). This feature may be accounted for by a potential reduction in neuroplasticity, which is corroborated by studies on neurotrophic factors in BD. Moreover, other cellular mechanisms, such as the endoplasmic reticulum (ER) stress, may be responsible for the increased cell vulnerability to stress. For instance, peripheral blood mononuclear cells from patients at an early stage responded better to in-vitro-induced ER stress (with induction of glucose-regulated protein of 78 kDa (GRP78) and phosphorylated eukaryotic initiation factor 2 (eIF2α-P), both essential proteins in activating ER stress response signalling), when compared to late-stage patients (Pfaffenseller et al. 2014). The mechanisms leading to these intracellular alterations may be linked to peripheral alterations, such as in neurotrophic factors, oxidative stress, and inflammation. Differences in cellular resilience might also be programmed by genetic and epigenetic mechanisms, in a way that genes and environmental stimuli interact to predict differential cell responses in response to stressors.

Neurotrophins

The family of neurotrophins is composed of several regulatory factors that mediate neuronal survival and differentiation, as well as modulate synaptic transmission and plasticity. Family members in mammals include neural growth factor (NGF), glial cell-derived neurotrophic factor (GDNF), brain-derived neurotrophic factor (BDNF), neurotrophin-3 (NT-3), and neurotrophin-4/5 (NT-4/5). Among them, BDNF is the most abundant neurotrophic factor in the adult human central nervous system, and it is able to induce long-term neurotrophic and neuroprotective effects. Brain BDNF levels reduce in rats after chronic stress (Gray et al. 2013), and its expression is increased in different brain regions after chronic treatment with mood stabilizers and antidepressants (Hunsberger et al. 2009). Moreover, learning tasks are associated with an increase in BDNF levels, and it also plays a key role in long-term potentiation (Gómez-Palacio-Schjetnan and Escobar 2013). These actions are mediated by BDNF's ability to bind tyrosine kinase receptor B (TrkB), which upon binding activates protective cell signalling cascades, including phospholipase C gamma, extracellular-regulated protein kinase (Erk), and phosphatidylinositol 3 kinase (PI3K) pathways (Grande et al. 2010).

Evidence suggests that there is an imbalance in peripheral BDNF levels in BD. Serum BDNF levels have been shown to be reduced in patients with BD during manic and depressive episodes, and its levels have been negatively correlated with the severity of symptoms (Cunha et al. 2006; Machado-Vieira et al. 2007a; Fernandes et al. 2011). In addition, symptom remission has been associated with normalization of serum BDNF levels (Tramontina et al. 2009), suggesting that this protein may be a marker of illness activity in BD. In this sense, its levels have been shown to be reduced in late-stage patients when compared to early-stage patients, being negatively correlated with the number of episodes (Kauer-Sant'Anna et al. 2009). These data have led to the hypothesis that the changes related to the increase in the number of episodes may explain at least in part some of the structural changes observed in patients with BD. BDNF levels have also been negatively correlated with the length of illness on the same study, suggesting a key role of this neurotrophin in the progression of BD. Of note, some recent studies have found opposite results, in which BDNF levels were increased in manic patients and also in patients with long-term BD (Barbosa et al. 2010; Barbosa et al. 2013a). This suggests that BDNF levels may be differentially modulated in different populations, and likely depend on the type of medications patients are on. In this same vein, other neurotrophins have been found to be altered in acute mood episodes as well, such as GDNF (Rosa et al. 2006; Barbosa et al. 2011), NT-3 (Walz et al. 2007; Fernandes et al. 2010), and NT-4/5 (Walz et al. 2009), but their involvement in BD neuroprogression still needs to be examined.

Oxidative stress

As discussed in the previous sections, mitochondrial dysfunction may play a key role in BD pathophysiology, mostly by impairing energy metabolism, cellular resilience, among other vital cellular functions. In fact, energy metabolism has been shown to be impaired in patients with BD (Kato 2007). Brain energy metabolism was reported to be increased in patients during manic episodes and decreased during depression (Baxter et al. 1985), which is further supported by evidences of an increased basal metabolic rate in mania and a higher VO_2 max, independent of caloric intake (Caliyurt and Altiay 2009).

Among the functions of mitochondria, they have been identified as the main sites of production of free radicals in the cell, especially the complex I (NADH: ubiquinone oxidoreductase) of the mitochondrial electron transfer chain (ETC). Post-mortem studies have shown that the activity of complex I of the ETC is reduced in the prefrontal cortex of patients with BD (Andreazza et al. 2010). In addition, lithium has been shown to be able to increase the activity of mitochondrial complexes I/II and II/III in human brain tissue (Maurer et al. 2009), which further corroborates the hypothesis of a mitochondrial dysfunction in BD.

Once reactive oxygen and nitrogen species are formed they can react with organic molecules in the cell and induce damages in lipids (and consequently in membranes), DNA, and proteins. This scenario is hindered by the action of antioxidant molecules, which act as scavengers of free radicals and thus reduce their toxicity. In this sense, an increase in the activity of the enzyme superoxide dismutase (SOD) has been reported in patients during the manic and depressive episodes, but not in euthymia (Andreazza et al. 2007b; Kunz et al. 2008). This same result has been replicated in another study assessing SOD activity in unmedicated manic patients with BD (Machado-Vieira et al. 2007b). Moreover, catalase activity has been shown to be decreased in euthymic patients and increased in unmedicated manic patients (Andreazza et al. 2007b; Machado-Vieira et al. 2007b), which suggests an imbalance in the production and control of reactive species. As a consequence, increased lipid peroxidation products have been reported in patients with BD in manic, depressive, or euthymic states (Andreazza et al. 2007b; Kunz et al. 2008). Of note, treatment of patients with N-acetylcysteine (NAC), which is a glutathione precursor and is able to scavenge free radicals, reduces depressive symptoms and improves functioning and quality of life in patients (Berk et al. 2011c).

Regarding illness progression, the activities of glutathione reductase and glutathione S-transferase have been shown to be increased in late-stage patients compared to early-stage patients (Andreazza et al. 2009), which are suggested to be part of a progressive failure of compensatory mechanisms over time. Nonetheless, the same study found increased levels of 3-nitrotyrosine, a marker of protein nitration, in both early and late stages. A more recent study has also reported an increase in protein carbonylation in early-stage patients (Magalhães et al. 2012a). In fact, oxidative changes in early-stage patients seem to be more subtle than those at late stages (Magalhães et al. 2012a). This suggests that some alterations regarding oxidative stress are already present at the first stages of illness, including protein oxidative damage, whereas others only take place as a means of BD neuroprogression.

Inflammation

Several studies have linked BD's pathophysiology with inflammation, in which immune alterations are associated with symptom severity, acute mood episodes, illness progression, metabolic disturbances, drug effects, increased prevalence of autoimmune and allergic disorders, as well as with neurotrophic alterations in patients (Berk et al. 2011b; Stertz et al. 2013). Most of the published data are related to illness activity and acute episodes, and little is actually known concerning BD progression itself. Nonetheless, the sum of findings on acute episodes help proposing mechanisms by which cumulative episodes can be so deleterious, as discussed below.

Acute episodes have been characterized as pro-inflammatory states based on findings of increased peripheral levels of pro-inflammatory cytokines on depression, such as interleukin (IL)-6 and tumour necrosis factor alpha (TNF-α), and of IL-2, IL-4, IL-6, and TNF-α in mania (Kim et al. 2007; Ortiz-Domínguez et al. 2007; Brietzke et al. 2009). Moreover, meta-analyses have reported an increase in the levels of TNF-α, soluble TNF receptor type 1, soluble IL-2 receptor, and IL-1 receptor antagonist in manic patients, whereas euthymic patients were found to present altered levels of IL-1 receptor antagonist compared to controls (Munkholm et al. 2012; Modabbernia et al. 2013). Patients with BD have also been shown to present increased levels of acute phase proteins, such as C-reactive protein and haptoglobin (Maes et al. 1997; Cunha et al. 2008), whose production is normally induced by pro-inflammatory cytokines. In this same vein, complement factors, such as C3 and C4, have also been associated with BD (Wadee et al. 2002). In summary, peripheral studies strongly indicate that BD can be characterized as a systemic inflammatory disease, even though the exact mechanisms by which these peripheral alterations take place are not yet known. Of note, it has been suggested that sleep and circadian rhythm alterations, stress, immune activation by retrovirus infection of autoimmune dysfunctions, unhealthy lifestyle, as well as long-term exposure to drugs may contribute to BD-associated inflammatory status (Goldstein et al. 2009).

These inflammatory alterations may play a key role in the development of several comorbidities reported in patients, and may likely contribute to the illness progression, as well. The pro-inflammatory cytokines IL-6 and TNF-α have been shown to be elevated in both early- and late-stage disorder, whereas the anti-inflammatory cytokine IL-10 was increased only in the early stage of the disorder (Kauer-Sant'Anna et al. 2009; Magalhães et al. 2012b). Moreover, increased plasma levels of CCL11, CCL24, and CXCL10, and decreased plasma levels of CXCL8 have been reported in late-stage BD patients when compared to healthy controls (Barbosa et al. 2013b). Based on these findings, it has been hypothesized that an increase in pro-inflammatory cytokines in the initial phases of disease could be part of the disease process itself or represent an adaptive response to insult. Whereas the anti-inflammatory response may be effective in the early course of the disease, it becomes less effective after multiple episodes. As a consequence of the continued elevations in pro-inflammatory cytokines, the deleterious effects of those would become more apparent as the disorder progresses.

Epigenetic mechanisms

Increasing evidence suggests that modulation of gene expression and gene versus environment interactions may play key roles in BD (Petronis 2003; Pregelj 2011). This indicates the importance of chromatin structure modulation by epigenetic mechanisms in the pathophysiology of BD, given that this is the main avenue by which environmental factors end up modulating gene activities. Studies have shown that early-life events, such as childhood trauma and abuse, can induce long-term epigenetic markers on specific genes, which can also interact with genetic alterations (polymorphisms) and ultimately lead to a pathological phenotype (Szyf 2013). The most studied epigenetic marker is DNA methylation, which can inhibit gene transcription by inducing the formation of heterochromatin around a gene's promoter. DNA methylation is also the most stable epigenetic marker, and several preclinical studies have shown that early-life events-induced DNA methylation can actually last until adulthood in animals (Champagne 2013). Based on the allostatic load hypothesis, it seems reasonable to assume that cumulative stressors (i.e. acute episodes) might act as environmental stimuli able to induce specific alterations in epigenetic markers, ultimately interfering with the ability of a patient to respond and cope to a novel stressor. These markers would then be responsible for differences in resilience among patients, possibly shedding light into the mechanisms by which some of them end up developing severe functioning impairments after a few episodes, whereas others manage to surpass the stressor effects and properly cope with them.

In fact, patients with BD have been shown to present alterations in DNA methylation within several genes. A recent study has found that patients with BD type II present a hypermethylation of the *BDNF* promoter region compared with controls, which was accompanied by a significant BDNF gene expression downregulation (D'Addario et al. 2012). Moreover, DNA derived from both the brain and saliva was shown to present a hypomethylation of the membrane-bound catechol-O-methyltransferase (MB-COMT) promoter in patients (Nohesara et al. 2011), and an increased DNA methylation of the serotonin receptor 5HTR1A gene promoter has also been reported in leukocytes (Carrard et al. 2011). Of note, global leukocyte methylation was not altered in euthymic patients with BD when compared to controls (Bromberg et al. 2009), which suggests that such epigenetic alterations are exclusive to specific genes in different tissues. These alterations may be related to the altered expression of DNA methyltransferases (DNMTs), whose expression is altered in a state-dependent way in patients with BD (Higuchi et al. 2011). So far, no study has ever assessed differences in methylation levels between early- and late-stage patients.

The relevance of epigenetics in the pathophysiology and progression of BD are also corroborated by the known mechanisms of action of mood stabilizers and antidepressants, which are able to modulate several enzymes and pathways associated with chromatin remodelling. For instance, sodium valproate can inhibit the enzyme histone deacetylase, ultimately inducing the formation of euchromatin around specific promoters (Monti et al. 2009; Machado-Vieira et al. 2011). Moreover, this drug has been shown to induce DNA demethylation in nuclear extracts from adult mouse brain (Dong et al. 2010), suggesting a novel mechanism of epigenetic alteration. Antidepressants have also been shown to reverse histone alterations induced by chronic stress paradigms in rats (Tsankova et al. 2006), which show the ability of these psychotropic drugs to reverse environment-induced alterations. Considering that BD progression has been associated with reduced response to certain treatments, one can speculate that these drugs' abilities to modify chromatin might get compromised along with illness progression.

Based on the effects of chronic stress on epigenetic markers, we hypothesize that specific epigenetic alterations may determine one's resilience to stress and to other environmental stimuli. This may not only be crucial in determining the genesis of BD in ultra-high-risk individuals, but also in modulating the natural history of one's disease. That is to say that epigenetic markers may regulate the detrimental effects of recurrent episodes, which fit the staging hypothesis of BD.

Conclusions

The biological mechanisms associated with BD neuroprogression appear to be complex, involving several systems in the central nervous system and in the periphery (Fig. 4.1). Although the means by which each of these systems individually articulate to generate the disorder are not known, we hypothesize that cellular resilience impairments are initially induced by chronic stress, which makes cells more vulnerable to stressful stimuli. In addition, the reduced trophic signalling and increase in oxidative stress seen in late-stage patients may also work as feedforward mechanisms in amplifying cellular dysfunction, eventually making them more vulnerable to stressors and inducing apoptosis and inflammation. These systems may interact and ultimately mediate the clinical outcomes associated with illness progression, such as increased comorbidity, lower responsiveness to treatment, impaired cognitive and functional parameters, among others.

Once the biological mechanisms of BD progression have been clarified, these will be able to assist in a biologically based clinical staging of patients. Different staging models for BD have already been proposed (Berk et al. 2007; Kapczinski et al. 2009a), but the use of biomarkers for clinical staging still lacks stronger biological evidence and consistency (Kapczinski et al. 2009b; Fries et al. 2012). To that end, future research should further explore these differences in longitudinal studies. Moreover, the field would also significantly benefit from the assessment of these biomarkers in adolescents and young adults with BD, in addition to the analysis of the effects of treatment on the same parameters. Among all of the previously mentioned alterations, epigenetic mechanisms seem to be of a special relevance, given that it can itself modulate all of the other systems, including neurotrophins, inflammation, and oxidative stress.

As previously discussed, current data available on the use of biomarkers in BD focus mostly on illness activity, and little is known regarding these parameters and the progression of BD. Moreover, the staging models that have been proposed so far differ from each other, as well as the concept of illness progression itself (some focus on the number of episodes, while others take the length of illness or the functional outcome into account), which might explain inconsistencies between studies for the same measurements.

In sum, the further study of the biological underpinnings of BD neuroprogression may hold the key to the discovery of biomarkers with prognostic value, as well as the development of novel drugs aimed at hindering the patients' progressive functioning and cognitive impairments, ultimately improving their quality of life.

References

Altshuler LL, Bartzokis G, Grieder T, et al. (2000) An MRI study of temporal lobe structures in men with bipolar disorder or schizophrenia. Biol Psychiat 48(2):147–162.

Anand A, Verhoeff P, Seneca N, et al. (2000) Brain SPECT imaging of amphetamine-induced dopamine release in euthymic bipolar disorder patients. Am J Psychiat 157(7):1108–1114.

Andreazza AC, Cassini C, Rosa AR, et al. (2007a) DNA damage in bipolar disorder. Psychiat Res 153(1):27–32.

Andreazza AC, Frey BN, Erdtmann B, et al. (2007b) Serum S100B and antioxidant enzymes in bipolar patients. J Psychiat Res 41(6):523–529.

Andreazza AC, Kapczinski F, Kauer-Sant'Anna M, et al. (2009) 3-Nitrotyrosine and glutathione antioxidant system in patients in the early and late stages of bipolar disorder. J Psychiat Neurosci 34(4):263–271.

Andreazza AC, Shao L, Wang JF, and et al. (2010) Mitochondrial complex I activity and oxidative damage to mitochondrial proteins in the prefrontal cortex of patients with bipolar disorder. Arch Gen Psychiat 67(4):360–368.

Barbosa IG, Huguet RB, Mendonça VA, et al. (2010) Increased plasma levels of brain-derived neurotrophic factor in patients with long-term bipolar disorder. Neurosci Lett 475(2):95–98.

Barbosa IG, Huguet RB, Sousa LP, et al. (2011) Circulating levels of GDNF in bipolar disorder. Neurosci Lett 502(2):103–106.

Barbosa IG, Rocha NP, Miranda AS, et al. (2013a) Increased BDNF levels in long-term bipolar disorder patients. Rev Bras Psiquiatr 35(1):67–69.

Barbosa IG, Rocha NP, Bauer ME, et al. (2013b) Chemokines in bipolar disorder: trait or state? Eur Arch Psy Clin N 263(2):159–165.

Baxter LR Jr, Phelps ME, Mazziotta JC, et al. (1985) Cerebral metabolic rates for glucose in mood disorders. Studies with positron emission tomography and fluorodeoxyglucose F18. Arch Gen Psychiat 42(5):441–447.

Benes FM, Matzilevich D, Burke RE, et al. (2006) The expression of proapoptosis genes is increased in bipolar disorder, but not in schizophrenia. Mol Psychiatr 11(3):241–251.

Berk M (2009) Neuroprogression: pathways to progressive brain changes in bipolar disorder. Int J Neuropsychoph 12(4):441–445.

Berk M, Brnabic A, Dodd S, et al. (2011a) Does stage of illness impact treatment response in bipolar disorder? Empirical treatment data and their implication for the staging model and early intervention. Bipolar Disord 13(1):87–98.

Berk M, Kapczinski F, Andreazza AC, et al. (2011b) Pathways underlying neuroprogression in bipolar disorder: focus on inflammation, oxidative stress and neurotrophic factors. Neurosci Biobehav R 35(3):804–817.

Berk M, Dean O, Cotton SM, et al. (2011c) The efficacy of N-acetylcysteine as an adjunctive treatment in bipolar depression: an open label trial. J Affect Disorders 135(1–3):389–394.

Berk M, Conus P, Kapczinski F, et al. (2010) From neuroprogression to neuroprotection: implications for clinical care. Med J Australia 193(4 Suppl):S36–40.

Berk M, Hallam KT, and McGorry PD (2007) The potential utility of a staging model as a course specifier: a bipolar disorder perspective. J Affect Disorders 100(1–3):279–281.

Bora E, Fornito A, Yücel M, et al. (2010) Voxelwise meta-analysis of gray matter abnormalities in bipolar disorder. Biol Psychiat 67(11):1097–1105.

Brietzke E, Stertz L, Fernandes BS, et al. (2009) Comparison of cytokine levels in depressed, manic and euthymic patients with bipolar disorder. J Affect Disorders 116(3):214–217.

Bromberg A, Bersudsky Y, Levine J, et al. (2009) Global leukocyte DNA methylation is not altered in euthymic bipolar patients. J Affect Disorders **118**(1–3):234–239.

Brown KM and Tracy DK (2013) Lithium: the pharmacodynamic actions of the amazing ion. Ther Adv Psychopharmacol **3**(3):163–176.

Caliyurt O and Altiay G (2009) Resting energy expenditure in manic episode. Bipolar Disord **11**(1):102–106.

Carrard A, Salzmann A, Malafosse A, et al. (2011) Increased DNA methylation status of the serotonin receptor 5HTR1A gene promoter in schizophrenia and bipolar disorder. J Affect Disorders **132**(3):450–453.

Champagne FA, (2013) Early environments, glucocorticoid receptors, and behavioral epigenetics. Behav Neurosci **127**(5):628–636.

Cousins DA, Butts K, Young AH (2009) The role of dopamine in bipolar disorder. Bipolar Disord **11**(8):787–806.

Cunha AB, Andreazza AC, Gomes FA, et al. (2008) Investigation of serum high-sensitive C-reactive protein levels across all mood states in bipolar disorder. Eur Arch Psy Clin N **258**(5):300–304.

Cunha AB, Frey BN, Andreazza AC, et al. (2006) Serum brain-derived neurotrophic factor is decreased in bipolar disorder during depressive and manic episodes. Neurosci Lett **398**(3):215–219.

Daban C, Vieta E, Mackin P, et al. (2005) Hypothalamic-pituitary-adrenal axis and bipolar disorder. Psychiat Clin N Am **28**(2):469–480.

D'Addario C, Dell'Osso B, Palazzo MC, et al. (2012) Selective DNA methylation of BDNF promoter in bipolar disorder: differences among patients with BDI and BDII. Neuropsychopharmacology **37**(7):1647–1655.

Dong E, Chen Y, Gavin DP, et al. (2010) Valproate induces DNA demethylation in nuclear extracts from adult mouse brain. Epigenetics **5**(8):730–735.

Du J, Wang Y, Hunter R, et al. (2009) Dynamic regulation of mitochondrial function by glucocorticoids. Proc Natl Acad Sci U S A **106**(9):3543–3548.

Eastwood SL and Harrison PJ (2001) Synaptic pathology in the anterior cingulate cortex in schizophrenia and mood disorders. A review and a Western blot study of synaptophysin, GAP-43 and the complexins. Brain Res Bull **55**(5):569–578.

Evans DL and Nemeroff CB (1983) The dexamethasone suppression test in mixed bipolar disorder. Am J Psychiat **140**(5):615–617.

Fernandes BS, Gama CS, Cereser KM, et al. (2011) Brain-derived neurotrophic factor as a state-marker of mood episodes in bipolar disorders: a systematic review and meta-regression analysis. J Psychiat Res **45**(8):995–1004.

Fernandes BS, Gama CS, Walz JC, et al. (2010) Increased neurotrophin-3 in drug-free subjects with bipolar disorder during manic and depressive episodes. J Psychiat Res **44**(9):561–565.

Frey BN, Andreazza AC, Cereser KM, et al. (2006) Effects of mood stabilizers on hippocampus BDNF levels in an animal model of mania. Life Sci **79**(3):281–286.

Frey BN, Zunta-Soares GB, Caetano SC, et al. (2008) Illness duration and total brain gray matter in bipolar disorder: evidence for neurodegeneration? Eur Neuropsychopharm 18(10):717–722.

Fries GR, Pfaffenseller B, Stertz L, et al. (2012) Staging and neuroprogression in bipolar disorder. Curr Psychiat Rep 14(6):667–675.

Fries GR, Vasconcelos-Moreno MP, Gubert C, et al. (2014) Early apoptosis in peripheral blood mononuclear cells from patients with bipolar disorder. J Affect Disorders 152–154: 474–477.

Fries GR, Vasconcelos-Moreno MP, Gubert C, et al. (2014) Hypothalamic-pituitary-adrenal axis dysfunction and illness progression in bipolar disorder. Int J Neuropsychoph 18.

Frye MA, Watzl J, Banakar S, et al. (2007) Increased anterior cingulate/medial prefrontal cortical glutamate and creatine in bipolar depression. Neuropsychopharmacology 32(12):2490–2499.

Galigniana NM, Ballmer LT, Toneatto J, et al. (2012) Regulation of the glucocorticoid response to stress-related disorders by the Hsp90-binding immunophilin FKBP51. J Neurochem 122(1):4–18.

Gigante AD, Lafer B, and Yatham LN (2014) 1H-MRS of hippocampus in patients after first manic episode. World J Biol Psychiat 15(2):145–154.

Godwin CD (1984) The dexamethasone suppression test in acute mania. J Affect Disorders 7(3–4):281–286.

Goldstein BI, Kemp DE, Soczynska JK, et al. (2009) Inflammation and the phenomenology, pathophysiology, comorbidity, and treatment of bipolar disorder: a systematic review of the literature. J Clin Psychiat 70(8):1078–1090.

Gómez-Palacio-Schjetnan A and Escobar ML (2013) Neurotrophins and synaptic plasticity. Curr Top Behav Neurosci 15:117–136.

Gong Y, Chai Y, Ding JH, et al. (2011) Chronic mild stress damages mitochondrial ultrastructure and function in mouse brain. Neurosci Lett 488(1):76–80.

Grande I, Fries GR, Kunz M, et al. (2010) The role of BDNF as a mediator of neuroplasticity in bipolar disorder. Psychiat Invest 7(4):243–250.

Gray JD, Milner TA, and McEwen BS (2013) Dynamic plasticity: the role of glucocorticoids, brain-derived neurotrophic factor and other trophic factors. Neuroscience 239:214–227.

Griesinger W (1867) Mental Pathology and Therapeutics. London: The New Sydenham Society.

Hashimoto R, Hough C, Nakazawa T, et al. (2002) Lithium protection against glutamate excitotoxicity in rat cerebral cortical neurons: involvement of NMDA receptor inhibition possibly by decreasing NR2B tyrosine phosphorylation. J Neurochem 80(4):589–597.

Herberth M, Koethe D, Levin Y, et al. (2011) Peripheral profiling analysis for bipolar disorder reveals markers associated with reduced cell survival. Proteomics 11(1):94–105.

Higuchi F, Uchida S, Yamagata H, et al. (2011) State-dependent changes in the expression of DNA methyltransferases in mood disorder patients. J Psychiat Res 45(10):1295–1300.

Hunsberger JG, Austin DR, Chen G, et al. (2009) Cellular mechanisms underlying affective resiliency: the role of glucocorticoid receptor- and mitochondrially-mediated plasticity. Brain Res 1293:76–84.

Jakobsson J, Zetterberg H, Blennow K, et al. (2013) Altered concentrations of amyloid precursor protein metabolites in the cerebrospinal fluid of patients with bipolar disorder. Neuropsychopharmacology 38(4):664–672.

Javadapour A, Malhi GS, Ivanovski B, et al. (2010) Hippocampal volumes in adults with bipolar disorder. J Neuropsych Clin N 22(1):55–62.

Joyce PR, Fergusson DM, Woollard G, et al. (1995) Urinary catecholamines and plasma hormones predict mood state in rapid cycling bipolar affective disorder. J Affect Disorders 33(4):233–243.

Kapczinski F, Dias VV, Kauer-Sant'Anna M, et al. (2009a) Clinical implications of a staging model for bipolar disorders. Exp Rev Neurother 9(7):957–966.

Kapczinski F, Dias VV, Kauer-Sant'Anna M, et al. (2009b) The potential use of bio-markers as an adjunctive tool for staging bipolar disorder. Prog Neuro-Psychoph 33(8):1366–1371.

Kapczinski F, Vieta E, Andreazza AC, et al. (2008) Allostatic load in bipolar disorder: implications for pathophysiology and treatment. Neurosci Biobehav R 32(4):675–692.

Kato T (2007) Mitochondrial dysfunction as the molecular basis of bipolar disorder: therapeutic implications. CNS Drugs 21:1–11.

Kauer-Sant'Anna M, Kapczinski F, Andreazza AC, et al. (2009) Brain-derived neuro-trophic factor and inflammatory markers in patients with early- vs. late-stage bipolar disorder. Int J Neuropsychoph 12(4):447–458.

Kessing LV and Andersen PK (1998) Clinical definitions of sensitisation in affective disorder: a case register study of prevalence and prediction. J Affect Disorders 47:31–39.

Kim YK, Jung HG, Myint AM, et al. (2007) Imbalance between pro-inflammatory and anti-inflammatory cytokines in bipolar disorder. J Affect Disorders 104(1–3):91–95.

Krishnan RR, Maltbie AA, and Davidson JR (1983) Abnormal cortisol suppression in bipolar patients with simultaneous manic and depressive symptoms. Am J Psychiat 140(2):203–205.

Kunz M, Gama CS, Andreazza AC, et al. (2008) Elevated serum superoxide dismutase and thiobarbituric acid reactive substances in different phases of bipolar disorder and in schizophrenia. Prog Neuro-Psychoph 32(7):1677–1681.

Linkowski P, Kerkhofs M, Van Onderbergen A, et al. (1994) The 24-hour profiles of cortisol, prolactin, and growth hormone secretion in mania. Arch Gen Psychiat 51(8):616–624.

López-Jaramillo C, Lopera-Vásquez J, Gallo A, et al. (2010) Effects of recurrence on the cognitive performance of patients with bipolar I disorder: implications for relapse prevention and treatment adherence. Bipolar Disord 12(5):557–567.

López-Larson MP, DelBello MP, Zimmerman ME, et al. (2002) Regional prefrontal gray and white matter abnormalities in bipolar disorder. Biol Psychiat 52(2):93–100.

Machado-Vieira R, Dietrich MO, Leke R, et al. (2007a) Decreased plasma brain derived neurotrophic factor levels in unmedicated bipolar patients during manic episode. Biol Psychiat 61(2):142–144.

Machado-Vieira R, Andreazza AC, Viale CI, et al. (2007b) Oxidative stress parameters in unmedicated and treated bipolar subjects during initial manic episode: a possible role for lithium antioxidant effects. Neurosci Lett 421(1):33–36.

Machado-Vieira R, Ibrahim L, and Zarate CA Jr (2011) Histone deacetylases and mood disorders: epigenetic programming in gene-environment interactions. CNS Neurosci Ther 17(6):699–704.

Maes M, Delange J, Ranjan R, et al. (1997) Acute phase proteins in schizophrenia, mania and major depression: modulation by psychotropic drugs. Psychiat Res 66(1):1–11.

Magalhães PV, Jansen K, Pinheiro RT, et al. (2012a) Peripheral oxidative damage in early-stage mood disorders: a nested population-based case-control study. Int J Neuropsychoph 15(8):1043–1050.

Magalhães PV, Jansen K, Pinheiro RT, et al. (2012b) A nested population-based case-control study on peripheral inflammation markers and brain-derived neurotrophic factor in early-stage mood disorders. Presented at the 5th Biennial Conference of the International Society for Bipolar Disorders. Istambul, Turkey.

Maurer IC, Schippel P, and Volz HP (2009) Lithium-induced enhancement of mitochondrial oxidative phosphorylation in human brain tissue. Bipolar Disord 11:515–522.

McCurdy RD, Féron F, Perry C, et al. (2006) Cell cycle alterations in biopsied olfactory neuroepithelium in schizophrenia and bipolar I disorder using cell culture and gene expression analyses. Schizophr Res 82(2–3):163–173.

McEwen BS and Stellar E (1993) Stress and the individual. Mechanisms leading to disease. Arch Intern Med 153(18):2093–2101.

Mills NP, Delbello MP, Adler CM, et al. (2005) MRI analysis of cerebellar vermal abnormalities in bipolar disorder. Am J Psychiat 162(8):1530–1532.

Modabbernia A, Taslimi S, Brietzke E, et al. (2013) Cytokine alterations in bipolar disorder: a meta-analysis of 30 studies. Biol Psychiat 74(1):15–25.

Monkul ES, Hatch JP, Sassi RB, et al. (2008) MRI study of the cerebellum in young bipolar patients. Prog Neuro-Psychoph 32(3):613–619.

Monti B, Polazzi E, and Contestabile A (2009) Biochemical, molecular and epigenetic mechanisms of valproic acid neuroprotection. Curr Mol Pharmacol 2(1):95–109.

Moorhead TW, McKirdy J, Sussmann JE, et al. (2007) Progressive gray matter loss in patients with bipolar disorder. Biol Psychiat 62(8):894–900.

Munkholm K, Vinberg M, Berk M, et al. (2012) State-related alterations of gene expression in bipolar disorder: a systematic review. Bipolar Disord 14(7):684–696.

Nohesara S, Ghadirivasfi M, Mostafavi S, et al. (2011) DNA hypomethylation of MB-COMT promoter in the DNA derived from saliva in schizophrenia and bipolar disorder. J Psychiat Res 45(11):1432–1148.

Ortiz-Dominguez A, Hernandez ME, Berlanga C, et al. (2007) Immune variations in bipolar disorder: phasic differences. Bipolar Disord 9(6):596–602.

Perova T, Wasserman MJ, Li PP, et al. (2008) Hyperactive intracellular calcium dynamics in B lymphoblasts from patients with bipolar I disorder. Int J Neuropsychoph 11(2):185–196.

Petronis A (2003) Epigenetics and bipolar disorder: new opportunities and challenges. Am J Med Genet C Semin Med Genet 123C(1):65–75.

Pfaffenseller B, Fries GR, Wollenhaupt-Aguiar B, et al. (2013) Neurotrophins, inflammation and oxidative stress as illness activity biomarkers in bipolar disorder. Exp Rev Neurother 13(7):827–842.

Pfaffenseller B, Wollenhaupt-Aguiar B, Fries GR, et al. (2014) Impaired endoplasmic reticulum stress response in bipolar disorder: cellular evidence of illness progression. Int J Neuropsychoph 17(9):1453–1463.

Politi P, Brondino N, and Emanuele E (2008) Increased proapoptotic serum activity in patients with chronic mood disorders. Arch Med Res 39(2):242–245.

Post RM (1992) Transduction of psychosocial stress into the neurobiology of recurrent affective disorder. Am J Psychiat 149(8):999–1010.

Post RM (2007) Kindling and sensitization as models for affective episode recurrence, cyclicity, and tolerance phenomena. Neurosci Biobehav R 31(6):858–873.

Post RM, Fleming J, and Kapczinski F (2012) Neurobiological correlates of illness progression in the recurrent affective disorders. J Psychiat Res 46(5):561–573.

Pregelj P (2011) Gene environment interactions in bipolar disorder. Psychiat Danubia 23(Suppl 1):S91–93.

Ra, JS, Harry GJ, Rapoport SI, et al. (2010) Increased excitotoxicity and neuroinflammatory markers in postmortem frontal cortex from bipolar disorder patients. Mol Psychiatr 15(4):384–392.

Reinares M, Colom F, Rosa AR, et al. (2010) The impact of staging bipolar disorder on treatment outcome of family psychoeducation. J Affect Disorders 123(1–3): 81–86.

Rosa AR, Frey BN, Andreazza AC, et al. (2006) Increased serum glial cell line-derived neurotrophic factor immunocontent during manic and depressive episodes in individuals with bipolar disorder. Neurosci Lett 407(2):146–150.

Rosa AR, González-Ortega I, González-Pinto A, et al. (2012) One year psychosocial functioning in patients in the early vs. late stage of bipolar disorder. Acta Psychiat Scand 125 (4):335–341.

Sassi RB, Brambilla P, Hatch JP, et al. (2004) Reduced left anterior cingulate volumes in untreated bipolar patients. Biol Psychiat 56(7):467–475.

Schmider J, Lammers CH, Gotthardt U, et al. (1995) Combined dexamethasone/corticotropin-releasing hormone test in acute and remitted manic patients, in acute depression, and in normal controls: I. Biol Psychiat 38(12):797–802.

Shao L, Martin MV, Watson SJ, et al. (2008) Mitochondrial involvement in psychiatric disorders. Ann Med 40(4):281–295.

Shao L, Young LT, and Wang JF (2005) Chronic treatment with mood stabilizers lithium and valproate prevents excitotoxicity by inhibiting oxidative stress in rat cerebral cortical cells. Biol Psychiat 58(11):879–884.

Stertz L, Magalhães PV, and Kapczinski F (2013) Is bipolar disorder an inflammatory condition? The relevance of microglial activation. Curr Opin Psychiatr 26(1):19–26.

Stork C and Renshaw PF (2005) Mitochondrial dysfunction in bipolar disorder: evidence from magnetic resonance spectroscopy research. Mol Psychiatr 10(10):900–919.

Strakowski SM, DelBello MP, Zimmerman ME, et al. (2002) Ventricular and periventricular structural volumes in first- versus multiple-episode bipolar disorder. Am J Psychiat 159(11):1841–1847.

Swann AC, Stokes PE, Casper R, et al. (1992) Hypothalamic-pituitary-adrenocortical function in mixed and pure mania. Acta Psychiat Scand 85(4):270–274.

Szyf M (2013) DNA methylation, behavior and early life adversity. J Genet Genom 40(7):331–338.

Torres IJ, Boudreau VG, and Yatham LN (2007) Neuropsychological functioning in euthymic bipolar disorder: a meta-analysis. Acta Psychiat Scand Suppl 434:17–26.

Tramontina JF, Andreazza AC, Kauer-Sant'anna M, et al. (2009) Brain-derived neurotrophic factor serum levels before and after treatment for acute mania. Neurosci Lett 452(2):111–113.

Tsankova NM, Berton O, Renthal W, et al. (2006) Sustained hippocampal chromatin regulation in a mouse model of depression and antidepressant action. Nat Neurosci 9(4):519–525.

Usher J, Leucht S, Falkai P, et al. (2010) Correlation between amygdala volume and age in bipolar disorder—a systematic review and meta-analysis of structural MRI studies. Psychiat Res 182(1):1–8.

Varghese FP and Brown ES (2001) The hypothalamic-pituitary-adrenal axis in major depressive disorder: a brief primer for primary care physicians. The Primary Care Companion—J Clin Psychiat 3(4):151–155.

Vieta E, Martínez-De-Osaba MJ, Colom F, et al. (1999) Enhanced corticotropin response to corticotropin-releasing hormone as a predictor of mania in euthymic bipolar patients. Psychol Med 29(4):971–978.

Wadee AA, Kuschke RH, Wood LA, et al. (2002) Serological observations in patients suffering from acute manic episodes. Hum Psychopharm 17(4):175–179.

Walz JC, Andreazza AC, Frey BN, et al. (2007) Serum neurotrophin-3 is increased during manic and depressive episodes in bipolar disorder. Neurosci Lett 415(1):87–89.

Walz JC, Magalhães PV, Giglio LM, et al. (2009) Increased serum neurotrophin-4/5 levels in bipolar disorder. J Psychiat Res **43**(7):721–723.

Watson S, Gallagher P, Ritchie JC, et al.(2004) Hypothalamic-pituitary-adrenal axis function in patients with bipolar disorder. Brit J Psychiat **184**:496–502.

Yatham LN, Liddle PF, Shiah IS, et al. (2002) PET study of [(18)F]6-fluoro-L-dopa uptake in neuroleptic- and mood-stabilizer-naive first-episode nonpsychotic mania: effects of treatment with divalproex sodium. Am J Psychiat **159**(5):768–774.

Yoon SJ, Lyoo IK, Haws C, et al. (2009) Decreased glutamate/glutamine levels may mediate cytidine's efficacy in treating bipolar depression: a longitudinal proton magnetic resonance spectroscopy study. Neuropsychopharmacology **34**(7):1810–1818.

Zarate C Jr, Machado-Vieira R, Henter I, et al. (2010) Glutamatergic modulators: the future of treating mood disorders? Harv Rev Psychiat **18**(5):293–303.

Chapter 5

Functioning and illness progression in bipolar disorder

Adriane R. Rosa, Clarissa S. Gama, and Eduard Vieta

Introduction

Bipolar disorder is a chronic and severe mental disorder. It is the sixth leading cause of disability-adjusted life years in the world among people aged 15–44 (Catalá-López et al. 2013). Bipolar disorder represents a major public health problem, with severe psychosocial disruptions, in addition to an increased mortality (Baldessarini et al. 2006; Rosa et al. 2008). Although early studies reported that functional impairment is associated with acute mood episodes (Altshuler et al. 2006; Rosa et al. 2010), modern studies have shown that such impairment persists even during remission (Strakowski et al. 1998; Tohen et al. 2005). Moreover, psychosocial dysfunctions in bipolar disorder are not limited to symptomatic periods, but may be enduring or result in sustained disability, which contributes to high personal suffering and socioeconomic costs to society (Gardner et al. 2006; González-Pinto et al. 2010).

Concept of functioning

Psychosocial functioning is a complex concept that involves a person's ability to perform the tasks of daily life and to engage in relationships with other people in ways that are gratifying to the individual and others, and that meet the needs of the community in which the person lives (Zarate et al. 2000). The assessment of psychosocial functioning, therefore, should ideally involve evaluation across one or more behavioural domains, such as the individual's ability to function socially or occupationally, or to live independently, with functional recovery typically being defined as restoration of normal role functioning in multiple domains (Mintz et al. 1992; Üstün and Kennedy 2009). However, researchers have traditionally measured one or two elements of functioning and typically fail to take into account all the other elements necessary for *optimal functioning*. The Global Assessment of Functioning scale (GAF), for example, is often used to assess disability, although the original GAF instructions call for rating symptoms as well as overall functioning (Martínez-Arán et al. 2007). Beyond the GAF, there are other instruments to assess functioning in psychiatric disorders such as Social Adjustment Scale (SAS), the Life Functioning Questionnaire (LFQ), the Short Form-36 (SF-36), and the World Health Organization (WHO-DAS). In bipolar disorder, a novel brief 24-item interviewer administered instrument was developed in order to assess psychosocial functioning in distinct life domains. The Functioning Assessment Short Test (FAST) provides strong psychometric properties and it seems to be sensitive to detect minimal changes in functioning in the short and long term (Rosa et al. 2008, 2011). The FAST is available in distinct languages and has been also validated in several psychiatric disorders such as bipolar disorder, schizophrenia, and in patients with a first psychotic episode (Cacilhas et al. 2009; González-Ortega et al. 2010).

Evidence of functional impairment in bipolar disorder

Emerging evidence has shown that functional and symptomatic recoveries do not occur at the same time in many cases of bipolar disorder. For instance, a study conducted by Tohen et al. (2000) in the United States reported that 98% of first-episode manic patients had a clinical remission within 2 years, whereas only 38% of them achieved functional recovery (defined by the proportion of patients who regained premorbid level of functioning). Keck (2004) found that only 24% of patients with bipolar I disorder achieved functional recovery at some time during the interval between hospital discharge and 12-month follow-up. Results from the European Mania in Bipolar Longitudinal Evaluation of Medication (EMBLEM) study showed that only about 20% of patients returned to normal levels of functioning within 12 months after an acute episode, even when they were not suffering from subsyndromal symptoms (Montoya et al. 2007). In a 10-year follow-up period, Goldberg and Harrow (2004) showed that about 50% of bipolar patients had sustained remissions or patterns of improvement, while 30–40% experienced some degree of social disability. Similarly, our previous findings showed greater disability associated with bipolar disorder as only one-quarter of patients who attained symptomatic remission within 6 months of continuous treatment achieved favourable functioning (Rosa et al. 2010). Patients with bipolar disorder experience serious dysfunction in distinct life domains (Strakowski et al. 1998; Goetz et al. 2007; Rosa et al. 2012); such dysfunctions may begin early in the course of illness (see Fig. 5.1).

Although bipolar disorder seems to affect several areas of psychosocial functioning, impairment in the occupational domain seems to be highly pronounced (MacQueen et al. 2000). In this regard, a research conducted by the Stanley Foundation Bipolar Network showed that 62% of outpatients with bipolar disorder had moderate to severe impact of the illness on occupational functioning (Suppes et al. 2001). The EMBLEM study reported that only 40% of patients were able to work after 2 years of continuous treatment for mania (Goetz et al. 2007). Assessing employment rates in a Spanish sample,

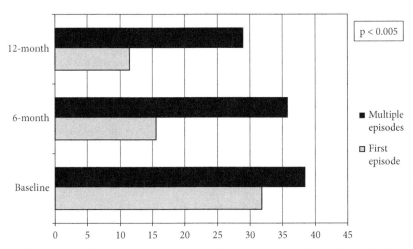

Fig. 5.1 Functional impairment in patients in first episode vs. patients with multiple episodes.

we found that 20% of patients had a permanent disability. In addition, among those who were employed, a quarter had lower-qualification jobs, around 20% had lower incomes for the same jobs than non-bipolar subjects, almost 60% reported having problems in finishing their tasks promptly, and a quarter of them mentioned difficulties in achieving the expected performance. This is consistent with previous studies showing that one-third of patients who have a full-time or part-time job experience frequent problems at work (Michalak et al. 2007). All these data indicate that bipolar disorder is associated with a decline in job status and income, which may be a consequence of the progression of the illness. Furthermore, occupational impairment is not only bad per se, as it has also been associated with a short time to relapse (Fagiolini et al. 2005).

Although the basis for such limited functional recovery is not entirely clear, it may be associated with progressive course of the illness. Recently, we showed that there is a strong linear association between functional impairment and clinical stages of bipolar disorder, with FAST scores increasing from early to late stages. Patients in stage I had greater work functioning than those in stage II, whereas patients in stage IV were more impaired on autonomy than patients in stage III, followed by the stage II group. These findings suggest that bipolar disorder is associated with progressive functional changes from early to late stages, with a greater impairment on stage IV (Rosa et al. 2014). (Fig. 5.2).

Some clinical variables, such as number of previous episodes, longer duration of illness, subclinical depressive symptoms, hospitalizations, mixed episodes, psychosis, and substance use disorder have been identified as predictors of functional impairment in bipolar patients. In addition, sociodemographic factors including male sex, older age at onset, unmarried status, low socioeconomic level, environmental factors (lack of social supports or life events), and pharmacological factors (e.g. side effects, treatment adherence) may contribute to poor functioning (Sánchez-Moreno et al. 2009). Additionally, neurocognitive deficits have emerged as an important predictor to poor functioning in bipolar disorder (Martínez-Arán et al. 2007; Bonnín et al. 2010). The following sections discuss the relevance of some variables on functioning.

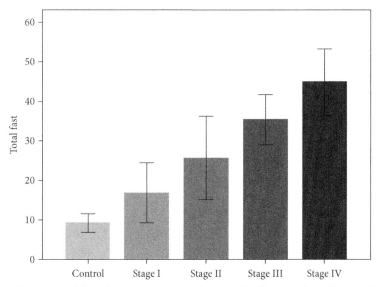

Fig. 5.2 Mean total functioning assessment short test (FAST) scores in patients in distinct stages and healthy controls.

Rosa et al. *Clinical Staging in Bipolar Disorder: Focus on Cognition and Functioning, The Journal of Clinical Psychiatry*, 75(5), 450–456, Copyright 2014, Physicians Postgraduate Press, Reprinted by Permission.

Clinical factors

Number of episodes

There is a body of evidence reporting that poor functioning may, in part, be explained by the severity of their illness (i.e. the number of episodes). For instance, MacQueen et al. (2000) found that patients with a greater number of episodes, especially past depressions, were more likely to experience poor global functioning, as measured by GAF. In addition, past depressions were associated with impairment on the mental health and social functioning subscales of the Mood Outcome Questionnaire (MOS), highlighting the negative impact of number of episodes on functioning (MacQueen et al. 2000). Using the FAST instrument, we demonstrated that the number of previous mixed episodes was associated with poor functioning mainly on social functioning, cognition, and financial issues (Rosa et al. 2009). Furthermore, a recent 1-year follow-up study compared functioning between patients with first versus multiple episodes showing a greater functional and symptomatic recovery in the former. In particular, patients with a first episode showed a higher level of autonomy, better work performance, and greater capacity to enjoy their relationships and leisure time as compared to those with multiple episodes (Rosa et al. 2012). Together, these data give support to the model of staging in bipolar disorder, suggesting that the number of episodes is an important contributor to the stage progression of the illness from less to more severe presentations, with consequently poor outcome.

Furthermore, it has been documented that the degree of functional impairment can vary according to the nature of mood episodes (Simon et al. 2007). Comparing functional impairment and disability across mood states, we found higher FAST scores in patients who were in a depressive episode, followed by patients in a hypo(manic) episode and finally the euthymic group (Rosa et al. 2010). In particular, patients with depression presented greater difficulties on work performance and interpersonal relationships than did manic patients (Rosa et al. 2010). Simon et al. (2007) found a strong association between the severity of depression and work impairment, measured by probability of employment and days missed from work due to illness. Nevertheless, associations between manic changes and work performance were less consistent (Simon et al. 2008). Moreover, some reports have shown the negative impact of number of manic episodes on neurocognitive performance and consequently poor functioning (Robinson and Ferrier 2006; Lopez-Jaramillo et al. 2010). This is consistent with previous studies showing an association between reduced grey matter and the number of manic episodes in the prefrontal cortex of subjects with bipolar disorder; such alterations may contribute to executive dysfunctions (Lyoo et al. 2004).

A large epidemiological survey conducted in United States showed that patients with mixed state were more likely to experience work impairment and problems with marital relationships than those without symptoms (Goldberg et al. 1995). Additionally, an independent study found that patients with mixed/cycling episodes required a longer time (40 weeks) to respond to treatment compared to those with bipolar depression (24 weeks), and finally to stabilize patients with mania

(11 weeks) (Chengappa et al. 2005). Likewise, it has been demonstrated that patients with depressive episode and mixed components, and especially subjects with bipolar II disorder, are more likely to experience suicide attempts and have a poor prognosis (Rihmer 2005).

Depressive symptoms

It has been documented that subjects with bipolar disorder spend approximately one-third of their adult lives with depressive symptoms (Judd et al. 2003). The depressive symptomatology at syndromal or sub-syndromal levels has been consistently associated with poor functioning (Fagiolini et al. 2005; Altshuler et al. 2006; Simon et al. 2008; Marangell et al. 2009). A British study involving patients with unipolar depression demonstrated that 34% of them suffer from residual depressive symptoms after the index episode of depression. In addition, patients with residual symptoms were more likely to experience poor functioning in terms of marital status, leisure time, social relationships, work functioning, and overall functioning at follow-up (Coryell et al. 1993). Data from the National Institute of Mental Health Treatment of Depression Collaborative Research Program showed an apparently linear relation between increasing depressive symptoms and increased disability, including when the symptoms were not severe enough to fulfil criteria for a depressive episode (Judd et al. 2005). Another independent work reported that an improvement of one level in depression severity was associated with 22-point improvement in the Role-Emotional subscale of the Medical Outcomes Survey 36-item SF-36, and with an additional 3.8 days per 3 months of being able to participate in usual activities (Simon et al. 2007). The subsyndromal depressive symptoms have been strongly related to impairment in multiple domains of functioning such as duties at work/school, duties at home, and relationships with family/friends among bipolar patients (Simon et al. 2007). Likewise, our previous studies showed that residual depressive symptoms, albeit minimal, were the best predictor of cognitive and occupational impairment (Rosa et al. 2008). Furthermore, ongoing depressive symptoms are strongly associated with relapses (Keller et al. 1992; Atkinson et al. 1997). Given the negative impact of depressive symptoms on functioning, there is a need to introduce therapeutic interventions focused on treating such symptoms in order to improve psychosocial functioning, and also to prevent relapses.

Age at onset

The impact of age at onset on outcome has been well documented in a large Systematic Treatment Enhancement Program for Bipolar Disorder (STEP-BD) study conducted by Perlis et al. (2009). The authors reported that patients with onset before age 13 experience poorer functioning and quality of life as well as fewer days of euthymia than those with onset of mood symptoms after 18 years (Perlis et al. 2009). These findings are consistent with a recent report by Baldessarini et al. (2012) showing greater social and functional outcomes in patients with older onset (≥19 years), compared to those with onset in childhood (<12 years) and in adolescence (12–18 years). Patients with earlier-age onset are more likely to have family history and high rates of psychotic symptoms, comorbidities, and rapid cycling. Investigating potential clinical differences between patients with treatment-related switches versus the nonswitch group, Valentí et al. (2012) found that age at onset was strongly associated with the occurrence of an antidepressant-related switch. Additionally, a recent review of existing evidence related to age at onset in bipolar disorder has emphasized the importance of the time of onset in terms of prognosis of the illness. Patients with early and late onset of bipolar disorder seem to present significant differences on some clinical aspects, family history, neurocognition, and anatomical profile (Geoffroy et al. 2013). Taken together, all these studies point out that bipolar disorder with juvenile onset may be associated with a more virulent form of the illness, highlighting the importance of recognition, early diagnosis, and accurate treatments for the early onset bipolar subgroup.

Cognitive deficits

Cognitive impairment seems to be related to a worse clinical course and poor psychosocial functioning (Tabarés-Seisdedos et al. 2008). Greater cognitive deficits are also associated with the severity of the illness (Robinson and Ferrier 2006; Martínez-Arán et al. 2007), and especially with the cumulative mood episodes (Torres et al. 2007). Indeed, the number of manic episodes seems to predict cognitive impairment (Robinson and Ferrier 2006). In this regard, Lopez-Jaramillo et al. (2010) found a lower neurocognitive performance in euthymic patients who had at least three manic episodes compared to those with only one mania. Other clinical features such as hospitalizations (Lopez-Jaramillo et al. 2010), duration of the illness (Martínez-Arán et al. 2007), and psychiatric comorbidities (Sánchez-Moreno et al. 2009) appear to contribute to the cognitive impairment. Deficits of memory, attention, and executive function have been consistently reported in euthymic bipolar patients (Torrent et al. 2006); such deficits may lead to functional impairment (Delbello et al. 2007; Jaeger et al. 2007). In particular, verbal learning and memory impairment were identified as the best predictors of long-term functioning (Bonnín et al. 2012). Similarly, other longitudinal studies demonstrated that patients with greater executive dysfunctions tend to experience more difficulties with their daily activities (Tabarés-Seisdedos et al. 2008; Martino et al. 2011). Martínez-Arán et al. (2007) compared neurocognitive performance in patients with low and high functioning showing that patients with low functioning were significantly more impaired in memory and executive functions. The authors suggest that patients with memory dysfunctions experience difficulties with remembering long-term information, which may be associated with poor functioning, especially, with work productivity, and interpersonal relationships (Martínez-Áran et al. 2007).

Some studies have investigated the role of neuropsychological deficits on psychosocial functioning in a young population with bipolar disorder. For instance, one of these studies showed that a subgroup of patients with greater cognitive deficits tend to have an increased risk for placement in a special class and lower academic achievement. However, the authors did not find a relationship between neuropsychological impairment and psychosocial impairment in this specific population (Biederman et al. 2011). Henry et al. (2013) analysed everyday functional ability, by means of the Performance-Based Skills Assessment, in manic, depressed, and euthymic adults with bipolar disorder. The authors found that bipolar patients experience poorer functioning in all domains (including planning, recreational activities, finance, communication skills, transportation, household skills, and medication management) compared to healthy controls, and particularly manic patients had significantly lower performance on the overall functioning as well as on the medication management portion of the task compared to other groups. Investigating predictors of prognosis in bipolar disorder, Reinares et al. (2013) showed that four clinical features including episode density, residual depressive symptoms, estimated verbal intelligence, and inhibitory control were strongly associated with a worse course of the illness (Reinares et al. 2013). Recently, the impact of cognitive deficits on psychosocial functioning has been investigated in a longer 6-year follow-up study. The authors found that cognitive deficits, particularly executive functioning, inhibition, processing speed, and verbal memory, persist over time and they are strongly associated with cognitive and occupational impairment measured by the FAST tool. In addition, the study showed that cognitive deficits persist in the mid-late stages of the bipolar disorder, and it was more marked in patients with longer duration of the illness (Mora et al. 2013). To sum up, this evidence pointed out that there is a strong relationship between cognitive deficits and poor functioning and that greater impairment may be a consequence of longer duration of illness and higher number of episodes. (Fig. 5.3).

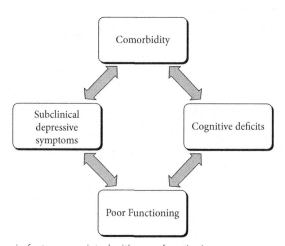

Fig. 5.3 The main factors associated with poor functioning.

Other factors (age, weight gain, stressful events, and stigma)

Many other factors have been investigated as potential predictors of functioning bipolar disorder. For instance, an association between older age and poor functioning has been reported by two independent studies (Depp et al. 2006; Rosa et al. 2009). This association could be explained due to the fact that older patients, in general, experience more comorbid physical illness and polypharmacy therapy, which may contribute to a more chronicity and psychosocial dysfunctions. On the other hand, ageing is also associated with marked cognitive deficits, particularly in processing speed and executive functions, which seem to be related to functional impairment (Depp et al. 2007; Gildengers et al. 2008).

Weight gain is another factor that may contribute to functional impairment as patients who gained more than 7% of their weight had significantly greater impairment in global functioning (over the previous 30 days) than those without weight gain (Bond et al. 2010). Finally, some reports have identified the stressful events (Yan-Meier et al. 2011), and stigma (Vázquez et al. 2011) may have an impact on functioning among bipolar patients.

Targets for functional recovery

Given the negative impact of cognitive deficits on functioning, the development of specific psychosocial interventions for the treatment of bipolar disorder would be particularly useful. In this regard, the Barcelona Bipolar Disorders Programme developed a 'functional remediation programme', focused not only on cognition but also on functioning. This programme includes education about cognitive deficits and their impact on daily life, providing strategies to manage cognitive deficits in multiple domains—mainly in attention, memory, and executive function.

Murray et al. (2011) identified specific self-management strategies used for 'high functioning individuals with bipolar disorder' to maintain or regain wellness. These self-management strategies consisted of actions, routines, and processes that would help individuals with bipolar disorder to cope better with illness and get on with the job of living. Colom et al. (2003) showed that the efficacy of psychoeducation programme in bipolar disorder can vary according to the number of previous episodes. The authors found that patients with fewer than eight episodes at study entry had better treatment response (time to recurrence) with the psychoeducation programme than those with more than seven episodes. In the same line, Reinares et al. (2010) compared the efficacy of psychoeducation for caregivers for the treatment of patients at early stages (stage I) and patients at advanced stages (stages II, III, and IV). This study reported that patients at stage I had better outcome, in terms of time to recurrence, compared to patients at advanced stages (Reinares et al. 2010). Together, these findings support the staging model in bipolar disorder emphasizing that response to treatment is generally better when it is introduced early in the course of the illness, with the only exception of functional remediation.

Conclusion and clinical considerations

- Taking into account the literature, the assessment of functioning should be used routinely in the assessment of bipolar patients;

- The functioning assessment short test (FAST) scale has been so far the most extensive used and may provide an easy and rapid overview of functioning in bipolar disorder patients. It is an interviewer-administered 24-item instrument, which allows assessment of functioning in distinct life domains in psychiatric disorders. The total FAST score is obtained when the scores of each item are added up (maximum 72); the higher the score, the more serious the difficulties.

- Some bipolar patients experience a progressive functional decline from early to late stages of the illness; such decline may be a consequence of increased severity of the illness.

- A model of functional staging in bipolar disorder may be useful to guide treatments according to individual needs.

References

Altshuler LL, Post RM, Black DO, et al. (2006) Subsyndromal depressive symptoms are associated with functional impairment in patients with bipolar disorder: results of a large, multisite study. J Clin Psychiat **67**:1551–1560.

Atkinson M, Zibin S, and Chuang H (1997) Characterizing quality of life among patients with chronic mental illness: a critical examination of the self-report methodology. Am J Psychiat **154**:99–105A.

Baldessarini RJ, Tondo L, Davis P, et al. (2006) Decreased risk of suicides and attempts during long-term lithium treatment: a meta-analytic review. Bipolar Disord **8**(5 Pt 2):625–639.

Baldessarini RJ, Tondo L, Vázquez GH, et al. (2012) Age at onset versus family history and clinical outcomes in 1,665 international bipolar-I disorder patients. World Psychiat **11**(1):40–46.

Biederman J, Petty CR, Wozniak J, et al. (2011) Impact of executive function deficits in youth with bipolar I disorder: a controlled study. Psychiat Res **186**(1):58–64.

Bond DJ, Kunz M, Torres IJ, et al. (2010) The association of weight gain with mood symptoms and functional outcomes following a first manic episode: prospective 12-month data from the Systematic Treatment Optimization Program for Early Mania (STOP-EM). Bipolar Disord **12**(6):616–626.

Bonnín CM, Martínez-Arán A, Torrent C, et al. (2010) Clinical and neurocognitive predictors of functional outcome in bipolar euthymic patients: a long-term, follow-up study. J Affect Disorders **121**(1–2):156–160.

Bonnín CM, Sánchez-Moreno J, Martínez-Arán A, et al. (2012) Subthreshold symptoms in bipolar disorder: impact on neurocognition, quality of life and disability. J Affect Disorders **136**(3):650–659.

Cacilhas AA, Magalhães PV, Ceresér KM, et al. (2009) Validity of a short functioning test (FAST) in Brazilian outpatients with bipolar disorder. Value Health **12**(4):624–627.

Catalá-López F, Gènova-Maleras R, Vieta E, et al. (2013) The increasing burden of mental and neurological disorders. Eur Neuropsychopharm **23**:1337–1339.

Chengappa KN, Hennen J, Baldessarini RJ, et al. (2005) Recovery and functional outcomes following olanzapine treatment for bipolar I mania. Bipolar Disord **7**(1):68–76.

Colom F, Vieta E, Martínez-Arán A, et al. (2003) A randomized trial on the efficacy of group psychoeducation in the prophylaxis of recurrences in bipolar patients whose disease is in remission. Arch Gen Psychiat **60**:402–407.

Coryell W, Scheftner W, Keller M, et al. (1993) The enduring psychosocial consequences of mania and depression. Am J Psychiat **150**(5):720–727.

Delbello MP, Hanseman D, Adler CM, et al. (2007) Twelve-month outcome of adolescents with bipolar disorder following first hospitalization for a manic or mixed episode. Am J Psychiat **164**:582–590.

Depp CA, Davis CE, Mittal D, et al. (2006) Health-related quality of life and functioning of middle-aged and elderly adults with bipolar disorder. J Clin Psychiat **67**:215–221.

Depp CA, Moore DJ, Sitzer D, et al. (2007) Neurocognitive impairment in middle aged and older adults with bipolar disorder: comparison to schizophrenia and normal comparison subjects. J Affect Disorders **101**:201–209.

Fagiolini A, Kupfer DJ, Masalehdan A, et al. (2005) Functional impairment in the remission phase of bipolar disorder. Bipolar Disord 7:281–285.

Gardner HH, Kleinman NL, Brook RA, et al. (2006) The economic impact of bipolar disorder in an employed population from an employer perspective. J Clin Psychiat 67:1209–1218.

Geoffroy PA, Etain B, Scott J, et al. (2013) Reconsideration of bipolar disorder as a developmental disorder: Importance of the time of onset. J Physiol Paris 107:278–285.

Gildengers AG, Whyte EM, Drayer RA, et al. (2008). Medical burden in late-life bipolar and major depressive disorders. Am J Geriat Psychiat 16:194–200.

Goetz I, Tohen M, Reed C, et al., and the EMBLEM Advisory Board (2007) Functional impairment in patients with mania: baseline results of the EMBLEM study. Bipolar Disord 9:45–52.

Goldberg JF and Harrow M (2004) Consistency of remission and outcome in bipolar and unipolar mood disorders: a 10-year prospective follow-up. J Affect Disorders 81(2):123–131.

Goldberg JF, Harrow M, and Grossman LS (1995) Course and outcome in bipolar affective disorder: a longitudinal follow-up study. Am J Psychiat 152(3):379–384.

González-Ortega I, Rosa A, Alberich S, et al. (2010) Validation and use of the functioning assessment short test in first psychotic episodes. J Nerv Ment Dis 198(11):836–840.

González-Pinto A, Reed C, Novick D, et al. (2010) Assessment of medication adherence in a cohort of patients with bipolar disorder. Pharmacopsychiatry (7):263–270.

Henry BL, Minassian A, and Perry W (2013) Everyday functional ability across different phases of bipolar disorder. Psychiat Res 210:850–856.

Jaeger J, Berns S, Loftus S, et al. (2007) Neurocognitive test performance predicts functional recovery from acute exacerbation leading to hospitalization in bipolar disorder. Bipolar Disord 9:93–102.

Judd LL, Akiskal HS, Schettler PJ, et al. (2005) Psychosocial disability in the course of bipolar I and II disorders: a prospective, comparative, longitudinal study. Arch Gen Psychiat 62:1322–1330.

Judd LL, Schettler PJ, Akiskal HS, et al. (2003) Long-term symptomatic status of bipolar I vs. bipolar II disorders. Int J Neuropsychoph 6(2):127–137.

Keck PE (2004) Defining and improving response to treatment in patients with bipolar disorder. J Clin Psychiat 65(Suppl 15):25–29.

Keller MB, Lavori PW, Kane JM, et al. (1992) Subsyndromal symptoms in bipolar disorder. A comparison of standard and low serum levels of lithium. Arch Gen Psychiat 49(5):371–376.

Lopez-Jaramillo C, Lopera-Vasquez J, Gallo A, et al. (2010) Effects of recurrence on the cognitive performance of patients with bipolar I disorder: implications for relapse prevention and treatment adherence. Bipolar Disord 12(5):557–567.

Lyoo IK, Kim MJ, Stoll AL, et al. (2004) Frontal lobe gray matter density decreases in bipolar I disorder. Biol Psychiat **55**(6):648–651.

MacQueen GM, Young LT, Robb JC, et al. (2000) Effect of number of episodes on wellbeing and functioning of patients with bipolar disorder. Acta Psychiat Scand **101**(5):374–381.

Marangell LB, Dennehy EB, Miyahara S, et al. (2009) The functional impact of subsyndromal depressive symptoms in bipolar disorder: data from STEP-BD. J Affect Disorders **114**(1–3):58–67.

Martínez-Arán A, Vieta E, Torrent C, et al. (2007) Functional outcome in bipolar disorder: the role of clinical and cognitive factors. Bipolar Disord **9**:103–113.

Michalak EE, Yatham LN, Maxwell V, et al. (2007) The impact of bipolar disorder upon work functioning: a qualitative analysis. Bipolar Disord **9**(1–2):126–143.

Mintz J, Mintz LI, Arruda MJ, et al. (1992) Treatments of depression and the functional capacity to work. Arch Gen Psychiat **49**:761–768.

Montoya A, Gilaberte I, Costi M, et al. (2007) Bipolar disorder in Spain: functional status and resource use on the basis of the Spanish sample of the observational, Pan European EMBLEM study. Vertex **18**(71): 13–19.

Mora E, Portella MJ, Forcada I, et al. (2013) Persistence of cognitive impairment and its negative impact on psychosocial functioning in lithium-treated, euthymic bipolar patients: a 6-year follow-up study. Psychol Med **43**(6):1187–1196.

Murray G, Suto M, Hole R, et al. (2011) Selfmanagement strategies used by 'high functioning' individuals with bipolar disorder: from research to clinical practice. Clin Psychol Psychother **18**(2):95–109.

Perlis RH, Dennehy EB, Miklowitz DJ, et al. (2009) Retrospective age at onset of bipolar disorder and outcome during two-year follow-up: results from the STEP-BD study. Bipolar Disord **11**(4):391–400.

Reinares M, Colom F, Rosa AR, et al. (2010) The impact of staging bipolar disorder on treatment outcome of family psychoeducation. J Affect Disorders **123**(1–3):81–86.

Reinares M, Papachristou E, Harvey P, et al. (2013) Towards a clinical staging for bipolar disorder: defining patient subtypes based on functional outcome. J Affect Disorders **144**(1–2):65–71.

Rihmer Z (2005) Prediction and prevention of suicide in bipolar disorder. Clin Neuropsychiat **2**:48–54.

Robinson LJ, Ferrier IN (2006) Evolution of cognitive impairment in bipolar disorder: a systematic review of cross-sectional evidence. Bipolar Disord **8**:103–116.

Rosa AR, Franco C, Martínez-Arán A, et al. (2008) Functional impairment in patients with remitted bipolar disorder. Psychother Psychosom **77**(6):390–392.

Rosa AR, González-Ortega I, González-Pinto A, et al. (2012) One-year psychosocial functioning in patients in the early vs. late stage of bipolar disorder. Acta Psychiat Scand **125**(4):335–341.

Rosa AR, Reinares M, Amann B, et al. (2011) Six-month functional outcome of a bipolar disorder cohort in the context of a specialized-care program. Bipolar Disord 13(7–8):679–686.

Rosa AR, Reinares M, Franco C, et al. (2009) Clinical predictors of functional outcome of bipolar patients in remission. Bipolar Disord 11(4):401–409.

Rosa AR, Reinares M, Michalak EE, et al. (2010) Functional impairment and disability across mood states in bipolar disorder. Value Health 13(8):984–988.

Sánchez-Moreno J, Martínez-Arán A, Tabares-Seisdedos R, et al. (2009) Functioning and disability in bipolar disorder: an extensive review. Psychother Psychosom 78(5):285–297.

Simon GE, Bauer MS, Ludman EJ, et al. (2007) Mood symptoms, functional impairment, and disability in people with bipolar disorder: specific effects of mania and depression. J Clin Psychiat 68:1237–1245.

Simon GE, Ludman EJ, Unützer J, et al. (2008) Severity of mood symptoms and work productivity in people treated for bipolar disorder. Bipolar Disord 10(6):718–725.

Strakowski SM, Keck PE Jr, McElroy SL, et al. (1998) Twelve-month outcome after a first hospitalization for affective psychosis. Arch Gen Psychiat 55(1):49–55.

Suppes T, Leverich GS, Keck PE, et al. (2001) The Stanley Foundation Bipolar Treatment Outcome Network. II. Demographics and illness characteristics of the first 261 patients. J Affect Disorders 67(1–3):45–59.

Tabarés-Seisdedos R, Balanza-Martinez V, Sanchez-Moreno J, et al. (2008) Neurocognitive and clinical predictors of functional outcome in patients with schizophrenia and bipolar I disorder at one-year follow-up. J Affect Disorders 109:286–299.

Tohen M, Greil W, Calabrese JR, et al. (2005) Olanzapine versus lithium in the maintenance treatment of bipolar disorder: a 12-month, randomized, double-blind, controlled clinical trial. Am J Psychiat 162(7):1281–1290.

Tohen M, Hennen J, Zarate Jr CM, et al. (2000) Two-year syndromal and functional recovery in 219 cases of first-episode major affective disorder with psychotic features. Am J Psychiat 157:220–228.

Torrent C, Martínez-Arán A, Daban C, et al. (2006) Cognitive impairment in bipolar II disorder. Brit J Psychiat 189:254–259.

Torres IJ, Boudreau VG, and Yatham LN (2007) Neuropsychological functioning in euthymic bipolar disorder: a meta-analysis. Acta Psychiat Scand Suppl 434:17–26.

Üstün B and Kennedy C (2009) What is 'functional impairment'? Disentangling disability from clinical significance. World Psychiat 8:82–85.

Valentí M, Pacchiarotti I, Bonnín CM, et al. (2012) Risk factors for antidepressant-related switch to mania. J Clin Psychiat 73(2):e271–276.

Vázquez GH, Kapczinski F, Magalhaes PV, et al., and the Ibero-American Network on Bipolar Disorders group (2011) Stigma and functioning in patients with bipolar disorder. J Affect Disorders 130(1–2):323–327.

Yan-Meier L, Eberhart NK, Hammen CL, et al. (2011) Stressful life events predict delayed functional recovery following treatment for mania in bipolar disorder. Psychiat Res **186**(2–3):267–271.

Zarate CA Jr, Tohen M, Land M, et al. (2000) Functional impairment and cognition in bipolar disorder. Psychiat Quart **71**:309–329.

Chapter 6

Cognition and illness progression in bipolar disorder

Anabel Martinez-Aran, Caterina del Mar Bonnin, Carla Torrent, Brisa Solé, Imma Torres, and Esther Jiménez

Introduction

Bipolar disorder (BD) is associated with cognitive impairment, which also occurs during euthymic periods. This statement is backed up by many publications. So far, six meta-analyses on the cognitive deficits associated with euthymic BD have been conducted (Robinson et al. 2006; Torres et al. 2007; Arts et al. 2008; Bora et al. 2009; Mann-Wrobel et al. 2011; Bourne et al. 2013). According to these studies, specific domains of impairment include executive control, verbal learning and memory, working memory, and sustained attention. Cognitive impairments are present already in the early course of BD (Torres et al. 2011). Moreover, a positive association between neurocognitive dysfunction and functional impairment has been shown in cross-sectional (Zubieta et al. 2001; Dickerson et al. 2004; Martinez-Aran et al. 2004b; Laes and Sponheim 2006) and longitudinal studies (Jaeger et al. 2007; Tabarés-Seisdedos et al. 2008; Martino et al. 2009; Bonnin et al. 2010). In any case, we have to bear in mind that recent studies have shown that the percentage of patients with clinically significant neurocognitive impairments fluctuates between 30% and 62% (Martino et al. 2008; Gualtieri and Morgan 2008; Reichenberg et al. 2009; Iverson et al. 2011), indicating that some people with BD might have neurocognitive functioning within normal limits.

Robinson and Ferrier (2006) provided a narrative review of studies that considered the relationship between illness variables and cognitive deficits. They found an association between the number of previous episodes, especially manic ones, and neurocognitive functioning suggesting that successive episodes might be related to a progressive neurocognitive decline. In the same line another recent review found that cognitive dysfunction increases as a function of prior number of mood episodes (Post et al. 2012). However, these results contrast with the few and small longitudinal studies about neurocognitive functioning published to date (see 'Follow-up studies and staging models' section). On the contrary, Martino and colleagues (2013) did not find that the experience of successive episodes is related to a progressive neurocognitive decline, rather it is just that cognitive impairment could be the cause more than the consequence of poorer clinical course; likewise Depp et al. (2012) suggested the relative independence of mood symptom severity and cognitive abilities.

Clinical and functioning implications

There are different factors that, directly or indirectly, may influence cognitive functioning in BD: the previous *history of psychotic symptoms* could be associated with poorer cognitive functioning in bipolar patients (Martinez-Aran et al. 2004b; Albus et al. 2006; Daban et al. 2006; Martinez-Aran et al. 2008). However, other recent reports suggest that the presence of prior history of psychotic symptoms was not related to more cognitive dysfunctions (Selva et al. 2007; Brissos et al. 2011). This factor warrants further investigation since research on this issue in BD is still very scant.

Regarding the bipolar subtype, bipolar I and II subtypes show cognitive dysfunction; nonetheless, bipolar I subjects are generally more impaired than those with bipolar II disorder (Harkavy-Friedman et al. 2006; Torrent et al. 2006; Sole et al. 2012; Kessler et al. 2013).

Subdepressive symptomatology has also a negative impact on overall functioning (Bauwens et al. 1991) and specifically on occupational functioning and cognitive functioning (Kessing 1998; Martinez-Aran et al. 2000, 2002; Bonnin et al. 2010).

Neurobiological research shows that some correlations with cognitive function, such as elevated levels of homocysteine, have been associated with cognitive impairment in otherwise healthy older adults and, in particular, impairment in attention, language, and immediate recall (Dittmann et al. 2007). *Hormonal factors* may be also associated with neurocognitive dysfunctions (Prohaska et al. 1996) together with *hypercortisolaemia*. Hypercortisolaemia can occur in the depressed and manic phases of BD. Some studies have suggested that high levels of cortisol may produce damage to the hippocampus and could partially explain the impaired performance found in neuropsychological measures of declarative learning and memory (Altshuler et al. 1998; van Gorp et al. 1998). Despite that, a recent study on the neurocognitive performance of euthymic bipolar patients did not find any association between the cognitive measures and hypercortisolaemia (Thompson et al. 2005).

Lifetime duration of BD has been associated with cognitive dysfunction (Johnstone et al. 1985). The length of illness negatively correlated with scores on tests of executive function (Clark et al. 2002; Thompson et al. 2005), psychomotor speed (Martinez-Aran et al. 2004a; Thompson et al. 2005), and verbal memory (Cavanagh et al. 2002; Deckersbach et al. 2004). Verbal memory was the measure that was more consistently associated with the duration of illness. None of the studies have reported any significant associations between duration of euthymia and performance on cognitive tests (El-Badri et al. 2001; Clark et al. 2002; Thompson et al. 2005).

According to several studies cognitive deficits, particularly in the domains of attention, memory, and executive functioning, are related to the number of prior mood episodes (Post et al. 2012); the effects of manic symptomatology on cognition seem stronger than the effects of depressive symptoms (Lopez-Jaramillo et al. 2010; Aminoff et al. 2013). Most studies have reported that those patients with a higher number of hospitalizations showed poorer performance on cognitive measures (Zubieta et al. 2001; Clark et al. 2002; Thompson et al. 2005); it is probable that the number of admissions may constitute an indirect measure of the severity of episodes, as well as of the illness course.

Other factors such as substance abuse (van Gorp et al. 1998; Sanchez-Moreno et al. 2009) and sleep disturbances (Cipolli 1995) have been found to influence negatively cognitive performance. Regarding medication, most of the current evidence suggests that the impairment effect appears more related to the illness itself rather than from the effects of pharmacotherapy.

Neurodevelopment or neuroprogression?

Some evidence suggests that individuals with BD have developmental and progressive neuropsychological alterations, BD can be considered as a developmental disorder, starting early in life, and resulting in pathological conditions during adulthood (Geoffroy et al. 2013). Patients with BD experience a chronic course of the disorder, characterized by progressive cognitive impairment, residual symptoms, sleep and circadian rhythm disturbances, emotional dysregulation, and increased risk for psychiatric and medical comorbidity between mood episodes (Leboyer and Kupfer 2010).

Following a *neurodevelopmental hypothesis*, some cognitive deficits may be present before illness onset, probably in a lesser degree or in a small subgroup of bipolar patients. For instance, both neural development and prefrontal cortex function are known to be abnormal in schizophrenia and BD. Tabarés-Seisdedos et al. (2006) tried to test the hypothesis that these features may be related with genes that regulate neuronal migration, their preliminary findings suggest that mutations on genes involved in neural migration observed in bipolar and schizophrenic patients may lead to poorer performance on tests of executive function. In all likelihood, some cognitive deficits are present before the onset of the illness but, to our knowledge, very few studies have been carried out with high-risk populations. Gourovitch et al. (1999) have reported cognitive deficits in a high-risk group of unaffected siblings of monozygotic twins discordant for BD, such as mild impairments in overall learning and retrieval. Several studies have reported some impairment in unaffected first-degree relatives of bipolar patients (Zalla et al. 2004; Antila et al. 2007; Schulze et al. 2011) compared to controls. These findings are in favour of cognitive dysfunction as an endophenotypic marker for BD.

Regarding emotional cognitive functions, early onset BD cases show greater reactivity to emotional stimuli and stronger reactions to threatening situations (Grillon et al. 2005). Compared with healthy controls both children with BD and those with a high familial risk of BD show poorer recognition of facial emotional expressions, and this deficit seems to predict progression to BD in the at-risk children (Brotman et al. 2008).

Impairments in working memory, visual-motor skills, and inhibitory control seem to be particularly marked in young BD patients when compared with healthy, age- and gender-matched adolescents (Lera-Miguel et al. 2011).

A recent meta-analysis from studies of early onset schizophrenia and paediatric BD found that individuals with paediatric BD demonstrate deficits in verbal learning and memory, processing speed, and executive control. Interestingly, these deficits are quantitatively less marked, but qualitatively similar, to those found in patients with early onset schizophrenia (Nieto and Castellanos 2011).

Following the *neuroprogressive hypothesis*, a poorer clinical course of the illness may also have a negative influence on cognition. This means that a higher number of episodes, especially the manic type, the duration of illness, and the number of hospitalizations may be related to more cognitive impairment.

Another interesting finding came from a study by Kessing and Andersen (2004), who suggested that the risk of dementia seemed to increase with the number of episodes in depressive and bipolar affective disorders. On average, the rate of dementia tended to increase 13% with every episode leading to admission for unipolar patients, and 6% with every episode leading to admission for bipolar patients. Further research is needed to examine whether cognitive decline in BD is different or not what would be expected from normal ageing. Nevertheless, disturbance progress following repeated episodes is not entirely clear, since other authors did not find significant differences between first- and multi-episode bipolar patients on cognitive functioning (Nehra et al. 2006). These contradictory findings suggest that further research is needed to elucidate the impact of chronicity.

Longitudinal studies are required to assess the evolution of cognitive impairment in bipolar patients, in order to determine the stability or progression of cognitive deficit, regarding these two hypotheses. Probably, with respect to BD both hypotheses are complementary.

Follow-up studies and staging models

Recently, a growing body of evidence of longitudinal studies confirms the findings stated in the prior cross-sectional studies.

The first longitudinal studies were of 1-year follow-up (Martino et al. 2009; Bonnín et al. 2010) and they found that neurocognitive impairment was related to poor psychosocial outcome. However, these studies only evaluated neurocognitive performance at baseline but not at follow-up.

The first 2-year follow-up study was published in 2008. Neurocognition was evaluated twice: at baseline and 2 years after, and it was found that patients treated with lithium presented with poor performance in processing speed and executive functions. These authors found that the impairment is stable across time; however, it is worth mentioning that only few patients had a relapse during the follow-up period (Mur et al. 2008). Similar results were found in a longitudinal study at 6-year follow-up by the same group: executive functioning, inhibition, processing speed, and verbal memory being the domains more affected, with its residual effect on the psychosocial adaptation of patients (Mora et al. 2013).

A 3-year follow-up study comparing schizophrenic and bipolar patients suggested that both patient groups were more impaired in several neuropsychological measures than the healthy controls (Balanza-Martinez et al. 2005).

In general, longitudinal studies of neurocognitive functioning published so far have found a stable pattern of cognitive impairment over time; the exception being a 9-year longitudinal study that found a worsening in executive functioning. Later analyses revealed that illness duration and subdepressive symptoms were associated with poorer performance in executive functions (Torrent et al. 2013).

Other studies suggest the effect of the clinical course on neurocognition and psychosocial functioning. For instance, Lopez-Jaramillo et al. (2010) assessed three groups of bipolar euthymic patients according to the number of previous manic episodes. Although this was not a follow-up study, the evidence pointed that the recurrence of mania in the long term had an impact on neurocognition. Those patients who had experienced three or more episodes were more impaired in attention and executive functions when compared to patients who had suffered only one episode.

The literature shows that BD patients present good premorbid neurocognitive functioning before illness onset (Lewandowski et al. 2011). However, after illness onset, and especially after the first episode of mania, meaningful pathophysiological changes start occurring (Andreazza et al. 2009; Kauer-Sant'anna et al. 2009). These changes (decrease in brain-derived neurotrophic factor, increase in inflammatory cytokines), which can be detected in serum levels, may mediate dysfunction, affecting neuropsychological performance. In fact, many studies point out the neurotoxic effect of manic episodes on neurocognition, and in particularly on executive functions (Thompson et al. 2005; Elshahawi et al. 2010; Lopez-Jaramillo et al. 2010). Hence, manic episodes seem to be more consistently related to neurocognitive impairment (especially verbal memory and executive functions) whereas depressive episodes relate less consistently to a broader range of impairments (Savitz et al. 2005).

When compared to schizophrenia, one 5-year longitudinal study suggests that neurocognition declines steadily over the early course of schizophrenia, but in BD it seems to be more stable. Burdick and colleagues found that schizophrenic patients exhibited significant deterioration in executive functioning, but no significant changes in other domains, while patients with BD showed stability over time in attention measures, but greater variability in other domains (Burdick et al. 2006).

A recent meta-analysis (Mann-Wrobel et al. 2011) subdivided the studies based on clinical course variables (e.g. number of episodes, insight, psychosis, etc.) in order to evaluate the impact of the clinical course on neurocognition. Their results suggested that the poor clinical course group performed modestly worse when compared to the good clinical course. In the same line, Bora et al. (2009) found that earlier age of onset was associated with verbal memory impairment and psychomotor slowing. Another meta-analysis found that neurocognitive function was negatively related to certain illness features, such as duration of illness (Robinson et al. 2006). Finally, Arts et al. (2008) found an effect for sex, age, and education. Specifically, larger effect sizes were found for education in tests measuring span, fluency, and card sorting variables in studies in which the participants' average level of education was higher. Similarly, Mann-Wrobel et al. (2011) found that cognitive impairment effect size decreased as a function of education. The authors hypothesized that education could be a marker related to the onset and severity of illness, since an early and severe illness interferes with educational attainment.

These results are in line with the hypothesis of neuroprogression (Goodwin et al. 2008) and staging models (Kapczinski et al. 2009), then it is possible that neuroprogression is as shown in Table 6.1.

Nevertheless, some data in older euthymic patients do not support the idea of greater impairment with ageing and illness progression. For instance, Delaloye et al. (2009) evaluated a sample of 17 euthymic elderly patients compared to age-, gender-, and education-matched healthy individuals. They found that BD patients had lower performances in tests measuring processing speed, working memory, and episodic memory when compared with healthy controls. Moreover, the observed effect size falls within the moderate-to-large difference to that reported in studies focusing on younger patients with BD. Finally, the BD group

Table 6.1 Clinical staging in bipolar disorder (source data from Kapczinski et al. 2009)

Stage	Clinical features	Cognition
Latent	At risk for developing BD, positive family history, mood or anxiety, symptoms without criteria for threshold BD	No impairment
I	Well-defined periods of euthymia without overt psychiatric symptoms	No impairment
II	Symptoms in interepisodic periods related to comorbidities	Transient impairment
III	Marked impairment in cognition and functioning	Severe cognitive impairment associated with functioning impairment (unable to work or very impaired performance)
IV	Unable to live autonomously owing to cognitive and functional impairment	Cognitive impairment prevents patients from living independently

did not display significant vascular or volumetric brain abnormalities. A further longitudinal study confirmed the lack of distinction between BD patients and controls in respect to the 2-year changes in cognition and magnetic resonance imaging findings (Delaloye et al. 2011).

However, as suggested by Robinson et al. (2006), it could be hypothesized that the differential between patients and controls would be expected to be greatest at younger ages until age-related decline in healthy subjects begins to narrow the gap.

Despite the research efforts in this area, the neurocognitive outcome in BD is still unclear. The heterogeneity in the neurocognitive impairment and its link with staging models presents one of the challenges in the upcoming years.

The prevention of relapses will be essential to reduce their negative impact on the cognitive functioning of bipolar patients. In this case, clinicians should try to improve the clinical course of patients by optimizing the pharmacological treatment and including psychoeducation.

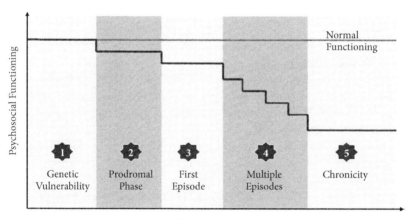

Fig 6.1 Functional impairment according to the staging model.

There is a genetic vulnerability for the development of BD (1); however, before illness onset there is no evidence of functional impairment. In the prodromal phase (2), patients may start to present minimal difficulties in their outcome. After the first episode, the functional impairment may be transient and related to acute phases (3). Nevertheless, every relapse provokes a marked impairment in the outcome (4). Finally (5), the accumulative impact of the recurrent episodes leads to chronicity and inadequate functional recovery.

Adapted from Martínez-Arán et al. 2011 and reproduced under the Creative Commons License 3.0.

Bipolar patients showing persistent cognitive impairment may also benefit from cognitive rehabilitation in order to improve, not only cognitive functioning, but also their general functioning (Fig. 6.1).

References

Albus M, Hubmann W, Mohr F, et al. (2006) Neurocognitive functioning in patients with first-episode schizophrenia: results of a prospective 5-year follow-up study. Eur Arch Psy Clin N **256**:442–451.

Altshuler LL, Bartzokis G, Grieder T, et al. (1998) Amygdala enlargement in bipolar disorder and hippocampal reduction in schizophrenia: an MRI study demonstrating neuroanatomic specificity. Arch Gen Psychiat **55**:663–664.

Aminoff SR, Hellvin T, Lagerberg TV, et al. (2013) Neurocognitive features in subgroups of bipolar disorder. Bipolar Disord **15**:272–283.

Andreazza AC, Kapczinski F, Kauer-Sant'anna M, et al. (2009) 3-Nitrotyrosine and glutathione antioxidant system in patients in the early and late stages of bipolar disorder. J Psychiat Neurosci **34**:263–271.

Antila M, Tuulio-Henriksson A, Kieseppa T, et al. (2007) Cognitive functioning in patients with familial bipolar I disorder and their unaffected relatives. Psychol Med **37**:679–687.

Arts B, Jabben N, Krabbendam L, et al. (2008) Meta-analyses of cognitive functioning in euthymic bipolar patients and their first-degree relatives. Psychol Med **38**:771–785.

Balanza-Martinez V, Tabarés-Seisdedos R, Selva-Vera G, et al. (2005) Persistent cognitive dysfunctions in bipolar I disorder and schizophrenic patients: a 3-year follow-up study. Psychother Psychosom **74**:113–119.

Bauwens F, Tracy A, Pardoen D, et al. (1991) Social adjustment of remitted bipolar and unipolar out-patients. A comparison with age- and sex-matched controls. Brit J Psychiat **159**:239–244.

Bonnin CM, Martinez-Aran A, Torrent C, et al. (2010) Clinical and neurocognitive predictors of functional outcome in bipolar euthymic patients: a long-term, follow-up study. J Affect Disorders **121**:156–160.

Bora E, Yucel M, and Pantelis C (2009) Cognitive endophenotypes of bipolar disorder: a meta-analysis of neuropsychological deficits in euthymic patients and their first-degree relatives. J Affect Disorders **113**:1–20.

Bourne C, Aydemir O, Balanza-Martinez V, et al. (2013) Neuropsychological testing of cognitive impairment in euthymic bipolar disorder: an individual patient data meta-analysis. Acta Psychiat Scand **128**:149–162.

Brissos S, Dias VV, Soeiro-de-Souza MG, et al. (2011) The impact of a history of psychotic symptoms on cognitive function in euthymic bipolar patients: a comparison with schizophrenic patients and healthy controls. Rev Bras Psiquiatr **33**:353–361.

Brotman MA, Skup M, Rich BA, et al. (2008) Risk for bipolar disorder is associated with face-processing deficits across emotions. J Am Acad Child Adolesc Psy **47**:1455–1461.

Burdick KE, Goldberg JF, Harrow M, et al. (2006) Neurocognition as a stable endophenotype in bipolar disorder and schizophrenia. J Nerv Ment Dis **194**:255–260.

Cavanagh JT, Van Beck M, Muir W, et al. (2002) Case-control study of neurocognitive function in euthymic patients with bipolar disorder: an association with mania. Brit J Psychiat **180**:320–326.

Cipolli C (1995) Symposium: Cognitive processes and sleep disturbances. Sleep, dreams and memory: an overview. J Sleep Res **4**:2–9.

Clark L, Iversen SD, and Goodwin GM (2002) Sustained attention deficit in bipolar disorder. Brit J Psychiat **180**:313–319.

Daban C, Martinez-Aran A, Torrent C, et al. (2006) Specificity of cognitive deficits in bipolar disorder versus schizophrenia. A systematic review. Psychother Psychosom **75**:72–84.

Deckersbach T, Savage CR, Reilly-Harrington N, et al. (2004) Episodic memory impairment in bipolar disorder and obsessive-compulsive disorder: the role of memory strategies. Bipolar Disord **6**:233–244.

Delaloye C, de Bilbao F, Moy G, et al. (2009) Neuroanatomical and neuropsychological features of euthymic patients with bipolar disorder. Am J Geriat Psychiat **17**:1012–1021.

Delaloye C, Moy G, de Bilbao F, et al. (2011) Longitudinal analysis of cognitive performances and structural brain changes in late-life bipolar disorder. Int J Geriat Psychiat **26**:1309–1318.

Depp CA, Mausbach BT, Harmell AL, et al. (2012) Meta-analysis of the association between cognitive abilities and everyday functioning in bipolar disorder. Bipolar Disord **14**:217–226.

Dickerson F, Boronow JJ, Stallings C, et al. (2004) Cognitive functioning in schizophrenia and bipolar disorder: comparison of performance on the Repeatable Battery for the Assessment of Neuropsychological Status. Psychiat Res **129**:45–53.

Dittmann S, Seemuller F, Schwarz MJ, et al. (2007) Association of cognitive deficits with elevated homocysteine levels in euthymic bipolar patients and its impact on psychosocial functioning: preliminary results. Bipolar Disord **9**:63–70.

El-Badri SM, Ashton CH, Moore PB, et al. (2001) Electrophysiological and cognitive function in young euthymic patients with bipolar affective disorder. Bipolar Disord **3**:79–87.

Elshahawi HH, Essawi H, Rabie MA, et al. (2010) Cognitive functions among euthymic bipolar I patients after a single manic episode versus recurrent episodes. J Affect Disorders **130**:180–191. doi: 10.1016/j.jad.2010.10.027.

Geoffroy PA, Etain B, Scott J, et al. (2013) Reconsideration of bipolar disorder as a developmental disorder: Importance of the time of onset. J Physiol Paris.

Goodwin GM, Martinez-Aran A, Glahn DC, et al. (2008) Cognitive impairment in bipolar disorder: neurodevelopment or neurodegeneration? An ECNP expert meeting report. Eur Neuropsychopharm 18:787–793.

Gourovitch ML, Torrey EF, Gold JM, et al. (1999) Neuropsychological performance of monozygotic twins discordant for bipolar disorder. Biol Psychiat 45:639–646.

Grillon C, Warner V, Hille J, et al. (2005) Families at high and low risk for depression: a three-generation startle study. Biol Psychiat 57:953–960.

Gualtieri CT and Morgan DW (2008) The frequency of cognitive impairment in patients with anxiety, depression, and bipolar disorder: an unaccounted source of variance in clinical trials. J Clin Psychiat 69:1122–1130.

Harkavy-Friedman JM, Keilp JG, Grunebaum MF, et al. (2006) Are BPI and BPII suicide attempters distinct neuropsychologically? J Affect Disorders 94:255–259.

Iverson GL, Brooks BL, Langenecker SA, et al. (2011) Identifying a cognitive impairment subgroup in adults with mood disorders. J Affect Disorders 132:360–367.

Jaeger J, Berns S, Loftus S, et al. (2007) Neurocognitive test performance predicts functional recovery from acute exacerbation leading to hospitalization in bipolar disorder. Bipolar Disord 9:93–102.

Johnstone EC, Owens DG, Frith CD, et al. (1985) Institutionalisation and the outcome of functional psychoses. Brit J Psychiat 146:36–44.

Kapczinski F, Dias VV, Kauer-Sant'anna M, et al. (2009) Clinical implications of a staging model for bipolar disorders. Expert Rev Neurother 9:957–966.

Kauer-Sant'anna M, Kapczinski F, Andreazza AC, et al. (2009) Brain-derived neurotrophic factor and inflammatory markers in patients with early- vs. late-stage bipolar disorder. Int J Neuropsychoph 12:447–458.

Kessing LV (1998) Cognitive impairment in the euthymic phase of affective disorder. Psychol Med 28:1027–1038.

Kessing LV and Andersen PK (2004) Does the risk of developing dementia increase with the number of episodes in patients with depressive disorder and in patients with bipolar disorder? J Neurol Neurosurg Ps 75:1662–1666.

Kessler U, Schoeyen HK, Andreassen OA, et al. (2013) Neurocognitive profiles in treatment-resistant bipolar I and bipolar II disorder depression. BMC Psychiat 13:105.

Laes JR and Sponheim SR (2006) Does cognition predict community function only in schizophrenia?: a study of schizophrenia patients, bipolar affective disorder patients, and community control subjects. Schizophr Res 84:121–131.

Leboyer M and Kupfer DJ (2010) Bipolar disorder: new perspectives in health care and prevention. J Clin Psychiat 71:1689–1695.

Lera-Miguel S, Andres-Perpina S, Calvo R, et al. (2011) Early-onset bipolar disorder: how about visual-spatial skills and executive functions? Eur Arch Psy Clin N 261:195–203.

Lewandowski KE, Cohen BM, and Ongur D (2011) Evolution of neuropsychological dysfunction during the course of schizophrenia and bipolar disorder. Psychol Med 41:225–241.

Lopez-Jaramillo C, Lopera-Vasquez J, Gallo A, et al. (2010) Effects of recurrence on the cognitive performance of patients with bipolar I disorder: implications for relapse prevention and treatment adherence. Bipolar Disord 12:557–567.

Mann-Wrobel MC, Carreno JT, and Dickinson D (2011) Meta-analysis of neuro-psychological functioning in euthymic bipolar disorder: an update and investigation of moderator variables. Bipolar Disord 13:334–342.

Martínez-Arán A, Torrent C, Solé B, Bonnín CM, Rosa AR, Sánchez-Moreno J, Vieta E (2011) Functional remediation for bipolar disorder. Clin Pract Epidemiol Ment Health 7:112–116.

Martinez-Aran A, Torrent C, Tabarés-Seisdedos R, et al. (2008) Neurocognitive impairment in bipolar patients with and without history of psychosis. J Clin Psychiatry 69:233–239.

Martinez-Aran A, Vieta E, Colom F, et al. (2000) Cognitive dysfunctions in bipolar disorder: evidence of neuropsychological disturbances. Psychother Psychosom 69:2–18.

Martinez-Aran A, Vieta E, Colom F, et al. (2002) Neuropsychological performance in depressed and euthymic bipolar patients. Neuropsychobiology 46(Suppl 1):16–21.

Martinez-Aran A, Vieta E, Colom F, et al. (2004a) Cognitive impairment in euthymic bipolar patients: implications for clinical and functional outcome. Bipolar Disord 6:224–232.

Martinez-Aran A, Vieta E, Reinares M, et al. (2004b) Cognitive function across manic or hypomanic, depressed, and euthymic states in bipolar disorder. Am J Psychiat 161:262–270.

Martino DJ, Marengo E, Igoa A, et al. 2009. Neurocognitive and symptomatic pre-dictors of functional outcome in bipolar disorders: a prospective 1 year follow-up study. J Affect Disorders 116:37–42.

Martino DJ, Strejilevich SA, Marengo E, et al. (2013) Relationship between neurocog-nitive functioning and episode recurrences in bipolar disorder. J Affect Disorders 147:345–351.

Martino DJ, Strejilevich SA, Scapola M, et al. (2008) Heterogeneity in cognitive func-tioning among patients with bipolar disorder. J Affect Disorders 109:149–156.

Mora E, Portella MJ, Forcada I, et al. (2013) Persistence of cognitive impairment and its negative impact on psychosocial functioning in lithium-treated, euthymic bipo-lar patients: a 6-year follow-up study. Psychol Med 43:1187–1196.

Mur M, Portella MJ, Martinez-Aran A, et al. (2008) Long-term stability of cogni-tive impairment in bipolar disorder: a 2-year follow-up study of lithium-treated euthymic bipolar patients. J Clin Psychiat 69:712–719.

Nehra R, Chakrabarti S, Pradhan BK, et al. (2006) Comparison of cognitive functions between first- and multi-episode bipolar affective disorders. J Affect Disorders 93:185–192.

Nieto RG and Castellanos FX (2011) A meta-analysis of neuropsychological function-ing in patients with early onset schizophrenia and pediatric bipolar disorder. J Clin Child Adolesc Psychol 40:266–280.

Post RM, Fleming J, and Kapczinski F (2012) Neurobiological correlates of illness progression in the recurrent affective disorders. J Psychiat Res **46**:561–573.

Prohaska ML, Stern RA, Nevels CT, et al. (1996) The relationship between thyroid status and neuropsychological performance in psychiatric outpatients maintained on lithium. Neuropsychiatry Neuropsychol Behav Neurol **9**:30–34.

Reichenberg A, Harvey PD, Bowie CR, et al. (2009) Neuropsychological function and dysfunction in schizophrenia and psychotic affective disorders. Schizophr Bull **35**:1022–1029.

Robinson LJ and Ferrier IN (2006) Evolution of cognitive impairment in bipolar disorder: a systematic review of cross-sectional evidence. Bipolar Disord **8**:103–116.

Robinson LJ, Thompson JM, Gallagher P, et al. (2006) A meta-analysis of cognitive deficits in euthymic patients with bipolar disorder. J Affect Disorders **93**:105–115.

Sanchez-Moreno J, Martinez-Aran A, Tabarés-Seisdedos R, Torrent C, Vieta E, Ayuso-Mateos JL (2009) Functioning and disability in bipolar disorder: an extensive review. Psychother Psychosom **78**:285–297.

Savitz J, Solms M, and Ramesar R (2005) Neuropsychological dysfunction in bipolar affective disorder: a critical opinion. Bipolar Disord **7**:216–235.

Schulze KK, Walshe M, Stahl D, et al. (2011) Executive functioning in familial bipolar I disorder patients and their unaffected relatives. Bipolar Disord **13**:208–216.

Selva G, Salazar J, Balanza-Martinez V, et al. (2007) Bipolar I patients with and without a history of psychotic symptoms: do they differ in their cognitive functioning? J Psychiat Res **41**:265–272.

Sole B, Bonnin CM, Torrent C, et al. (2012) Neurocognitive impairment and psychosocial functioning in bipolar II disorder. Acta Psychiat Scand **125**:309–317.

Tabarés-Seisdedos R, Balanza-Martinez V, Sanchez-Moreno J, et al. (2008) Neurocognitive and clinical predictors of functional outcome in patients with schizophrenia and bipolar I disorder at one-year follow-up. J Affect Disorders **109**:286–299.

Tabarés-Seisdedos R, Escamez T, Martinez-Gimenez JA, et al. (2006) Variations in genes regulating neuronal migration predict reduced prefrontal cognition in schizophrenia and bipolar subjects from Mediterranean Spain: a preliminary study. Neuroscience **139**:1289–1300.

Thompson JM, Gallagher P, Hughes JH, et al. (2005) Neurocognitive impairment in euthymic patients with bipolar affective disorder. Brit J Psychiat **186**:32–40.

Torrent C, Del Mar BC, Martinez-Aran A, et al. (2013) Efficacy of functional remediation in bipolar disorder: a multicenter randomized controlled study. Am J Psychiat **170**:852–859.

Torrent C, Martinez-Aran A, Daban C, et al. (2006) Cognitive impairment in bipolar II disorder. Brit J Psychiat **189**:254–259.

Torres IJ, Boudreau VG, and Yatham LN (2007) Neuropsychological functioning in euthymic bipolar disorder: a meta-analysis. Acta Psychiat Scand Suppl **116**:17–26.

Torres IJ, DeFreitas CM, DeFreitas VG, et al. (2011) Relationship between cognitive functioning and 6-month clinical and functional outcome in patients with first manic episode bipolar I disorder. Psychol Med **41**:971–982.

van Gorp WG, Altshuler L, Theberge DC, et al. (1998) Cognitive impairment in euthymic bipolar patients with and without prior alcohol dependence. A preliminary study. Arch Gen Psychiat **55**:41–46.

Zalla T, Joyce C, Szoke A, et al. (2004) Executive dysfunctions as potential markers of familial vulnerability to bipolar disorder and schizophrenia. Psychiat Res **121**:207–217.

Zubieta JK, Huguelet P, O'Neil RL, et al. (2001) Cognitive function in euthymic bipolar I disorder. Psychiat Res **102**:9–20.

Chapter 7

Social cognition and staging in bipolar disorder

Sergio Strejilevich and Diego Martino

Introduction

Most of the characteristic symptoms of bipolar disorders (BD) are related to distortions or failures in behaviours, which are related to decision-making and emotional processing. Mistakes on economic, vocational, and social decisions due to underestimation or biased understanding of the feelings of other people are usual in manic episodes, and are probably amongst the most important sources of the burden of affective disorders. In addition, difficulties to take simple decisions—such as to choose which clothes to wear for work—or inadequate fears that may lead to avoiding everyday challenges are typical symptoms, which are in the core of BD. One of the most promising ways to address the physiological bases of this kind of symptomatology is through social cognition paradigms. Social cognition refers to the mental operations underlying social interactions, which could be relatively independent from other aspects of cognition and it is not assessed by traditional neurocognitive tasks (Pinkham et al. 2003).

One of the key aspects of social cognition is the cognitive ability to attribute mental states, such as beliefs, desires, and intents to oneself and others. These abilities have been conceptualized as theory of mind (ToM). ToM, also referred to as metalizing or mindreading, starts to develop after the acquisition of secondary representation in the second year of life (Suddendorf and Withen 2001). Another aspect of social cognition relates to the ability discriminate accurately between different facially expressed emotions. These emotions are thought to be innate, automatic, and universal (Darwin 1872; Ekman and Friesen 1971); and new research have shown that they may be modulated by tymoleptic drugs as antidepressants (Harmer et al. 2009). Most of the investigations assessing facial emotion recognition required subjects to either match (matching paradigms) or name (labelling paradigms) pictures of posed facial expressions according to the six basic emotions displayed (happiness, sadness, anger, disgust, fear, and surprise) (Young et al. 2002; Bozikas et al. 2006).

Finally, a domain closely related with social cognition is affective decision-making that implies weighing up choices associated with variable degrees of reward and punishment. Different paradigms were developed intending to simulate real-life decision-making processes that require subject to weigh short-term gains against potential long-term losses (Bechara et al. 1994; Rubinsztein et al. 2000). Research on social cognition in BD may help in achieving a better understanding of cognitive mechanisms involved in these disorders. However, despite the robust evidence supporting the impairment of different traditional neurocognitive domains in bipolar patients and the strong association between cognitive dysfunction and functional disability (Martino et al. 2009; Bourne et al. 2013), research on social and emotional cognition in BD is still scant.

In order to assess a possible role of social cognition in staging models of BD (Berk et al. 2007; Kapczinski et al. 2009), we review, in the present chapter, the evidence on: (1) social cognition in BD, (2) social cognition and functioning, and (3) social cognition and the course of BD. At the end of the chapter, the authors delineate the directions of future research in the field and assess a possible role of social cognition assessment in models of tagging in BD.

Social cognition in bipolar disorder

The first study designed specifically to assess ToM skills in BD found that both manic and depressive patients had impairments while euthymic patients had a performance comparable to controls (Kerr et al. 2003). Later studies showed consistently that euthymic BD patients show deficits in ToM tasks (Inoue et al. 2004; Bora et al. 2005; Olley et al. 2005; Lahera et al. 2008; Shamay-Tsoory et al. 2009; McKinnon et al. 2010; Montag et al. 2010; Wolf et al. 2010; Martino et al. 2011). These studies are summarized in Table 7.1. However, the three studies with larger sample

Table 7.1 Studies about theory of mind in euthymic patients with bipolar disorder

Study	Sample	Age (mean)	Euthymic measures	Main findings
Kerr et al. 2003	48 BD and 15 controls	43.9	Euthymic (13): BDI, NS Depression (15) Mania (20)	ToM deficits in mania and depression, preserved in euthymic
Inoue et al. 2004	16 BDI, 34 MDD, and 50 controls	44.5	Remitted depression: HDRS ≤ 7	ToM impairments both in BD and MDD
Bora et al. 2005	43 BDI and 30 controls	38.6	Euthymic: HDRS < 7, YMRS < 6	ToM deficits
Olley et al. 2005	15 BDI and 13 controls	39.2	Euthymic: HDRS < 12, YMRS < 12	ToM deficits
Lahera et al. 2008	75 BDI and 48 controls	48.2	Euthymic: YMRS < 8, HDRS < 8	ToM deficits
Shamay-Tsoory et al. 2009	19 BDI and 20 controls	40.2	Euthymic: HDRS ≤ 9, YMRS ≤ 7	ToM deficits Preserved facial emotion recognition
McKinnon et al. 2010	14 BD and 14 controls	47.5	Subclinical symptoms: HDRS ≥ 7, ≤ 15; YMRS < 10	ToM deficits
Montag et al. 2010	29 BDI and 29 controls	44	Euthymic: HDRS < 14, YMRS < 5	Impairments in cognitive ToM
Wolf et al. 2010	33 BDI and 29 controls	47.7	Euthymic (11): HDRS < 15, YMRS < 12 Mania (10) Depression (12)	ToM deficits regarding controls, without differences between mood states
Martino et al. 2011	45 BDI, 36 BDII, and 34 controls	39.7	Euthymic: HDRS < 8, YMRS < 6	ToM deficits. Impairments in recognition of fearful facial expression

BD: bipolar disorder; BDI: bipolar disorder type I; BDII: bipolar disorder type II; MDD: major depressive disorder; BDI: Beck Depression Inventory; HDRS: Hamilton Depression Rating Scale; YMRS: Young Mania Rating Scale; ToM: theory of mind.

sizes reported that impairments in ToM could be mediated, at least in part, by impairments in traditional neurocognitive domains (attention and executive functions) and exposure to psychoactive drugs (Bora et al. 2005; Lahera et al. 2008; Martino et al. 2011). Therefore, future studies are needed before concluding that ToM deficits are trait markers in BD.

More controversial findings come from studies in euthymic BD that assessed other aspects of social cognition as the ability to discriminate accurately between different facially expressed emotions. A small study reported that patients with BD type II (BDII) ($n = 8$) showed greater recognition of fear than those with BD type I (BDI) (Lembke and Ketter 2002), while Harmer et al. (2002) found a robust facilitation in the discrimination of disgusted facial expressions in patients with BD compared with matched controls. On the contrary, in a study by Venn et al. (2004) there were no differences in facial affect recognition between BD patients and healthy controls, although there was an evident statistical trend to lower recognition of fear amongst patients, suggesting that the lack of significance may be the result of a small sample size ($n = 17$). Similarly, Bora et al. (2005) showed similar facial affect recognition of basic emotions between patients with BD and healthy controls. Bozikas et al. (2006) reported a deficit in the matching of facial basic emotional expressions, in a small sample ($n = 19$) of remitted BDI patients. Martino et al. (2011) reported deficits in recognition of fearful facial expression amongst euthymic BD patients. The inconsistent findings of the studies in facial affect recognition may be partly explained by heterogeneity within BD, but also by several methodological limitations, such as the employment of different measures of emotional processing, the inclusion of poorly matched control groups, varying definitions of euthymia, and high probabilities of type II error due to small sample sizes in most investigations.

Regarding decision-making paradigms, research showed that both manic (Clark et al. 2001; Murphy et al. 2001; Adida et al. 2008) and depressive BD patients (Murphy et al. 2001; Rubinsztein et al. 2006) presented impairments in decision-making.

Nevertheless, the findings of studies in euthymic patients are controversial. In earlier studies, euthymic patients with BDI demonstrated a similar performance to that of healthy controls (Rubinsztein et al. 2000;

Clark et al. 2002), suggesting that decision-making impairments are state-dependent. In contrast, more recent studies on euthymic patients reported an Iowa Gambling Task (IGT) net score, an overall measure of performance in the task, in the impaired range (+1.0) (Christodoulou et al. 2006); and the studies also found that the diagnosis of BD was linked with low decision-making performance (Jollant et al. 2007), suggesting that it is a trait-maker of BD. Moreover, two studies published recently that used the same paradigm of decision-making in a large sample of euthymic patients reported contradictory findings (Martino et al. 2010; Adida et al. 2011). Studies in euthymic patients are summarized in Table 7.2. Recently, our group performed the first meta-analytic study on social cognition in euthymic patients with BD (Samamé et al. 2012).

Table 7.2 Studies about decision-making in euthymic patients with bipolar disorder

Study	Sample	Age (mean)	Euthymic measures	Main findings
Rubinsztein et al. 2000	18 BDI and 18 controls	42	Euthymic: HDRS < 8, YMRS < 8	No differences between groups in the CGT BD greater response latency
Clark et al. 2002	30 BDI and 30 controls	35.9	Euthymic: HDRS < 8, YMRS < 8	No differences between groups in the IGT
Christodoulou et al. 2006	25 BDI	48.3	Euthymic: MADS < 11, YMRS < 7	Average score of IGT in deficient range Relationship between deficits in IGT and impulsiveness
Jollant et al. 2007	66 BD	36.0	Euthymic: HDRS < 7	Diagnosis of BD was associated with deficits in the IGT
Martino et al. 2010	48 BDI, 37 BDII, and 34 controls	39.9	Euthymic: HDRS < 8, YMRS < 6	No differences between groups in the IGT
Adida et al. 2011	90 BDI and 150 controls	39.8	Euthymic: HDRS < 8, YMRS < 6	Patients performed worse on the IGT

BD: bipolar disorder; BDI: bipolar disorder type I; BDII: bipolar disorder type II; HDRS: Hamilton Depression Rating Scale; YMRS: Young Mania Rating Scale; CGT: Cambridge Gamble Task; IGT: Iowa Gambling Task.

This study found moderate effect size for ToM skills and differences of small magnitude for the recognition of facial affect expressions, whereas decision-making appears to be preserved.

Social cognition and functioning

Data about the relationship between social cognition dysfunctions and functional outcomes are scarce. Regarding emotional processing, only two studies have explored the impact on functionality: Harmer et al. (2002) did not find correlation between emotion processing and social adjustment, while Martino et al. (2011) found that psychosocial functioning correlated positively with performance in facial recognition of disgust and fear. However, these variables did not contribute to the variance, neither were they independent predictors of psychosocial functioning, after controlling for the effect of traditional neurocognitive deficits. Similarly, two studies have evaluated the impact of failures in ToM on functional evolution and reported negative findings (Olley et al. 2005; Martino et al 2011).

Social cognition and the course of bipolar disorder

Currently, no longitudinal studies have assessed evaluated static or progressive nature of social cognition deficits. Cross-sectional studies have not found a relationship between performance in ToM tasks and number of previous episodes (Inoue et al. 2004; Bora et al. 2005; McKinnon et al. 2010; Martino et al. 2011), though this association was not assessed in some other works (Kerr et al. 2003; Olley et al. 2005; Lahera et al. 2008; Sharma-Tsoory et al. 2009; Wolf et al. 2010). Only one study found a correlation between the number of hypo/manic episodes and ToM skills, although statistical significance was not maintained after Bonferroni corrections (Montag et al. 2010). Similarly, most of the work found no relationship between ToM performance with measures of chronicity (Inoue et al. 2004; Bora et al. 2005; Martino et al. 2011), with the exception of McKinnon et al. (2010) who reported a correlation with length of illness.

Regarding emotion processing, only one study explored the association between recognition of facial expressions and number of previous episodes, with negative findings (Martino et al. 2011). Further, both Bozikas et al. (2006) and Martino et al. (2011) did not show any relationship between recognition of facial expressions and length of illness. Finally, the three studies that researched a relationship between decision-making performance and number of previous episodes, or length of illness, did not find any positive result (Clark et al. 2002; Martino et al. 2010; Adida et al. 2011).

Conclusions and future directions

Evidence suggests that the impairment in ToM tasks and emotional processing may be smaller in magnitude (in terms of effect size) as compared to that observed in traditional neurocognitive functions such as verbal memory, attention, and executive functions (Robinson et al. 2006; Torres et al. 2007). Moreover, it has been proposed that social cognition impairments could be mediated, at least in part, by attention and executive deficits and exposure to psychotropic drugs. Finally, existing impairments in social cognition in BD patients may have less impact on the functional outcome of affected patients as compared to other cognitive domains such as verbal memory (Bonnin et al. 2014). Additionally, data on decisions paradigms suggest a relative preservation in this domain (Samamé et al. 2012). Taken together, these data suggest the need to control confounding biases in studies assessing the performance in social cognition tasks as well as in those exploring the relationship between social cognitive flaws and psychosocial functioning in BD.

In addition, cross-sectional data available suggest that alterations in social cognition measures could be relatively independent of the number of previous episodes and other measures of chronicity such as length of illness. This pattern, unlike the one observed in traditional neurocognitive domains, would suggest that social cognition tasks might be of limited utility in the development of models of staging. However, these data should be considered cautiously because they are supported by few studies. Moreover, the data revised above do not exclude the presence of a subgroup of bipolar patients on which there were social cognition dysfunctions. As an example, in the study of Martino et al. (2011), patients with antecedents of suicide attempts had a lower performance in a decision-making paradigm (IGT) than those who do not.

Further assessment of the role of social cognition in the progression of BD should focus on longitudinal studies with serial cognitive assessments. This approach would clarify whether or not changes in social cognition reported amongst bipolar patients are progressive. It should be mentioned that evidence gathered so far does not support the notion of a progressive decline in social cognition in BD. This is in line with recent findings from our group which suggest that cognitive impairment may not be a consequence, but rather a risk factor for recurrent episodes (Martino et al. 2013). A pragmatic approach to the notion of staging would suggest that patients with poorer performance in tests of social cognition may be placed amongst those with a more severe and late-stage type of disorder. To that, we add as a final comment that clinicians should bear in mind that cognitive impairment as an endophenotype of BD has been traditionally associated with poorer outcomes. However, the direction of the association (cause or consequence) remains to be determined.

References

Adida M, Clark L, Pomietto P, et al. (2008) Lack of insight may predict impaired decision making in manic patients. Bipolar Disord **10**:829–837.

Adida M, Jollant F, Clark TL (2011) Trait-related decision-making impairment in the three phases of bipolar disorder. Biol Psychiat **70**:357–365.

Bechara A, Damasio A, Damasio H, et al. (1994) Insensitivity to future consequences following damage to human prefrontal cortex. Cognition **50**:7–15.

Berk M, Hallam KT, and McGorry PD (2007) The potential utility of a staging model as a course specifier: a bipolar disorder perspective. J Affect Disorders **100**:279–281.

Bonnín CDM, González-Pinto A, et al. (2014) Verbal memory as a mediator in the relationship between subthreshold depressive symptoms and functional outcome in bipolar disorder. J Affect Disorders **160**:50–54.

Bora E, Vahip S, Gonul A, et al. (2005) Evidence of theory of mind deficits in euthymic patients with bipolar disorder. Acta Psychiat Scand **112**:110–116.

Bourne C, Aydemir Ö, Balanzá-Martínez V, et al. (2013) Neuropsychological testing of cognitive impairment in euthymic bipolar disorder: an individual patient data meta-analysis. Acta Psychiat Scand **128**(3):149–162.

Bozikas V, Tonia T, Fokas K, et al. (2006) Impaired emotion processing in remitted patients with bipolar disorder. J Affect Disorders **91**(1):53–56.

Christodoulou T, Lewis M, Ploubidis G, et al. (2006) The relationship of impulsivity to response inhibition and decision-making in remitted patients with bipolar disorder. Eur Psychiat **21**:270–273.

Clark L, Iversen S, and Goodwin G (2001) A neuropsychological investigation of prefrontal cortex involvement in acute mania. Am J Psychiat **158**:1605–1611.

Clark L, Iverson SD, and Goodwin GM (2002) Sustained attention deficit in bipolar disorder. Brit J Psychiat **180**:313–319.

Darwin C (1965) The Expression of Emotions in Man and Animals (1872). Chicago IL: University of Chicago Press.

Ekman P and Friesen WV (1971) Constants across cultures in the face and emotion. J Pers Soc Psychol **17**:124–129.

Harmer CJ, Goodwin GM, and Cowen PH (2009) Why do antidepressants take so long to work? A cognitive neuropsychological model of antidepressant drug action. Brit J Psychiat **195**:102–108.

Harmer C, Grayson M, and Goodwin G (2002) Enhanced recognition of disgust in bipolar illness. Biol Psychiat **51**:298–304.

Inoue Y, Tonooka W, Yamada K, et al. (2004) Deficiency of theory of mind in remitted mood disorder. J Affect Disorders **82**:403–409.

Jollant F, Guillaume S, Jaussent I, et al. (2007) Psychiatric diagnoses and personality traits associated with disadvantageous decision-making. Eur Psychiat **22**:455–461.

Kapczinski F, Dias VV, Kauer-Sant'Anna M, et al. (2009) Clinical implications of a staging model for bipolar disorders. Expert Rev Neurother **9**:957–966.

Kerr N, Dunbar R, and Bentall R (2003) Theory of mind deficits in bipolar affective disorder. J Affect Disorders **73**:253–259.

Lahera G, Montes J, Benito A, et al. (2008) Theory of mind deficits in bipolar disorder: Is it related to a previous history of psychotic symptoms? Psychiat Res **161**:309–317.

Lembke A and Ketter T (2002) Impaired recognition of facial emotion in mania. Am J Psychiat **159**:302–304.

Martino DJ, Marengo E, Igoa A, et al. (2009) Neurocognitive and symptomatic predictors of functional outcome in bipolar disorder: a prospective 1 year follow-up study. J Affect Disorders **116**:37–42.

Martino DJ, Strejilevich SA, Fassi G, et al. (2011) Theory of mind and facial emotion recognition in euthymic bipolar I and bipolar II disorders. Psychiat Res **189**(3):379–384.

Martino DJ, Strejilevich SA, Marengo E, et al. (2013) Relationship between neurocognitive functioning and episode recurrences in bipolar disorder Affect Disord **147**(1–3):345–351.

Martino DJ, Strejilevich SA, Torralva T, et al. (2010) Decision making in euthymic bipolar I and bipolar II disorders. Psychol Med **22**:1–9.

McKinnon MC, Cusi AM, and MacQueen GM (2010) Impaired theory of mind performance in patients with recurrent bipolar disorder: moderating effect of cognitive load. Psychiat Res **177**:261–262.

Montag C, Ehrlich A, Neuhaus K, et al. (2010) Theory of mind impairments in euthymic bipolar patients. J Affect Disorders **123**:464–469.

Murphy F, Rubinsztein J, Michael A, et al. (2001) Decision making cognition in mania and depression. Psychol Med **31**:679–693.

Olley A, Malhi G, Bachelor J, et al. (2005) Executive functioning and theory of mind in euthymic bipolar disorder. Bipolar Disord **7**(s5):43–52.

Pinkham A, Penn D, Perkins D, et al. (2003) Implications for the neural basis of social cognition for the study of schizophrenia. Am J Psychiat **160**:815–824.

Robinson L, Thompson J, Gallagher P, et al. (2006) A meta-analysis of cognitive deficits in euthymic patients with bipolar disorder. J Affect Disorders **93**:105–115.

Rubinsztein JS, Michael A, Paykel ES, et al. (2000) Cognitive impairment in remission in bipolar affective disorder. Psychol Med **30**:1025–1036.

Rubinsztein JS, Michael A, Underwood B, et al. (2006) Impaired cognition and decision-making in bipolar depression but not 'affective bias' evident. Psychol Med **36**:629–639.

Samamé C, Martino DJ, and Strejilevich SA (2012) Social cognition in euthymic bipolar disorder: systematic review and meta-analytic approach. Acta Psychiat Scand **125**(4):266–280.

Shamay-Tsoory S, Harari H, Szepsenwol O, et al. (2009) Neuropsychological evidence of impaired cognitive empathy in euthymic bipolar disorder. J Neuropsych Clin N **21**:59–67.

Suddendorf T and Withen A (2001) Mental evolution and development: evidence for secondary representations in children, great ages, and other animals. Psychol Bull **127**:629–650.

Torres IJ, Boudreau VG, and Yatham LN (2007) Neuropsychological functioning in euthymic bipolar disorder: a meta-analysis. Acta Psychiat Scand **116**(s434):17–26.

Venn H, Gray J, Montagne B, et al. (2004) Perception of facial expressions of emotion in bipolar disorder. Bipolar Disord **6**:286–293.

Wolf F, Brune M, and Assion H (2010) Theory of mind and neurocognitive functioning in patients with bipolar disorder. Bipolar Disord **12**:657–666.

Young A, Perret D, and Calder A (2002) Facial expression of emotion-stimuli and tests (FEEST). Bury St Edmunds, UK: Thames Valley Test Company.

Chapter 8

Affective temperaments: potential latent stages of bipolar disorders

Gustavo H. Vázquez and Xenia Gonda

Introduction

In order to be able to better diagnose psychiatric illnesses and to identify conditions that fall between categories, there has been a shift towards the spectrum concept of psychiatric illness in general, and of affective and bipolar disorders in particular. This view may help to extend our understanding of the continuity of related pathological states into the domain of non-clinical and subclinical presentations, and to those manifestations which, although falling below the definition of bipolar illness, constitute a high risk or prodromal state, or may already cause significant suffering or increase the risk of worsening and later development of more serious forms of illness; these will require professional attention, and, possibly, specific treatment. This spectrum concept of affective and bipolar illness also means extending the continuum to mental health and identifying those who carry the potential of later laying the base for developing illness possibly on a genetic, personality, or behavioural basis. Also, understanding both ends and the whole span of this spectrum provides us with the opportunity to perform research on bipolar disorder in a continuum approach instead of a case–control perspective, which later could lead to ignoring important associations. Therefore identifying the healthier, non-affected and subclinical portion of the bipolar spectrum, which may also constitute latent stages of the illness, is crucial for understanding, treating, predicting, and also possibly preventing these severely debilitating illnesses.

Akiskal and colleagues have proposed the concept of the soft bipolar spectrum, which includes different manifestations of hypomania, in addition to depressive states, and also builds on the underlying temperamental dysregulation in the background of affective manifestations. This approach has the potential to contribute to a more sophisticated differentiation of subtypes of bipolar illness with the introduction of new more detailed clinical descriptions (Akiskal and Mallya 1987). Later on, besides the description of subtypes, the concept of affective temperaments was also introduced in order to further investigate the less pathologically affected end of the bipolar spectrum.

Besides the classical spectrum model, the staging model of bipolar illness also argues for a continuum approach, in order to predict evolution and prognosis and outcomes and to determine the most appropriate treatment at a given stage (Grande et al. 2013). Staging of bipolar illness is based on clinical assessment and functionality, especially in the interval between major episodes. Currently, in this theoretical model, there are five stages, with four clinical stages and a latent phase for those manifesting non-specific affective symptoms (Grande et al. 2013). The latent stage includes those individuals who can be considered at an extremely high risk of developing bipolar illness but do not have yet any specific symptoms, only atypical prodromal signs including positive family history, anxiety, hyperphagia and hypersomnia, seasonal mood fluctuations, mood lability and irritability, as well as psychomotor retardation, in addition to hyperthymic or cyclothymic temperamental traits (Balanza-Martinez et al. 2008). As symptoms at this phase can be highly unspecific and the later course and outcome of illness unpredictable, it is strongly controversial if pharmacological treatment should be recommended, although it may be useful in the treatment of subthreshold symptomatology (Grande et al. 2013).

Although at this point there is no study yet available to test the definitive validity of the staging model the description of the latent stage (Grande et al. 2013) closely resembles the states characterized by the presence of predominant affective temperaments. There are several factors that link affective temperaments with affective illness, which posits for searching manifestations of affective temperaments as a possible risk factor or precursor state for the development of major affective illnesses. In this sense, affective temperaments would be part of what Grande et al. (2013) describe as the latent stage.

Overview of the development of the affective temperament model

Putative traits underlying those for bipolar disorders represent an adequate paradigm to conceptualize the potential connection between mental disorders and adaptive temperamental attributes (Akiskal and Akiskal 2005). Temperaments refer to temporally stable behavioural traits with strong affective reactivity and have been associated with the biological foundations of personality, such as activity levels, rhythms, moods, cognition, and their variability. Affective temperaments not only could have a relevant role in the predisposition to major affective disorders but also represent the most prevalent phenotypic expression of the genes underlying bipolar disorders (Akiskal and Akiskal 1992; Kelsoe 2003). Origins of the modern concept for affective temperaments can be traced back to the humoural theories described by Hippocrates (Akiskal 1996). Later on, the German psychiatrist Emil Kraepelin described four basic affective dispositions (depressive, manic, cyclothymic, and irritable), basing his temperamental hypothesis on the classic works of Galen, who previously stated the melancholic, choleric, phlegmatic, and sanguine humors, and their imbalance and dysbalance, as the major origin of the different human illnesses. Kraepelin considered these basic affective temperaments as the subclinical forms of manic–depressive insanity—nowadays known as major affective disorders—which could be found not only in mental illness patients but also among their healthy relatives (Kraepelin 1921). Both Kraepelin and his German colleague Ernst Kretschmer considered that affective temperaments could predispose to endogenous psychosis or mood episodes; however, the latter postulated that the presence of a dominant temperament should be considered a variation of normal affectivity, which could potentially lead to mental illness.

Combining these foundational ideas with the use of extensive modern scientific and clinical observation and field research, Akiskal and collaborators developed the modern concept of affective temperaments to encompass the whole spectrum of affective disturbances from healthy emotional reactivity types to major affective illnesses. The model includes the four classical temperamental types, supplemented with a fifth one, the anxious temperament. A detailed clinical description for each temperament and their assessment with a psychometrically valid instrument (TEMPS-A) can be found elsewhere (Akiskal and Akiskal 2005).

Akiskal considers the five affective temperaments as spectrums stretching from health to pathology, involved in characteristic patterns of healthy emotional reactivity on one end and different types of major affective disorders on the other (Akiskal and Akiskal 2007). In between it can be found that the so-called predominant affective temperaments, which expressed in a marked form, can constitute the subclinical and subaffective manifestation of affective illnesses, and can be considered precursor or latent states which could represent high-risk conditions, corresponding to latent phases of mood disorders.

Clinical aspects of affective temperaments

As described earlier, affective temperaments are conceptualized as part of the affective disorder spectrum, a notion which is widely supported by familial, genetic, biological, and clinical studies. The affective spectrum describes a continuum between cyclothymia, bipolar II disorder, and bipolar I disorder (Akiskal et al. 1977; Evans et al. 2008), as well as subsyndromal depression, minor depression, dysthymia, and unipolar major depression (Akiskal et al. 1978; Judd and Akiskal 2000; Lewinsohn et al. 2003). Affective temperaments, besides constituting latent illness phases extending these spectrums towards the states of mental health, could play a pathoplastic role. In this manner, affective temperaments would have an important role in determining and modelling the emergence and clinical evolution of affective disorders. That would include several important characteristics, such as predominant polarity, symptomatic expression, long-term course and consequences, response and adherence to treatment, as well as treatment outcomes (Vazquez and Gonda 2013). The relationship between affective temperaments and affective illness could be, however, rather more complex.

Predominant affective temperaments are present in up to 20% of the healthy general population, ranging from 13% in Argentina to 20% in Germany (Vazquez et al. 2012). Affective temperaments show a characteristic gender distribution, with both depressive and anxious temperaments being more common among females while hyperthymia is found more commonly among males in most large-scale national studies (Vazquez et al. 2012). The higher prevalence of depressive and anxious temperaments among females in the general population correlates with the higher prevalence for unipolar major depression and anxiety disorders in women (Kuehner 2003; Somers et al. 2006). Conversely, higher prevalence of hyperthymic temperament among men is in line with the higher proportion of manic episodes reported in males (Baldassano et al. 2005). These findings also support the hypothesis that affective temperaments could be subclinical forms or precursors of those major psychiatric disorders which clearly display a particularly different gender distribution (Vazquez et al. 2012).

According to different studies in clinical samples, depressive temperament is usually more prevalent among major depressive patients, and hyperthymic as well as cyclothymic temperaments are a particular affective characteristic for bipolar illness. Moreover, some studies have reported that cyclothymic temperament was found to be present in both bipolar I and bipolar II presentations as well as in recurrent depressive disorder. In addition no difference in the prevalence of irritable temperament scores was found among these affective disorders (Gassab et al. 2008). As clinical studies report more subtle and complex association between affective temperaments and affective illness, it is increasingly noted that affective temperaments show important within-illness variations besides the well-known between-illness pattern. A more complex approach to detection and identification of affective temperaments within the basic constellations, as described earlier, may allow for performing a more sophisticated classification of affective illness, predicting and determining subtypes and characteristics (Mazzarini et al. 2009).

Even in the case of unipolar major depression, presence of other affective temperaments besides the depressive temperament has a crucial role in determining the clinical picture, and the presence of other affective temperaments in patients with a major depressive episode may be valuable in predicting the course illness and bipolar conversion. The presence of cyclothymic temperament in those cases of major depression has been related to atypical clinical features (Perugi et al. 2003). In patients with recurrent major unipolar depression, higher scores of cyclothymic temperament are also associated with earlier age of onset, a higher number of previous depressive episodes, more psychotic and melancholic features, as well as suicidal ideations and attempts, which are predictive factors of bipolarity in recurrent depression (Mechri et al. 2011).

Temperament may be one of the major factors influencing features in the clinical evolution of bipolar disorder. In this vein, the number of episodes has been associated with higher depressive and lower hyperthymic temperament scores. In addition, depressive temperament has been associated with a higher ratio of depressive episodes whereas hyperthymic temperament has been associated with manic episodes (Henry et al. 1999). Affective temperaments have been also shown to be related to age of onset in bipolar disorder (Oedegaard et al. 2009). Depressive temperament may prevail among bipolar I disorder patients with predominant depressive polarity, and hyperthymic temperament is commonly present in those bipolar disorder patients with manic predominant polarity (Henry et al. 1999). Bipolar disorder patients with predominant cyclothymic and hyperthymic temperament are significantly different from other groups in relevant clinical and course features, including gender ratio, episode polarity and number of episodes, hospitalizations, suicidality, comorbid anxiety disorders, and personality disorders (Perugi et al. 2012). Furthermore, hyperthymic temperament has been associated with psychotic features both in bipolar I and bipolar II illness (Gassab et al. 2008; Mazzarini et al. 2009). As for illness course, cyclothymic temperament has been related with a higher number for all types of affective bipolar episodes (Kochman et al. 2005) and is also related to poorer outcome (Cassano et al. 1992). Manic switches occur more commonly in bipolar disorder patients with hyperthymic temperament, while psychotic features among those subjects with an irritable temperament. Comorbidities among affective patients with a cyclothymic temperament are frequent, and irritable temperament is significantly associated with a manic first episode of the illness (Kesebir et al. 2005a). Higher scores of hyperthymic temperament are associated with higher risks for antidepressant-induced mania in bipolar depressives (Henry et al. 2001; Tondo et al. 2013).

While in the case of bipolar I disorder many different temperamental constellations may lie in the background, bipolar II disorder is more specifically related to cyclothymic temperament (Hantouche et al. 1998). The cyclothymic temperament not only is present in the majority of bipolar II patients, but also has a predictive value for bipolar conversion from unipolar depression (Akiskal et al. 1995; Kochman et al. 2005). Among bipolar I patients, but not bipolar II, hyperthymic and depressive temperament scores were found to have a negative correlation. Hyperthymic temperament was negatively correlated with the number of depressive episodes and seasonal features in bipolar disorder type II patients (Gassab et al. 2008).

Depressive, cyclothymic, irritable, and anxious temperaments are significantly more frequent in affective patients with mixed episodes indicating a relationship between mixed affective episodes and simultaneous presence of inverse temperamental types (Rottig et al. 2007). The presence of depressive temperament could also help distinguishing between mixed and pure manic states (Hantouche et al. 2001).

Genetic and neurochemical background of affective temperaments

An important feature of the staging model is assigning genetic, neurochemical, neuroanatomical, neurobiological, and neurocognitive characteristics that differentiate between different stages of the illness (Berk et al. 2007; Kapczinski et al. 2009; Grande et al. 2013). Although we have limited findings to support the association of such factors with affective temperaments, there are some positive results reported, which also argue for affective temperaments as being latent phases of affective illness.

By definition, temperaments have a strong biological and genetic base (Bouchard 1994; Cloninger 1994), and this also seems to be the case for affective temperaments (Chiaroni et al. 2005; Evans et al. 2005). A more recent approach to bipolar disorder conceptualizes the bipolar spectrum as a quantitative genetic trait with a continuous distribution instead of a qualitative one, as suggested by a categorical approach (Evans et al. 2005). In this vein, bipolar disorder is most likely a polygenic trait emerging as a result of interactions between environmental factors and multiple genes, each with only a small effect on its own (Evans et al. 2005; Craddock and Sklar 2013). Those genes predisposing to bipolar disorders may give rise to phenotypes that continuously blend into normally seen constellations in healthy non-clinical populations, which can be described as normal variations of affective temperaments. As mentioned earlier, affective illnesses are genetic reservoirs for adaptive temperaments and traits (Akiskal and Akiskal 2007).

Several studies have demonstrated that healthy relatives of bipolar probands exhibit a higher degree of temperamental dysregulation than normal controls (Evans et al. 2005; Mendlowicz et al. 2005). Also, it has been put forward that those temperamental traits may have a common genetic basis with bipolar disorder (Kelsoe 2003). Familial genetic studies of patients with affective disorders identified a strong aggregation of affective temperaments, mainly cyclothymic and, to a lesser degree, hyperthymic and anxious temperaments, among healthy first-degree relatives of bipolar I patients, supporting the genetic basis of affective temperaments (Chiaroni et al. 2005; Evans et al. 2005, 2008; Kesebir et al. 2005b; Mendlowicz et al. 2005; Vazquez et al. 2008; Mazzarini et al. 2009). These subaffective cyclothymic traits could serve as a potential vulnerability marker, and give support for the subthreshold forms and the softest end of the bipolar spectrum (Akiskal and Pinto 1999). There are reasonable arguments that cyclothymic temperament could contribute to a broad phenotypic definition of the bipolar condition (Chiaroni et al. 2005; Kochman et al. 2005) and would be considered as a preliminary or latent stage for full-blown bipolar disorder.

Notwithstanding the increasing attention for affective temperaments both in clinical and personality research fields, our knowledge concerning their genetic background needs further investigation. In a seminal study, Gonda and coworkers reported a significant association between the s allele of the *5-HTTLPR* polymorphism of the serotonin transporter gene and affective temperaments carrying a depressive component (depressive, cyclothymic, irritable, and anxious) (Gonda et al. 2006), which was not confirmed by some subsequent studies (Kang et al. 2008; Landaas et al. 2011). The possible correlation of the *5-HTTLPR* allele and affective temperaments was not surprising, since this allele has been found to be associated with anxiety- (Sen et al. 2004; Homberg and Lesch 2011) and neuroticism-related traits (Gonda et al. 2009) as well as unipolar (Clarke et al. 2010) and bipolar affective disorders (Levinson 2006). The *5-HTTLPR* s allele is thought to exert its influence on the emergence of depression by mediating the effect of life stress and adverse life events (Caspi et al. 2003, 2010; Karg et al. 2011). Accordingly, emotional reactivity is an important feature encompassed by affective temperaments. Moreover, a significant interaction effect between the *5-HTTLPR* and the cannabinoid 1 receptor gene promoter polymorphism (*CNR1*) was later reported for anxious temperament (Lazary et al. 2009) further supporting the strong genetic determination of affective temperaments as well as their claim for constituting latent stages for affective illness.

Besides genes encoding for elements of the serotonergic system, other monoaminergic genes often emerge as potential candidates for playing a role in determining temperaments. A Korean study reported a positive association between the *DRD4* gene and irritable and cyclothymic temperaments in healthy male subjects (Kang et al. 2008). Both the irritable and cyclothymic temperaments are classically conceptualized as mixed temperamental subtypes, incorporating both depressive and hyperthymic features, simultaneously in case of the irritable, and alternatively in case of the cyclothymic temperament (Kraepelin 1921), so the association with the *DRD4* gene may suggest a potential link between this receptor and the hyperthymic traits, such as in the Gonda et al (2006) study the *5-HTTLPR* s allele was associated with the depressive component of affective temperaments. The depressive temperament was also significantly associated with the most frequent haplotype of the oxytocin receptor gene in a healthy Japanese sample (Kawamura et al. 2010). One study reported a positive association between cyclothymic temperament and a chromosomal locus on 18p11 in bipolar disorder families, and other linkage peaks with potential regions of interest were also detected on chromosomes 3 and 7 (Evans et al. 2008).

The remaining few studies addressing the genetic background of affective temperaments yielded negative findings. There is increasing attention concerning the association of brain-derived neurotrophic factor (BDNF) and affective disorders with some positive results (Neves-Pereira et al. 2002; Sklar et al. 2002; Lohoff 2010), and there are similarly emerging results for the glycogen synthase kinase 3β (GSK3β) rs6782799 polymorphism (Zhang et al. 2010) and the rs2267665 polymorphism of the PPARD (peroxisome proliferative activated receptor delta) gene in the *Wnt* signalling pathway, which may also be implicated in the pathophysiology of affective disorders (Zandi et al. 2008). However, a recent study found no association between these polymorphisms and affective temperaments in a healthy population (Tsutsumi et al. 2011). It should be noted that this study applied a small sample on a Japanese subjects, and it must be kept in mind that genetic associations are ethnicity specific, and also that the distribution of affective temperament scores in Japan markedly differs from those in other countries, with typically much lower scores (Matsumoto et al. 2005).

The evidence described earlier indicates that there may be a common genetic heterogeneity in the background of affective temperaments and different major affective illness manifestations and syndromes. Thus, the delineation of the genetic correlates of affective temperaments would help to understand the genetic contributors and thus the etiopathogenic foundation of affective disorders. However, selecting candidate genes simply by extrapolating from polymorphisms known to be associated with affective disorders yielded mixed results, possibly because both the genetic background and the phenotypic expression of affective temperaments are present in a more diluted form among healthy samples (Akiskal and Akiskal 2005).

The potential association between affective temperaments and neurotransmitter function and neuroanatomical structures has been also understudied so far. In one study in patients with major mood disorders, predominantly depressive temperamental profiles characterized by high depressive, cyclothymic, anxious, and irritable as well as low hyperthymic temperament scores were found to be associated with different patterns of white matter hyperintensities in the brain, indicating a positive association between some affective temperament subtypes and specific alterations on subcortical brain regions (Serafini et al. 2011).

In another recent series of papers an association between affective temperaments and date of birth has been reported with characteristic patterns (Rihmer et al. 2011). Interestingly, this pattern of association corresponds to the birth season pattern earlier reported for bipolar I and II patients in a small clinical sample (Rihmer 1980). Birth season is an important marker and a proxy variable for several environmental factors varying with seasons and active during the time of conception, gestation, or birth (Chotai et al. 2002). It is not yet known which of the possible varying factors exert an effect and during which period of importance, but an association with season of birth has already been reported in case of various somatic and neuropsychiatric illnesses as well as healthy psychological traits (Rihmer et al. 2011). One likely explanation is that birth season exerts its influence via influencing monoaminergic neurotransmission neurodevelopment (Chotai et al. 2006).

Several biomarkers have been found to be associated with progression of bipolar disorder but not with the latent phase; therefore, it is believed that polymorphisms conferring increased susceptibility for bipolar illness may be important as biomarkers signalling this phase (Kapczinski et al. 2009). However, biochemical changes associated with the clinical features of the latent phase including mood and anxiety symptoms and temperamental dysregulation may be important already in this early stage.

Conclusions

The theoretical construct of affective temperaments was developed from a combination of ancient concepts with modern scientific and clinical observations. Affective temperaments encompass the complete domain of emotional reactivity from affective pathology to health. It is thought that affective temperaments emerge from genetic and neurochemical bases, which were developed and preserved over evolution due to evolutional and social advantages. Affective temperaments may constitute the subclinical manifestation of major affective illnesses. In this sense, affective temperaments can be considered a precursor state, or the latent phase, for the development of mood disorders.

Moreover, affective temperaments are not only risk factors or precursors of affective disorders, but also play an important pathoplastic role, therefore could constitute valuable tools for predicting the emergence of affective illness in high-risk healthy population or potential conversion from unipolar to bipolar disorders among patients with mood disorders; for more sophisticated diagnosis of affective, and especially bipolar illness subtypes; and for predicting illness course, therapeutic response, treatment adherence, prognosis, and outcomes including suicide. On the other hand, affective temperaments in the healthy population can be considered as an important foundation of personality. The further study of affective temperaments together with their neuroanatomical, biochemical, and genetic background would help us to understand the inner mechanisms underlying human affectivity.

The idea of a unified theoretical model that would include affective temperaments as early-stage manifestations of bipolar disorder may help to bridge the ideas developed by Akiskal (1996) with those put forward by Berk et al. (2007) and Kapczinski et al. (2009). A unifying model was proposed using the concept of allostatic load and cumulative impairments developing over time with the progression of bipolar illness (Kapczinski et al. 2008). However, the latent stage concept put forward by Kapczinski et al (2009) deserves further studies, both in terms of biological and phenotypical features. A better characterization of the latent phase of bipolar disorder would be an important step for early detection, intervention, and maybe prevention. The detailed study of affective temperaments as precursors of affective disorders may provide the staging model with important insights in terms of future research and clinical use of the concept.

Acknowledgement

Xenia Gonda is recipient of the Janos Bolyai Research Fellowship of the Hungarian Academy of Sciences.

References

Akiskal HS (1996) The temperamental foundations of affective disorders. London: Gaskell.

Akiskal HS and Akiskal KK (1992) Cyclothymic, hyperthymic and depressive temperaments as subaffective variants of mood disorders. In: Tasman A and Riba MB, eds. Annual Review, vol. II. Washington, D.C.: American Psychiatric Press.

Akiskal HS and Akiskal KK (2007) In search of Aristotle: temperament, human nature, melancholia, creativity and eminence. J Affect Disorders 100:1–6.

Akiskal HS, Bitar AH, Puzantian VR, et al. (1978) The nosological status of neurotic depression: a prospective three- to four-year follow-up examination in light of the primary-secondary and unipolar-bipolar dichotomies. Arch Gen Psychiat 35:756–766.

Akiskal HS, Djenderedjian AM, Rosenthal RH, et al. (1977) Cyclothymic disorder: validating criteria for inclusion in the bipolar affective group. Am J Psychiat 134:1227–1233.

Akiskal HS and Mallya G (1987) Criteria for the 'soft' bipolar spectrum: treatment implications. Psychopharmacol Bull 23:68–73.

Akiskal HS, Maser JD, Zeller PJ, et al. (1995) Switching from unipolar to bipolar-Ii—an 11-year prospective-study of clinical and temperamental predictors in 559 patients. Arch Gen Psychiat 52:114–123.

Akiskal HS and Pinto O (1999) The evolving bipolar spectrum—prototypes I, II, III, and IV. Psychiat Clin N Am 22:517–534.

Akiskal KK and Akiskal HS (2005) The theoretical underpinnings of affective temperaments: implications for evolutionary foundations of bipolar disorder and human nature. J Affect Disorders 85:231–239.

Balanza-Martinez V, Rubio C, Selva-Vera G, et al. (2008) Neurocognitive endophenotypes (Endophenocognitypes) from studies of relatives of bipolar disorder subjects: a systematic review. Neurosci Biobehav R 32:1426–1438.

Baldassano CF, Marangell LB, Gyulai L, et al. (2005) Gender differences in bipolar disorder: retrospective data from the first 500 STEP-BD participants. Bipolar Disord 7:465–470.

Berk M, Conus P, Lucas N, et al. (2007) Setting the stage: from prodrome to treatment resistance in bipolar disorder. Bipolar Disord 9:671–678.

Bouchard TJ Jr (1994) Genes, environment, and personality. Science 264:1700–1701.

Caspi A, Hariri AR, Holmes A, et al. (2010) Genetic sensitivity to the environment: the case of the serotonin transporter gene and its implications for studying complex diseases and traits. Am J Psychiat 167:509–527.

Caspi A, Sugden K, Moffitt TE, et al. (2003) Influence of life stress on depression: moderation by a polymorphism in the 5-HTT gene. Science 301:386–389.

Cassano GB, Akiskal HS, Savino M, et al. (1992) Proposed subtypes of bipolar II and related disorders: with hypomanic episodes (or cyclothymia) and with hyperthymic temperament. J Affect Disorders 26:127–140.

Chiaroni P, Hantouche EG, Gouvernet J, et al. (2005) The cyclothymic temperament in healthy controls and familially at risk individuals for mood disorder: endophenotype for genetic studies? J Affect Disorders **85**:135–145.

Chotai J, Jonasson M, Hagglof B, et al. (2002) The Temperament Scale of Novelty Seeking in adolescents shows an association with season of birth opposite to that in adults. Psychiat Res **111**:45–54.

Chotai J, Murphy DL, and Constantino JN (2006) Cerebrospinal fluid monoamine metabolite levels in human newborn infants born in winter differ from those born in summer. Psychiat Res **145**:189–197.

Clarke H, Flint J, Attwood AS, et al. (2010) Association of the 5- HTTLPR genotype and unipolar depression: a meta-analysis. Psychol Med **40**:1767–1778.

Cloninger CR (1994) Temperament and personality. Curr Opin Neurobiol **4**:266–273.

Craddock N and Sklar P (2013) Genetics of bipolar disorder. Lancet **381**:1654–1662.

Evans L, Akiskal HS, Keck PE, et al. (2005) Familiality of temperament in bipolar disorder: support for a genetic spectrum. J Affect Disorders **85**:153–168.

Evans LM, Akiskal HS, Greenwood TA, et al. (2008) Suggestive linkage of a chromosomal locus on 18p11 to cyclothymic temperament in bipolar disorder families. Am J Med Genet B **147B**:326–332.

Gassab L, Mechri A, Bacha M, et al. (2008) [Affective temperaments in the bipolar and unipolar disorders: distinctive profiles and relationship with clinical features]. Encephale **34**:477–482.

Gonda X, Fountoulakis KN, Juhasz G, et al. (2009) Association of the s allele of the 5-HTTLPR with neuroticism-related traits and temperaments in a psychiatrically healthy population. Eur Arch Psy Clin N **259**:106–113.

Gonda X, Rihmer Z, Zsombok T, et al. (2006) The 5HTTLPR polymorphism of the serotonin transporter gene is associated with affective temperaments as measured by TEMPS-A. J Affect Disorders **91**:125–131.

Grande I, Frey BN, Vieta E, et al. (2013) Soft bipolar spectrum and staging in bipolar disorder. Curr Psychiatry Rev **9**:33–40.

Hantouche EG, Akiskal HS, Lancrenon S, et al. (1998) Systematic clinical methodology for validating bipolar-II disorder: data in mid-stream from a French national multi-site study (EPIDEP). J Affect Disorders **50**:163–173.

Hantouche EG, Allilaire JP, Bourgeois ML, et al. (2001) The feasibility of self-assessment of dysphoric mania in the French national EPIMAN study. J Affect Disorders **67**:97–103.

Henry C, Lacoste J, Bellivier F, et al. (1999) Temperament in bipolar illness: impact on prognosis. J Affect Disorders **56**:103–108.

Henry C, Sorbara F, Lacoste J, et al. (2001) Antidepressant-induced mania in bipolar patients: identification of risk factors. J Clin Psychiat **62**:249–255.

Homberg JR and Lesch KP (2011) Looking on the bright side of serotonin transporter gene variation. Biol Psychiat **69**:513–519.

Judd LL and Akiskal HS (2000) Delineating the longitudinal structure of depressive illness: beyond clinical subtypes and duration thresholds. Pharmacopsychiatry 33:3–7.

Kang JI, Namkoong K, and Kim SJ (2008) The association of 5-HTTLPR and DRD4 VNTR polymorphisms with affective temperamental traits in healthy volunteers. J Affect Disorders 109:157–163.

Kapczinski F, Dias VV, Kauer-Sant'anna M, et al. (2009) The potential use of bio-markers as an adjunctive tool for staging bipolar disorder. Prog Neuro-Psychoph 33:1366–1371.

Kapczinski F, Vieta E, Andreazza AC, et al. (2008) Allostatic load in bipolar disorder: Implications for pathophysiology and treatment. Neurosci Biobehav R 32:675–692.

Karg K, Burmeister M, Shedden K, et al. (2011) The serotonin transporter promoter variant (5-HTTLPR), stress, and depression meta-analysis revisited evidence of genetic moderation. Arch Gen Psychiat 68:444–454.

Kawamura Y, Liu XX, Akiyama T, et al. (2010) The association between oxytocin receptor gene (OXTR) polymorphisms and affective temperaments, as measured by TEMPS-A. J Affect Disorders 127:31–37.

Kelsoe JR (2003) Arguments for the genetic basis of the bipolar spectrum. J Affect Disorders 73:183–197.

Kesebir S, Vahip S, Akdeniz F, et al. (2005a) [The relationship of affective tempera-ment and clinical features in bipolar disorder]. Turk Psikiyatri Derg 16:164–169.

Kesebir S, Vahip S, Akdeniz F, et al. (2005b) Affective temperaments as measured by TEMPS-A in patients with bipolar I disorder and their first-degree relatives: a con-trolled study. J Affect Disorders 85:127–133.

Kochman FJ, Hantouche EG, Ferrari P, et al. (2005) Cyclothyrnic temperament as a prospective predictor of bipolarity and suicidality in children and adolescents with major depressive disorder. J Affect Disorders 85:181–189.

Kraepelin E (1921) Manic-Depressive Illness and Paranoia. Edinburgh: Livingstone.

Kuehner C (2003) Gender differences in unipolar depression: an update of epidemio-logical findings and possible explanations. Acta Psychiat Scand 108:163–174.

Landaas ET, Johansson S, Halmoy A, et al. (2011) No association between the seroto-nin transporter gene polymorphism 5-HTTLPR and cyclothymic temperament as measured by TEMPS-A. J Affect Disorders 129:308–312.

Lazary J, Lazary A, Gonda X, et al. (2009) Promoter variants of the cannabinoid recep-tor 1 gene (CNR1) in interaction with 5-HTTLPR affect the anxious phenotype. Am J Med Genet B 150B:1118–1127.

Levinson DF (2006) The genetics of depression: a review. Biol Psychiat 60:84–92.

Lewinsohn PM, Klein DN, Durbin EC, et al. (2003) Family study of subthreshold depressive symptoms: risk factor for MDD? J Affect Disorders 77:149–157.

Lohoff FW (2010) Overview of the genetics of major depressive disorder. Curr Psy-chiatry Rep 12:539–546.

Matsumoto S, Akiyama T, Tsuda H, et al. (2005) Reliability and validity of TEMPS-A in a Japanese non-clinical population: application to unipolar and bipolar depressives. J Affect Disorders 85:85–92.

Mazzarini L, Pacchiarotti I, Colom F, et al. (2009) Predominant polarity and temperament in bipolar and unipolar affective disorders. J Affect Disorders 119:28–33.

Mechri A, La Kerkeni N, Touati I, et al. (2011) Association between cyclothymic temperament and clinical predictors of bipolarity in recurrent depressive patients. J Affect Disorders 132:285–288.

Mendlowicz MV, Jean-Louis G, Kelsoe JR, et al. (2005) A comparison of recovered bipolar patients, healthy relatives of bipolar probands, and normal controls using the short TEMPS-A. J Affect Disorders 85:147–151.

Neves-Pereira M, Mundo E, Muglia P, et al. (2002) The brain-derived neurotrophic factor gene confers susceptibility to bipolar disorder: evidence from a family-based association study. Am J Hum Genet 71:651–655.

Oedegaard KJ, Syrstad VEG, Morken G, et al. (2009) A study of age at onset and affective temperaments in a Norwegian sample of patients with mood disorders. J Affect Disorders 118:229–233.

Perugi G, Toni C, Maremmani I, et al. (2012) The influence of affective temperaments and psychopathological traits on the definition of bipolar disorder subtypes: a study on Bipolar I Italian National sample. J Affect Disorders 136:E41–E49.

Perugi G, Toni C, Travierso MC, et al. (2003) The role of cyclothymia in atypical depression: toward a data-based reconceptualization of the borderline-bipolar II connection. J Affect Disorders 73:87–98.

Rihmer Z (1980) Season of birth and season of hospital admission in bipolar depressed female patients. Psychiat Res 3:247–251.

Rihmer Z, Erdos P, Ormos M, et al. (2011) Association between affective temperaments and season of birth in a general student population. J Affect Disorders 132:64–70.

Rottig D, Rottig S, Brieger P, et al. (2007) Temperament and personality in bipolar I patients with and without mixed episodes. J Affect Disorders 104:97–102.

Sen S, Burmeister M, and Ghosh D (2004) Meta-analysis of the association between a serotonin transporter promoter polymorphism (5-HTTLPR) and anxiety-related personality traits. Am J Med Genet B 127B:85–89.

Serafini G, Pompili M, Innamorati M, et al. (2011) Affective temperamental profiles are associated with white matter hyperintensity and suicidal risk in patients with mood disorders. J Affect Disorders 129:47–55.

Sklar P, Gabriel SB, Mcinnis MG, et al. (2002) Family-based association study of 76 candidate genes in bipolar disorder: BDNF is a potential risk locus. Brain-derived neurophic factor. Mol Psychiatr 7:579–593.

Somers JM, Goldner EM, Waraich P, (2006) Prevalence and incidence studies of anxiety disorders: a systematic review of the literature. Can J Psychiat 51:100–113.

Tondo L, Baldessarini RJ, Vazquez G, et al. (2013) Clinical responses to antidepressants among 1036 acutely depressed patients with bipolar or unipolar major affective disorders. Acta Psychiat Scand **127**:355–364.

Tsutsumi T, Terao T, Hatanaka K, et al. (2011) Association between affective temperaments and brain-derived neurotrophic factor, Glycogen synthase kinase 3 beta and Wnt signaling pathway gene polymorphisms in healthy subjects. J Affect Disorders **131**:353–357.

Vazquez GH and Gonda X (2013) Affective temperaments and mood disorders: a review of current knowledge. Curr Psychiatry Rev **9**:21–32.

Vazquez GH, Kahn C, Schiavo CE, et al. (2008) Bipolar disorders and affective temperaments: a national family study testing the 'endophenotype' and 'subaffective' theses using the TEMPS-A Buenos Aires. J Affect Disorders **108**:25–32.

Vazquez GH, Tondo L, Mazzarini L, et al. (2012) Affective temperaments in general population: a review and combined analysis from national studies. J Affect Disorders **139**:18–22.

Zandi PP, Belmonte PL, Willour VL, et al. (2008) Association study of Wnt signaling pathway genes in bipolar disorder. Arch Gen Psychiat **65**:785–793.

Zhang KR, Yang CX, Xu Y, et al. (2010) Genetic association of the interaction between the BDNF and GSK3B genes and major depressive disorder in a Chinese population. J Neural Transm **117**:393–401.

Chapter 9

Neuroimaging and illness progression

Benicio N. Frey, Luciano Minuzzi,
Bartholomeus C.M. Haarman, and
Roberto B. Sassi

Introduction

Staging is extensively used in several areas of medicine such as oncology and cardiology because of its utility in guiding treatment choice and/or prognosis. As reviewed in earlier chapters, the concept of staging has been applied to bipolar disorder (BD), largely driven by clinical, neuro-cognitive, and peripheral biomarkers research. Research on neuroimaging and illness progression is still limited, primarily due to a lack of long-term longitudinal imaging research. However, studies in offspring at higher risk for development of BD, paediatric bipolar disorder (PBD), adult, and elderly BD may shed light on which brain areas/circuits may be more relevant in illness progression in BD. Here, we critically review structural and functional neuroimaging studies in BD, with a focus on changes in brain circuits that may be associated with the course of BD.

Children at high risk of developing bipolar disorder

There are significant clinical challenges in the diagnosis of BD in pae-diatric samples. Often, a prodromal presentation of non-specific symp-toms such as sleep disturbances, anxiety, or irritability may precede the appearance of mania for many years, delaying the correct diagnosis and appropriate treatment (Duffy et al. 2010). In addition, clinicians may easily overestimate the risk of PBD if considering only these poorly defined symptoms, leading to an artificial rise in its prevalence (Moreno et al. 2007). Of all potential risk factors for the development of BD, family history seems to be the one of the most important ones, and can be used successfully to increase the accuracy of diagnosis (Jenkins et al. 2011). However, even though a family history of BD in a first-degree relative dramatically increases one's risk of developing BD (Rasic et al. 2013), most children with this risk factor will not develop the illness (Birmaher et al. 2009). Longitudinal studies with the offspring of parents with BD have shown that clinical presentation alone cannot effectively predict which children with anxiety or unipolar depression will eventually have a manic episode or not (Mesman et al. 2013). Thus, there has been renewed interest in finding potential markers that could accurately discriminate which children should be classified as going through a prodromal stage of the illness.

Neuroimaging studies over the last few years have started to explore this question. As discussed later in this chapter, there is convincing evidence that BD is associated with specific functional and structural changes in brain structures involved in emotional expression and regulation. Studies examining unaffected children at high risk of developing BD, usually defined as having a parent or another first-degree relative with the illness, have overall found some grey matter volume (GMV) differences in anterior cingulate cortex, ventral striatum, medial frontal gyrus, precentral gyrus, insular cortex, and medial orbital gyrus (Matsuo- et al. 2012; Nery et al. 2013). However, no differences were found in the volume of other structures usually associated to emotion regulation, such as hippocampal, thalamic, caudate, and subgenual cingulate volumes (Hajek et al. 2009, 2010; Karchemskiy et al. 2011). Amygdala volumes, in turn, seem to be reduced among youth at high risk who had mood symptoms and eventually did develop BD in a single study (Bechdolf et al. 2012). Therefore, in the absence of longitudinal studies, with the exception of amygdala volume, the volumes of other brain regions are unlikely to be useful as morphological endophenotypes for risk for BD among youth at familial risk for BD, unless we consider their symptomatic versus non-symptomatic state.

Regarding brain functioning, there is evidence of significant differences between unaffected youth at high risk to develop BD and healthy controls. Reduced frontal and exaggerated amygdala activation during face processing has been shown in at-risk youth, similar to what is seen among youth with diagnosis of BD (Olsavsky et al. 2012; Roberts et al. 2013). The amygdala is an area of key interest, given its relevance in emotional processing and its well-known role in other forms of psychopathology. For instance, amygdala hyperactivity is also observed in anxiety disorders (Beesdo et al. 2009). Moreover, anxiety seems to be a risk factor to develop BD among children with a family history of the illness (Duffy et al. 2013). Thus, amygdala functioning may be a promising candidate neuroimaging marker of prodromal staging. The absence of longitudinal studies tracking the correlations between amygdala hyperactivity, anxiety symptoms, and eventual first-onset manic episode among children at risk limits the usefulness of this marker at this time.

There is also evidence that white matter as a whole may go through abnormal developmental processes in children at high risk of developing BD (Sprooten et al. 2011). Diffusion tensor imaging (DTI) data suggest that the corpus callosum and the temporal associative tracts may show opposite patterns in age-related changes in fractional anisotropy (FA), a measure of white matter integrity, between healthy offspring of bipolar parents and healthy controls (Versace et al. 2010). Indeed, a meta-analysis of 27 structural and 10 functional imaging studies revealed significant correlations between genetic risk for BD and white matter abnormalities (Fusar-Poli et al. 2012), which has been suggested by other lines of evidence as well (Mahon et al. 2010). On the other hand, white matter hyperintensities (WMH)—that is, small non-specific white matter lesions associated with multiple aetiologies such as cardiovascular illness and demyelinating disorders—did not differ between youths at high risk of developing BD and controls (Gunde et al. 2011). Thus, it is still not clear whether it is widespread or localized white matter abnormalities that are associated with high familial risk for BD. Longitudinal studies with both broad and specific measures of white matter integrity are necessary to determine whether these findings will be valuable enough to be useful in determining illness staging in prodromal cases.

Paediatric bipolar disorder

Among young patients fully diagnosed with BD, most neuroimaging studies so far tend to find abnormalities in parallel with those found in older adults. Broadly, fronto-limbic-striatal dysfunction seems to be a common finding across affected youths and adults (Blond et al. 2012); using paradigms involving the processing of emotional faces, multiple studies confirmed amygdala hyperactivation and prefrontal hypoactivation in affected youths when compared to healthy controls (Chang et al. 2004; Rich et al. 2006; Brotman et al. 2010, 2013; Schneider al. 2012). Although there are very few studies directly comparing early onset with late onset bipolar illness, an important study compared the degree of amygdala hyperactivity in PBD and adult BD cases, and found that PBD cases showed a pattern of amygdala hyperactivity to a broader range of emotional faces (Kim et al. 2012), when compared to older patients with BD. This was a cross-sectional study, so a longitudinal study is still awaited to confirm the developmental aspects of amygdala functioning in BD.

Longitudinal studies have, however, been conducted for amygdala volumes. There is significant evidence of reduced amygdala volume in PBD in general, as confirmed by two meta-analyses (Pfeifer et al. 2008; Hajek et al. 2009). However, longitudinal studies on amygdala volume have provided conflicting results (Schneider et al. 2012), although the most recent studies suggest that amygdala volume decreases over time (Geller et al. 2009; Bitter et al. 2011). Moreover, there seems to be an inverse correlation between amygdala functioning and volume, that is, amygdala hyperactivation is associated with smaller volumes (Kalmar et al. 2009), suggesting that a possible loss of inhibitory neurons within the amygdala could explain both its progressively smaller volume and increased activation after emotional stimuli (Schneider et al. 2012). Nonetheless, these data, together with the exaggerated amygdala response to emotional faces found among youths at high risk of developing BD (albeit with normal volume), place the amygdala as a potentially key structure in the staging of the illness. Further studies will need to assess whether other functional magnetic resonance imaging (fMRI) paradigms capable of differentially activate the amygdala may allow us to better understand its role on the prodromal, early and late stages of the illness.

An important component of the imaging literature in PBD involves the comparison between youths with narrowly defined BD— type I or II—and 'severe mood dysregulation' (SMD)—chronic non-episodic irritability. SMD has been contentiously debated in the literature whether it represents a paediatric manifestation of BD or not (Biederman et al. 2000). Overall, both PBD and SMD present with abnormal labelling of facial emotional expression (Rich et al. 2008) and exaggerated amygdala activation to emotional faces (Thomas et al. 2013), but with prefrontal differences in the underlying neural activity mediating these deficits (Brotman et al. 2010; Thomas et al. 2013a, b).

White matter abnormalities, not surprisingly, have also been found in multiple regions in PBD cases, including genu, body, and splenium of the corpus callosum, corona radiate, and anterior commissure (Saxena et al. 2012; Lagopoulos et al. 2013). However, in the absence of longitudinal studies, we are not able to link these findings with staging or illness progression.

Adult bipolar disorder

Grey matter volume

A number of studies have applied repeated MRI acquisition in the investigation of GMV changes overtime in BD. Reduction in GMV in the dorsolateral prefrontal cortex (DLPFC) has been consistently observed over the course of BD (Lisy et al. 2011). This is consistent with three prospective studies that found a significant decrease in the nucleus accumbens (ACC) in BD subjects (Kalmar et al. 2009). Notably, there is evidence that lithium can increase GMV in the ACC, particularly the subgenual ACC, which makes this brain area an interesting candidate for investigation of illness progression and treatment response in BD (Lyoo et al. 2010).

On the other hand, other studies found an increase in the right ventrolateral prefrontal cortex and in the orbitofrontal cortex (OFC) in BD (Gogtay et al. 2007).

In contrast with reduced amygdala volume observed in paediatric BD, most longitudinal studies in adult and elderly BD did not show changes in amygdala volume over time (Moorhead et al. 2007; Bitter et al. 2011; Delaloye et al. 2011).

Much like the results from subgenual ACC, it is possible that the stability of amygdala volume in adult/elderly BD may be associated with treatment effects. Longitudinal studies looking at changes in hippocampal volume have provided inconsistent results. While studies have found a decrease in the left parahippocampal gyrus and left hippocampus over time (Moorhead et al. 2007), other studies have found opposite results (Delaloye et al. 2011; Lisy et al. 2011). Again, treatment differences may account for some of these discrepancies, since there is evidence that lithium may increase hippocampal volume (Yucel et al. 2007).

White matter hyperintensities

WMH are white matter areas of high intensity in human brain that are observed on T2-weighted MRI. WMH can be classified according to its anatomical localization: in the deep white matter (deep WMH) or contiguous to the lateral ventricles (periventricular WMH). The pathophysiology of WMH has been associated to localized vascular abnormalities such as ischaemic areas, infarctions, and enlarged perivascular spaces (Braffman et al. 1988; van Swieten et al. 1991; Chimowitz et al. 1992; Fazekas et al. 1993; Manolio et al. 1994), and also neurodegenerative processes such as demyelination, loss of axons, and necrosis (Thomas et al. 2002, 2003).

Although WMH have been found in healthy elderly individuals, some studies have reported an association between hyperintensities and cognitive deficits in healthy ageing (de Groot et al. 2001, 2002).

Dupont et al. (1987) reported for the first time the association between WMH and BD. The study consisted of 14 bipolar patients and 8 healthy controls (mean age 38 ± 8 and 41 ± 9 years old, respectively), and the WMH were associated with the number of hospitalizations. After that first report, several studies showed the association between hyperintensities and BD, being one of the most replicated imaging findings in mood disorder. Although not all studies have found higher WMH in bipolar patients compared to controls, three meta-analyses have examined the prevalence of WMH and BD and confirmed a positive association between hyperintensities and BD. The odds ratios of hyperintensities, which included deep, perivascular, and subcortical grey matter hyperintensities, were 2.9 (Altshuler et al. 1995), 3.29 (Videbech 1997), and 2.5 (Beyer et al. 2009). Another important finding in the meta-analyses was the significant heterogeneity of the hyperintensities across studies. Such variability might be explained by the inclusion of heterogeneous populations in different studies, differences in MRI procedures, and analysis techniques. Notably, no sex differences were found in WMH in BD (Aylward et al. 1994; Persaud et al. 1997; McDonald et al. 1999; Krabbendam et al. 2000; Ahn et al. 2004).

WMH have been strongly associated with ageing (de Leeuw et al. 2001; Sachdev et al. 2007; Wen et al. 2009). However, results showing the association between hyperintensities and age in bipolar patients have been conflicting. Some studies have not found a correlation between WMH and age in the bipolar population (Figiel et al. 1991; Strakowski et al. 1993; Dupont 1995; McDonald et al. 1999; Krabbendam et al. 2000). However, three studies found the association between hyperintensities and age was higher in older bipolar patients compared to healthy controls (Aylward et al. 1994; Altshuler et al. 1995; Moore et al. 2001). McDonald et al. (1999) recruited four groups for the study: bipolar patients younger and older than 50 years old, and healthy controls younger and older than 50. With this design, they found an association between periventricular WMH and age, but not diagnosis. Conversely Silverstone et al. (2003) found that only deep WMH were attributable to the effect of age, and no differences were found in periventricular WMH. A possible explanation for the discrepancy in the association between WMH and age might be related to a higher risk for cardiovascular events in the bipolar population (McIntyre et al. 2012). McDonald et al. (1999) found that bipolar subjects had more cardiovascular risk factors than healthy controls, but they were not statistically different between the groups. The same study did not find a correlation between the presence of WMH and cardiovascular risk factors.

Only a few studies have focused on the presence of WMH and illness progression of BD. Some studies have found an association between WMH and the number of psychiatric hospitalizations (Dupont et al. 1987, 1990; Dupont 1995; McDonald et al. 1999). In contrast, Altshuler et al. (1995) failed to find the same correlation in their sample of 29 bipolar type I and 26 bipolar type II patients. No correlation between WMH and history of psychotic episodes has been found in three studies (Dupont et al. 1990; Figiel et al. 1991; Altshuler et al. 1995). However, later McDonald et al. (1999) found in a group of 70 bipolar patients (38 younger and 32 older than 50 years old) that the older patients presented more WMH and were more likely to be psychotic on psychiatric admission. Only one study found association between WMH and history of suicide attempts (Pompili et al. 2007). Also, only one preliminary study with 16 patients reviewed the association between length of illness and WMH in bipolar patients, but no correlation was found (Kato et al. 2000). Also, conflicting results have been reported on increased WMH, treatment resistance, and response to treatment (Moore et al. 2001; Silverstone et al. 2003). In conclusion, while increased WMH is one of the most consistent finding in brain imaging research in BD, it is unclear at this point whether or how these abnormalities are related to disease progression.

White matter tracts: diffusion tensor imaging

DTI is an imaging technique that maps the dispersion of water molecules in biological tissue. The technique is based on the fact that water molecules move equally in all directions in space (isotropic diffusion) but when water is constrained by physical barriers (e.g. along the axon), the molecules move more along the long axis of the fibre than the perpendicular axis (anisotropic diffusion). FA expresses the degree of anisotropy, and it is zero when the diffusion is equal in all directions (e.g. in the cerebrospinal fluid) and close to one when the diffusion is only in one direction. FA has been considered as a marker of white matter integrity. Decreased FA has been described in tissues with inflammation, oedema, gliosis, and also in the demyelination process (Xekardaki et al. 2011).

Eight studies have used region of interest (ROI) analysis to obtain FA values from white matter tracts in bipolar patients. Decreased FA values (indicating localized abnormal white matter integrity) compared to healthy controls have been reported in frontal white matter (Adler et al. 2004b, 2006), occipital white matter (Macritchie et al. 2010), corpus callosum (Wang et al. 2008b; Macritchie et al. 2010), cingulate white matter (Wang et al. 2008a), internal capsule, and fronto-occipital fasciculus (Haznedar et al. 2005). Only two studies have shown increased FA values in anterior frontal white matter (Haznedar et al. 2005) and corpus callosum (Yurgelun-Todd et al. 2007).

Studies using voxel-based analysis have shown different patterns and distributions of FA across white matter tracts in bipolar patients. Two recent meta-analysis studies have used whole-brain voxel-based anatomical likelihood estimation (Turkeltaub et al. 2002) to obtain a localization probability distribution of the voxel-based results of the literature (Vederine et al. 2011; Nortje et al. 2013). Vederine et al. (2011) included 11 DTI voxel-based studies with total of 314 bipolar patients and 300 healthy controls. Voxel-based anatomical likelihood estimation analysis identified two white matter regions of low FA in bipolar patients compared to healthy controls. The clusters were located in the white matter near the right parahippocampal gyrus and right anterior cingulate cortex. The authors identified four white matter tracts crossing the parahippocampal gyrus: (1) the superior longitudinal fasciculus, (2) the inferior fronto-occipital fasciculus, (3) the inferior longitudinal fasciculus, and (4) the posterior thalamic radiations; and three white matter tracts that cross the anterior cingulate cortex: (1) the uncinate, (2) the inferior fronto-occipital fasciculus, and (3) the corpus callosum forceps minor. Those white matter tracts have been involved in the identification of facial emotion and emotional processing. Nortje et al. (2013) included 15 DTI voxel-based studies with total of 390 bipolar patients and 354 healthy controls. Anatomical likelihood estimation analysis identified three white matter regions of low FA in bipolar patients: the right temporoparietal white matter, left cingulate gyrus, and left anterior cingulate. White matter tracts connected to those regions are the inferior longitudinal fasciculus, the inferior fronto-occipital fasciculus, the middle and posterior cingulum, and the anterior thalamic radiation. Those white matter tracts have been also described to be involved in emotional regulation.

Two studies have examined the association of duration of illness and diffusion values in white matter tracts in bipolar patients compared to healthy controls. Longer length of illness was correlated with low FA in several brain regions of bipolar patients (Versace et al. 2008; Zanetti et al. 2009). Age was negatively correlated with FA values in different white matter regions in bipolar patients but not in healthy individuals (Versace et al. 2008). Only one study compared depressed with euthymic bipolar patients. Zanetti et al. (2009) reported that depressed patients presented lower FA values compared to euthymic patients. In summary, cross-sectional studies suggest that abnormalities in subcortical white matter tracts may be associated with illness progression in BD. While longitudinal studies are awaited to confirm this association, these results are in line with the notion that inflammation and other neurotoxic processes may affect white matter sheath in BD.

Resting state fMRI

fMRI is a non-invasive imaging technique that measures brain activity by detecting localized changes in blood flow. Resting state fMRI is an imaging technique that studies the function of the brain in the absence of specific task ('resting'). Anand et al. (2009) studied 11 bipolar patients using ROI analysis of resting state fMRI. They found decreased cortico-limbic connectivity (between pregenual anterior cingulated cortex (pgACC) and dorsomedial thalamus, between pgACC and amygdala, and between thalamus and palidoestriatum) in bipolar patients compared to healthy controls. Chepenik et al. (2010) studied 15 clinically heterogeneous bipolar patients. They found an increased correlation between left ventral prefrontal cortex (vPFC) and right hemisphere, and a decreased correlation between left ventral PFC and dorsofrontal and parietal regions. Ongür et al. (2010) studied 17 bipolar type I patients. They found reduced connectivity in the medial prefrontal cortex (mPFC) and abnormal recruitment of parietal cortex with DMN that was correlated with mania scores. Chai et al. (2011) studied 14 bipolar type I patients. They found positive correlations between mPFC and left insula, between mPFC and vlPFC, and between vlPFC and left amygdala in patients with mania. Anticevic et al. (2013) studied a large sample of 68 euthymic bipolar type I patients. They found increased connectivity between the mPFC and amygdala in euthymic patients. Meda et al. (2012) studied 64 psychotic bipolar patients and compared to 52 unaffected first-degree relatives and 118 healthy controls. They found increased connectivity between mesoparalimbic and fronto-temporal/paralimbic regions in bipolar patients.

The studies that have focused on default mode network changes in BD and progression of illness are still limited. Chai et al. (2011) found a positive correlation between the mPFC–DLPFC connectivity and age of onset of BD. Regarding symptomatology and severity, a decreased connectivity between the dlPFC and amygdala was found in euthymic patients with psychosis history compared to patients without psychosis history and healthy controls (Anticevic et al. 2013). In sum, at this point it is still early to assess the usefulness of resting state fMRI in staging/illness progression in BD.

Task-based fMRI

Only three studies have addressed sustained attention functioning in BD. Euthymic bipolar patients have shown less activation in the left medial frontal gyrus, and greater activation in vPFC, left amygdala, and parahippocampal regions during sustained attention task (Strakowski et al. 2004). Manic patients have showed less activation in the left striatum, left thalamus, and bilateral left frontal gyrus (LFG), and blunted activation in ventrolateral and dorsolateral PFC (Fleck et al. 2010; Strakowski et al. 2011).

Working memory functioning has been extensively investigated in BD using fMRI. Euthymic bipolar patients have consistently shown less activation in right dlPFC (Monks et al. 2004; Lagopoulos et al. 2007; Hamilton et al. 2009; Glahn et al. 2010; Townsend et al. 2010), less activation in the cingulate cortex (Adler et al. 2004a; Monks et al. 2004; Lagopoulos et al. 2007), and less activation of hippocampus/parahippocampus (Lagopoulos et al. 2007; Glahn et al. 2010) during working memory tasks. Despite these consistent results, three studies failed to show reduction of dlPFC during memory task in euthymic patients (Adler et al. 2004a; Frangou et al. 2008; Gruber et al. 2010). In contrast to the decreased activation in the dlPFC, euthymic bipolar patients presented higher activation in temporal regions during working memory tasks (Adler et al. 2004a; Lagopoulos et al. 2007; Townsend et al. 2010). Only one fMRI study has examined working memory in patients with mania. It has shown an important reduction of activation in right dlPFC and right parietal cortex, compared to healthy controls (Townsend et al. 2010). Consistent with mania, patients with bipolar depression have also shown reduced activation in right dlPFC and right parietal cortex during working memory tasks (Townsend et al. 2010).

Cognitive interference tasks (e.g. Stroop tasks) have evoked a robust activation of ACC and dlPFC in the healthy population (Minzenberg et al. 2009). Euthymic bipolar patients have consistently shown less activation in the ventral PFC compared to healthy controls during Stroop task (Blumberg et al. 2003; Strakowski et al. 2005; Kronhaus et al. 2006; Lagopoulos and Malhi 2007). Euthymic patients have also exhibited less activation in dlPFC (Kronhaus et al. 2006; Lagopoulos and Malhi 2007) during Stroop tasks; however, this finding was not replicated in three other studies (Blumberg et al. 2003; Malhi et al. 2005; Strakowski et al. 2005); in contrast, a single study found increased activation in dlPFC in euthymic patients compared to controls during cognitive interference tasks (Gruber et al. 2004). To date only one study has examined brain activation during cognitive interference tasks in mania. Blumberg et al. (2003) analysed 36 bipolar patients and found less activation in bilateral vPFC during mania compared to healthy controls. Consistent with mania, patients with bipolar depression have also shown reduced activation in left vPFC (Blumberg et al. 2003) during Stroop task. In depressed bipolar patients, cognitive interference tasks also evoked increased activation in the left OFC (Blumberg et al. 2003) and less activation in the posterior cingulate and occipital cortex (Marchand et al. 2007b), compared to controls.

Response inhibition tasks (e.g. GoNoGo tasks) have mainly evoked the activation of IFC in healthy controls (Horn et al. 2003). Euthymic bipolar subjects have shown less activation in bilateral striatum (Kaladjian et al. 2009) and left frontal cortex during GoNoGo tasks (Kaladjian et al. 2009) compared to controls using response inhibition tasks. Bipolar patients during mania have consistently shown reduced activation in IFC when responding to inhibition tasks (Elliott et al. 2004; Altshuler et al. 2005a; Mazzola-Pomietto et al. 2009). GoNoGo tasks during mania have also shown less activation in bilateral putamen (Kaladjian et al. 2009), bilateral thalamus (Strakowski et al. 2008), and less activation in ACC (Altshuler et al. 2005a; Strakowski et al. 2008). In depressed bipolar patients, response inhibition tasks have evoked increased activation in motor/sensory cortex (Caligiuri et al. 2003; Marchand et al. 2007a) compared to controls. Interestingly in contrast to mania, depressed bipolar patients showed increased activation in bilateral striatum and ACC (Marchand et al. 2007a) during motor GoNoGo tasks.

Emotional regulation tasks in healthy individuals have evoked activation of OFC, which is responsible for integrating and regulating the intensity of the emotional response with other limbic structures, as well as activation of amygdala and insula cortex (Hariri et al. 2000). Euthymic bipolar subjects have shown conflicting results regarding OFC function during emotional regulation tasks. Three studies have found less activation in left OFC during euthymia (Malhi et al. 2005; Lagopoulos and Malhi 2007; Jogia et al. 2008), and two studies gave reported increased activation in right OFC (Robinson et al. 2008; Chen et al. 2010) in euthymic patients compared to healthy controls. Euthymic bipolar patients have also shown conflicting results regarding amygdala activation during emotional regulation tasks. Six studies have found no difference in amygdala activation during euthymia (Malhi et al. 2007; Hassel et al. 2008, 2009; Robinson et al. 2008; Almeida et al. 2009a, b), and three studies have found increased activation in right amygdala (Lagopoulos and Malhi 2007; Chen et al. 2010; Surguladze et al. 2010). Bipolar patients during mania have consistently shown less OFC activation during emotional processing and regulation tasks (Yurgelun-Todd et al. 2000; Rubinsztein et al. 2001; Elliott et al. 2004; Malhi et al. 2004; Altshuler et al. 2005a; Killgore et al. 2008). Consistent with OFC activations in mania, other robust finding has been increased activation in left amygdala in response to emotional tasks (Yurgelun-Todd et al. 2000; Altshuler et al. 2005b; Chen et al. 2006; Bermpohl et al. 2009). Contrary to the findings in mania, depressive bipolar patients have shown heterogeneous results in response to emotional regulation tasks. Two studies have shown increased activation in left amygdala in response to emotional faces (Lawrence et al. 2004; Almeida et al. 2010) compared to healthy controls. In another study of depressed bipolar patients in response to emotional faces, it has been shown less activation in bilateral OFC and right DLPFC, increased activation in medial PFC, and no difference in amygdala activation compared to healthy individuals (Altshuler et al. 2008). Chen et al. (2006) found that depressed bipolar patients showed overactivation of fronto-striato-thalamic regions in response to fearful faces. Conversely, Malhi et al. (2004) found increased activation in right thalamus, striatum, hypothalamus, and amygdala in response to emotional regulation task in depressed bipolar patients.

To the best of our knowledge, no fMRI study has examined the association of cognitive and emotional functions and the progression/severity of BD. Neuropsychological studies suggest that euthymic bipolar patients display cognitive dysfunction in frontal executive tasks compared to healthy subjects, suggesting that these neurocognitive dysfunctions may represent a trait rather than a state (Goswami et al. 2006). Longitudinal fMRI studies are still required to better understand the pathophysiology and illness progression of BD.

Neuroimaging of microglia activation

The concept of an activated inflammatory response system (IRS) in mood disorders was first described by Maes in the 'monocyte-T-cell theory of mood disorders' (Maes et al. 1995). IRS activation has been considered an imbalance in immune regulatory processes. In BD, this theory is corroborated by altered concentrations of immune-related peripheral bioassays: for example, elevated cytokine levels (Modabbernia et al. 2013); aberrant expression of pro-inflammatory genes in peripheral monocytes (Padmos et al. 2008); an increase in C-reactive protein (CRP) (Dickerson et al. 2007; Cunha et al. 2008; Becking et al. 2013); alterations in the kynurenine pathway (Myint et al. 2007).

IRS activation is thought to correspond to neuroinflammation, which is histopathologically reflected by an increase of activated microglia (Beumer et al. 2012; Stertz et al. 2013). Microglia are the immunoactive resident macrophages of the brain. They scavenge the brain, engulf cellular debris, pathogens, and other foreign material, present antigens, and release cytotoxic compounds under inflammatory circumstances (Gehrmann et al. 1995). However, they do not only play a role in the immune defence of the central nervous system. Animal model studies have demonstrated that microglia also have an active role in brain development and homeostasis (Nimmerjahn et al. 2005). They steer development of mature synapses during embryogenesis, prune synapses postnatally (Schafer et al. 2012), regulate neurogenesis, and induce apoptosis when necessary (Sierra et al. 2010; Beumer et al. 2012).

In humans, microglia activation can be visualized by means of positron emission tomography (PET) with the radiopharmaceuticals [^{11}C]-PBR28 and [^{11}C]-(R)-PK11195. These radiopharmaceuticals bind to the translocator protein (TSPO), a receptor that is upregulated in the mitochondria of activated microglia cells (Doorduin et al. 2008). In various psychiatric and neurodegenerative disorders [^{11}C]-(R)-PK11195 PET and [^{11}C]-PBR28 PET have been used successfully for imaging neuroinflammation (Banati 2002; Van Berckel et al. 2008; Doorduin et al. 2009; Folkersma et al. 2011; Kreisl et al. 2013).

A recent PET imaging study found increased binding potential of [11C]-(R)-PK11195 in the right hippocampus of mostly euthymic bipolar type I disorder, and a trend in the left hippocampus (Haarman et al. 2014a, b). This in vivo molecular imaging finding is consistent with previous studies suggesting an increase in activated microglia in BD, such as increased interleukin (IL)-1β levels in the cerebrospinal fluid (Söderlund et al. 2011) and increased expression in pro-apoptotic genes and increased oxidative damage to nucleic acids in post-mortem brain in BD (Benes et al. 2006; Che et al. 2010; Rao et al. 2010).

In reviewing the brain imaging findings in BD, it is tempting to speculate that disturbances in microglia function and microglia–neuron interactions may be associated with the structural and functional disturbances described in this chapter. Recent studies tried to investigate the association between immune system and brain structure/function in BD. A study found a negative correlation between serum high sensitive CRP and orbitofrontal cortical volume in individuals with BD I (Chung et al. 2013). In another study, serum IL-10 correlated with serotonin transporter availability in the thalamus of BD I patients (Hsu et al. 2014). A study on mood disorder subjects found that mRNA expression of several inflammatory genes correlated with amygdala, vmPFC, and hippocampal activation when contrasting sad versus happy faces, as well as with thickness of the left subgenual ACC, and of the hippocampal and caudate volume (Savitz et al. 2013). Longitudinal studies and studies including affected and non-affected offspring of BD subjects are required to better understand the role of microglia in the pathophysiology and illness progression of BD.

Conclusions

Although there is considerable enthusiasm in using neuroimaging in the understanding of illness progression and staging in BD, the available literature is largely limited by the dearth of longitudinal studies. The findings of abnormal amygdala volume and functioning among high risk and PBD show that this brain area may be a potential imaging marker for early stages in BD, but given the cross-sectional nature of most studies we are not able to determine their association with risk, resilience, and illness progression. However, these studies are providing a good foundation for future longitudinal studies.

Prospective studies have consistently found a decrease in the GMV in the dlPFC and in sub-areas of the ACC, as well as an increase in the GMV in the vlPFC over time. These brain regions also emerge as potential candidates for future neuroimaging research in staging and illness progression in BD. Here it is worth mentioning that prospective studies assessing hippocampus and amygdala in adult BD may have been obscured by treatment effects. On the other hand, one may hypothesize that loss of GMV in the dlPFC and ACC may be more prominent and may be observed *despite* medication effects.

Increased WMH has been the most consistent neuroimaging finding in BD. Differences in WMH between bipolar subjects and matched controls have been observed primarily in adult and elderly but not in paediatric or offspring BD, which may suggest that the presence of WMH may be associated with illness progression in BD. While some studies have suggested an association between the presence of WMH and illness progression (e.g. number of hospitalizations, psychotic symptoms, and mood episodes), longitudinal studies are awaited to confirm this hypothesis. FA has been considered as valuable marker of in vivo white matter integrity. Neuroimaging studies in bipolar patients using DTI technique have shown low FA values in white matter regions related to emotional processing and emotional regulation. The few studies that investigated the association between FA values in white matter and course of the illness have shown preliminary evidence of a positive association between localized loss of white matter integrity and longer duration of the illness and mood episodes.

Results from resting state fMRI in bipolar patients have revealed abnormal frontal cortical connectivity especially with limbic regions. This is consistent with task-related fMRI studies showing abnormal activation patterns involving fronto-limbic circuitry which may correlate with phase of the illness and/or mood states. However, the usefulness of fMRI in staging/illness progression is still unclear and requires more longitudinal data.

Recent evidence of microglia activation in the CNS and peripheral cells further supports the hypothesis of inflammatory processes underlying structural and functional abnormalities in BD (Stertz et al. 2013). However, these studies require replication and the role of microglia activation in relation to disease progression in BD remains unclear.

In conclusion, several brain imaging methods have been used to uncover the neurobiological underpinnings of BD. Most data so far have converged to a model of frontal cortical-limbic abnormalities in BD. Future studies should try to identify exactly when this circuit becomes abnormal in BD and which are the successful and unsuccessful brain adaptation processes that follow over the course of this devastating illness.

Future trends

- ◆ Longitudinal studies following up children at risk and paediatric BD patients into adulthood may help to understand which brain changes are related to the emergence of the bipolar phenotype and which ones are related to illness progression.

- ◆ Anatomical changes such as WMH and reduced volume of PFC may help in identifying late-stage cases of BD.

- ◆ Amygdala dysfunction, abnormal white matter tracts, and microglia activation seem to play an important role in BD pathology; longitudinal studies involving different treatment modalities are required to evaluate if such structures can be used as biomarkers of staging, prognosis, or response to treatment.

- ◆ Long-term longitudinal anatomical, fMRI, and molecular imaging studies are critical next steps in the understanding of the pathophysiology and illness progression of BD.

References

Adler CM, Holland SK, Schmithorst V, et al. (2004a) Changes in neuronal activation in patients with bipolar disorder during performance of a working memory task. Bipolar Disord 6(6):540–549.

Adler CM, Holland SK, Schmithorst V, et al. (2004b) Abnormal frontal white matter tracts in bipolar disorder: a diffusion tensor imaging study. Bipolar Disord 6(3):197–203.

Adler CM, Adams J, DelBello MP, et al. (2006) Evidence of white matter pathology in bipolar disorder adolescents experiencing their first episode of mania: a diffusion tensor imaging study. Am J Psychiat 163(2):322–324.

Ahn KH, Lyoo IK, Lee HK, et al. (2004) White matter hyperintensities in subjects with bipolar disorder. Psychiat Clin Neuros 58(5):516–521.

Almeida JRC de, Versace A, Mechelli A, et al. (2009a) Abnormal amygdala-prefrontal effective connectivity to happy faces differentiates bipolar from major depression. Biol Psychiat 66(5):451–459.

Almeida JRC, Mechelli A, Hassel S, et al. (2009b) Abnormally increased effective connectivity between parahippocampal gyrus and ventromedial prefrontal regions during emotion labeling in bipolar disorder. Psychiat Res 174(3):195–201.

Almeida JRC, Versace A, Hassel S, et al. (2010) Elevated amygdala activity to sad facial expressions: a state marker of bipolar but not unipolar depression. Biol Psychiat 67(5):414–421.

Altshuler LL, Bookheimer SY, Proenza MA, et al. (2005a) Increased amygdala activation during mania: a functional magnetic resonance imaging study. Am J Psychiat 162(6):1211–1213.

Altshuler LL, Bookheimer SY, Townsend J, et al. (2005b) Blunted activation in orbitofrontal cortex during mania: a functional magnetic resonance imaging study. Biol Psychiat 58(10):763–769.

Altshuler L, Bookheimer S, Townsend J, et al. (2008) Regional brain changes in bipolar I depression: a functional magnetic resonance imaging study. Bipolar Disord 10(6):708–717.

Altshuler LL, Curran JG, Hauser P, et al. (1995) T2 hyperintensities in bipolar disorder: magnetic resonance imaging comparison and literature meta-analysis. Am J Psychiat 152(8):1139–1144.

Anand A, Li Y, Wang Y, Lowe MJ, et al. (2009) Resting state corticolimbic connectivity abnormalities in unmedicated bipolar disorder and unipolar depression. Psychiat Res 171(3):189–198.

Anticevic A, Brumbaugh MS, Winkler AM, et al. (2013) Global prefrontal and fronto-amygdala disconnectivity in bipolar I disorder with psychosis history. Biol Psychiat 73(6):565–573.

Aylward EH, Roberts-Twillie JV, Barta PE, et al. (1994) Basal ganglia volumes and white matter hyperintensities in patients with bipolar disorder. Am J Psychiat 151(5):687–693.

Banati RB (2002) Visualising microglial activation in vivo. Glia **40**(2):206–217.

Bechdolf A, Wood SJ, Nelson B, et al. (2012) Amygdala and insula volumes prior to illness onset in bipolar disorder: a magnetic resonance imaging study. Psychiat Res **201**(1):34–39.

Becking K, Boschloo L, Vogelzangs N, et al. (2013) The association between immune activation and manic symptoms in patients with a depressive disorder. Transl Psychiat **3**(10):e314.

Beesdo K., Lau JYF, Guyer AE, et al. (2009) Common and distinct amygdala-function perturbations in depressed vs anxious adolescents. Arch Gen Psychiat **66**:275–285.

Benes FM, Matzilevich D, Burke RE, et al. (2006) The expression of proapoptosis genes is increased in bipolar disorder, but not in schizophrenia. Mol Psychiat **11**(3):241–251.

Bermpohl F, Dalanay U, Kahnt T, et al. (2009) A preliminary study of increased amygdala activation to positive affective stimuli in mania. Bipolar Disord **11**(1):70–75.

Beumer W, Gibney SM, Drexhage RC, et al. (2012) The immune theory of psychiatric diseases: a key role for activated microglia and circulating monocytes. J Leukocyte Biol **92**:1–17.

Beyer JL, Young R, Kuchibhatla M, et al. (2009) Hyperintense MRI lesions in bipolar disorder: a meta-analysis and review. Int Rev Psychiatr **21**(4):394–409.

Biederman J, Mick E, Faraone SV, et al. (2000) Pediatric mania: a developmental subtype of bipolar disorder? Biol Psychiat **48**(6):458–466.

Birmaher B, Axelson D, Monk K, et al. (2009) Lifetime psychiatric disorders in school-aged offspring of parents with bipolar disorder: the Pittsburgh Bipolar Offspring study. Arch Gen Psychiat **66**:287–296.

Bitter SM, Mills NP, Adler CM, et al. (2011) Progression of amygdala volumetric abnormalities in adolescents after their first manic episode. J Am Acad Child Adolesc Psy **50**(10):1017–1026.

Blond BN, Fredericks CA, and Blumberg HP (2012) Functional neuroanatomy of bipolar disorder: structure, function, and connectivity in an amygdala-anterior paralimbic neural system. Bipolar Disord **14**(4):340–355.

Blumberg HP, Leung H-C, Skudlarski P, et al. (2003) A functional magnetic resonance imaging study of bipolar disorder: state- and trait-related dysfunction in ventral prefrontal cortices. Arch Gen Psychiat **60**(6):601–609.

Braffman BH, Zimmerman RA, Trojanowski JQ, et al. (1988) Brain MR: pathologic correlation with gross and histopathology. 2. Hyperintense white-matter foci in the elderly. AJR. Am J Roentgenol **151**(3):559–566.

Brotman MA, Rich BA, Guyer AE, et al. (2010) Amygdala activation during emotion processing of neutral faces in children with severe mood dysregulation versus ADHD or bipolar disorder. Am J Psychiat **167**:61–69.

Brotman MA, Tseng W-L, Olsavsky AK, et al. (2013) Fronto-limbic-striatal dysfunction in pediatric and adult patients with bipolar disorder: impact of face emotion and attentional demands. Psychol Med **44**:1639–1651.

Caligiuri MP, Brown GG, Meloy MJ, et al. (2003) An fMRI study of affective state and medication on cortical and subcortical brain regions during motor performance in bipolar disorder. Psychiat Res 123(3):171–182.

Chai XJ, Whitfield-Gabrieli S, Shinn AK, et al. (2011) Abnormal medial prefrontal cortex resting-state connectivity in bipolar disorder and schizophrenia. Neuropsychopharmacology 36(10):2009–2017.

Chang K, Adleman NE, Dienes K, et al. (2004) Anomalous prefrontal-subcortical activation in familial pediatric bipolar disorder: a functional magnetic resonance imaging investigation. Arch Gen Psychiat 61:781–792.

Che Y, Wang J-F, Shao L, et al. (2010) Oxidative damage to RNA but not DNA in the hippocampus of patients with major mental illness. J Psychiat Neurosci 35(5):296–302.

Chen C-H, Lennox B, Jacob R, et al. (2006) Explicit and implicit facial affect recognition in manic and depressed States of bipolar disorder: a functional magnetic resonance imaging study. Biol Psychiat 59(1):31–39.

Chen C-H, Suckling J, Ooi C, et al. (2010) A longitudinal fMRI study of the manic and euthymic states of bipolar disorder. Bipolar Disord 12(3):344–347.

Chepenik LG, Raffo M, Hampson M, et al. (2010) Functional connectivity between ventral prefrontal cortex and amygdala at low frequency in the resting state in bipolar disorder. Psychiat Res 182(3):207–210.

Chimowitz MI, Estes ML, Furlan AJ, et al. (1992) Further observations on the pathology of subcortical lesions identified on magnetic resonance imaging. Arch Neurol 49(7):747–752.

Chung K-H, Huang S-H, Wu J-Y, et al. (2013) The link between high-sensitivity C-reactive protein and orbitofrontal cortex in euthymic bipolar disorder. Neuropsychobiology 68(3):168–173.

Cunha AB, Andreazza AC, Gomes FA, et al. (2008) Investigation of serum high-sensitive C-reactive protein levels across all mood states in bipolar disorder. Eur Arch Psy Clin N 258(5):300–304.

De Groot JC, De Leeuw F-E, Oudkerk M, et al. (2002) Periventricular cerebral white matter lesions predict rate of cognitive decline. Ann Neurol 52(3):335–341.

De Groot JC, De Leeuw FE, Oudkerk M, et al. (2001) Cerebral white matter lesions and subjective cognitive dysfunction: the Rotterdam Scan Study. Neurology 56(11):1539–1545.

De Leeuw FE, De Groot JC, Achten E, et al. (2001) Prevalence of cerebral white matter lesions in elderly people: a population based magnetic resonance imaging study. The Rotterdam Scan Study. J Neurol Neurosur Psychiatr 70(1):9–14.

Delaloye C, Moy G, de Bilbao F, et al. (2011) Longitudinal analysis of cognitive performances and structural brain changes in late-life bipolar disorder. Int J Geriatr Psych 26(12):1309–1318.

Dickerson F, Stallings C, Origoni A, et al. (2007) Elevated serum levels of C-reactive protein are associated with mania symptoms in outpatients with bipolar disorder. Prog Neuro-Psychoph 31(4): 952–955.

Doorduin J, de Vries EF, Dierckx RA, et al. (2008) PET imaging of the peripheral benzodiazepine receptor: monitoring disease progression and therapy response in neurodegenerative disorders. Curr Pharm Design 14(31):3297–3315.

Doorduin J, de Vries EFJ, Willemsen ATM, et al. (2009) Neuroinflammation in schizophrenia-related psychosis: a PET study. J Nucl Med 50(11):1801–1807.

Duffy A, Alda M, Hajek T, et al. (2010) Early stages in the development of bipolar disorder. J Affect Disorders 121:127–135.

Duffy A, Horrocks J, Doucette S, et al. (2013) Childhood anxiety: an early predictor of mood disorders in offspring of bipolar parents. J Affect Disorders 150:363–369.

Dupont RM (1995) Magnetic resonance imaging and mood disorders: localization of white matter and other subcortical abnormalities. Arch Gen Psychiat 52(9):747.

Dupont RM, Jernigan TL, Butters N, et al. (1990) Subcortical abnormalities detected in bipolar affective disorder using magnetic resonance imaging. Clinical and neuropsychological significance. Arch Gen Psychiat 47(1):55–59.

Dupont RM, Jernigan TL, Gillin JC, et al. (1987) Subcortical signal hyperintensities in bipolar patients detected by MRI. Psychiat Res 21(4):357–358.

Elliott R, Ogilvie A, Rubinsztein JS, et al. (2004) Abnormal ventral frontal response during performance of an affective go/no go task in patients with mania. Biol Psychiat 55(12):1163–1170.

Fazekas F, Kleinert R, Offenbacher H, et al. (1993) Pathologic correlates of incidental MRI white matter signal hyperintensities. Neurology 43(9):1683–1689.

Figiel GS, Krishnan KR, Rao VP, et al. (1991) Subcortical hyperintensities on brain magnetic resonance imaging: a comparison of normal and bipolar subjects. J Neuropsych Clin N 3(1):18–22.

Fleck DE, Eliassen JC, Durling M, et al. (2010) Functional MRI of sustained attention in bipolar mania. Mol Psychiatr 17:325–336.

Folkersma H, Boellaard R, Yaqub M, et al. (2011) Widespread and prolonged increase in (R)-(11)C-PK11195 binding after traumatic brain injury. J Nucl Med 52(8):1235–1239.

Frangou S, Kington J, Raymont V, et al. (2008) Examining ventral and dorsal prefrontal function in bipolar disorder: a functional magnetic resonance imaging study. Eur Psychiat 23(4):300–308.

Fusar-Poli P, Howes O, Bechdolf A, et al. (2012) Mapping vulnerability to bipolar disorder: a systematic review and meta-analysis of neuroimaging studies. J Psychiatr Neurosci 37:110061.

Gehrmann J, Matsumoto Y, and Kreutzberg GW (1995) Microglia: intrinsic immuneffector cell of the brain. Brain Res Rev 20(3):269–287.

Geller B, Harms MP, Wang L, et al. (2009) Effects of age, sex, and independent life events on amygdala and nucleus accumbens volumes in child bipolar I disorder. Biol Psychiat 65:432–437.

Glahn DC, Robinson JL, Tordesillas-Gutiérrez D, et al. (2010) Fronto-temporal dysregulation in asymptomatic bipolar I patients: a paired associate functional MRI study. Hum Brain Mapp 31(7):1041–1051.

Gogtay N, Ordonez A, Herman DH, et al. (2007) Dynamic mapping of cortical development before and after the onset of pediatric bipolar illness. J Child Psychol Psyc 48(9):852–862.

Goswami U, Sharma A, Khastigir U, et al. (2006) Neuropsychological dysfunction, soft neurological signs and social disability in euthymic patients with bipolar disorder. Brit J Psychiat 188(4):366–373.

Gruber SA, Rogowska J, and Yurgelun-Todd DA (2004) Decreased activation of the anterior cingulate in bipolar patients: an fMRI study. J Affect Disorders 82(2):191–201.

Gruber O, Tost H, Henseler I, et al. (2010) Pathological amygdala activation during working memory performance: evidence for a pathophysiological trait marker in bipolar affective disorder. Hum Brain Mapp 31(1):115–125.

Gunde E, Novak T, Kopecek M, et al. (2011) White matter hyperintensities in affected and unaffected late teenage and early adulthood offspring of bipolar parents: a two-center high-risk study. J Psychiat Res 45:76–82.

Haarman BCM, Riemersma-Van der Lek RF, Burger H, et al. (2014a) Relationship between clinical features and inflammation-related monocyte gene expression in bipolar disorder—towards a better understanding of psychoimmunological interactions. Bipolar Disord 16(2):137–150.

Haarman BC, Riemersma-Van der Lek RF, Burger H, Netkova M, Drexhage RC, Bootsman F, Mesman E, Hillegers MH, Spijker AT, Hoencamp E, Drexhage HA, Nolen WA (2014) Relationship between clinical features and inflammation-related monocyte gene expression in bipolar disorder - towards a better understanding of psychoimmunological interactions. Bipolar Disord 16:137–150.

Hajek T, Gunde E, Slaney C, et al. (2009) Striatal volumes in affected and unaffected relatives of bipolar patients—high-risk study. J Psychiat Res 43:724–729.

Hajek T, Kopecek M, Kozeny J, et al. (2009) Amygdala volumes in mood disorders—meta-analysis of magnetic resonance volumetry studies. J Affect Disorders 115(3): 395–410.

Hajek T, Novak T, Kopecek M, et al. (2010) Subgenual cingulate volumes in offspring of bipolar parents and in sporadic bipolar patients. Eur Arch Psychiat Clin N 260:297–304.

Hamilton LS, Altshuler LL, Townsend J, et al. (2009) Alterations in functional activation in euthymic bipolar disorder and schizophrenia during a working memory task. Human Brain Mapp 30(12):3958–3969.

Hariri AR, Bookheimer SY, and Mazziotta JC (2000) Modulating emotional responses: effects of a neocortical network on the limbic system. Neuroreport 11(1):43–48.

Hassel S, Almeida JR, Frank E, et al. (2009) Prefrontal cortical and striatal activity to happy and fear faces in bipolar disorder is associated with comorbid substance abuse and eating disorder. J Affect Disorders 118(1–3):19–27.

Hassel S, Almeida JR, Kerr N, et al. (2008) Elevated striatal and decreased dorsolateral prefrontal cortical activity in response to emotional stimuli in euthymic bipolar disorder: no associations with psychotropic medication load. Bipolar Disord 10(8):916–927.

Haznedar MM, Roversi F, Pallanti S, and Baldini-Rossi N (2005) Fronto-thalamostriatal gray and white matter volumes and anisotropy of their connections in bipolar spectrum illnesses. Biol Psychiat 57:733–742.

Horn NR, Dolan M, Elliott R, et al. (2003) Response inhibition and impulsivity: an fMRI study. Neuropsychologia 41(14):1959–1966.

Hsu J-W, Lirng J-F, Wang S-J, et al. (2014) Association of thalamic serotonin transporter and interleukin-10 in bipolar I disorder: a SPECT study. Bipolar Disord 16(3): 241–248.

Jenkins MM, Youngstrom EA, Washburn JJ, et al. (2011) Evidence-based strategies improve assessment of pediatric bipolar disorder by community practitioners. Prof Psychol: Res PR Am Psychol Assoc 42:121–129.

Jogia J, Haldane M, Cobb A, et al. (2008) Pilot investigation of the changes in cortical activation during facial affect recognition with lamotrigine monotherapy in bipolar disorder. Brit J Psychiat 192(3):197–201.

Kaladjian A, Jeanningros R, Azorin J-M, et al. (2009) Remission from mania is associated with a decrease in amygdala activation during motor response inhibition. Bipolar Disord 11(5):530–538.

Kalmar JH, Wang F, Chepenik LG, et al. (2009) Relation between amygdala structure and function in adolescents with bipolar disorder. J Am Acad Child Adolesc Psy 48:636–642.

Karchemskiy A, Garrett A, Howe M, et al. (2011) Amygdalar, hippocampal, and thalamic volumes in youth at high risk for development of bipolar disorder. Psychiat Res 194:319–325.

Kato T, Fujii K, Kamiya A, et al. (2000) White matter hyperintensity detected by magnetic resonance imaging and lithium response in bipolar disorder: a preliminary observation. Psychiatry Clin Neuros 54(1):117–120.

Killgore WDS, Gruber SA, and Yurgelun-Todd DA (2008) Abnormal corticostriatal activity during fear perception in bipolar disorder. Neuroreport 19(15):1523–1527.

Kim P, Thomas LA, Rosen BH, et al. (2012) Differing amygdala responses to facial expressions in children and adults with bipolar disorder. Am J Psychiat 169:642–649.

Krabbendam L, Honig A, and Wiersma J (2000) Cognitive dysfunctions and white matter lesions in patients with bipolar disorder in remission. Acta Psychiat Scand 101:274–280.

Kreisl WC, Lyoo CH, McGwier M, et al. (2013) In vivo radioligand binding to translocator protein correlates with severity of Alzheimer's disease. Brain 136(Pt 7):2228–2238.

Kronhaus DM, Lawrence NS, Williams AM, et al. (2006) Stroop performance in bipolar disorder: further evidence for abnormalities in the ventral prefrontal cortex. Bipolar Disord 8(1):28–39.

Lagopoulos J, Hermens DF, Hatton SN, et al. (2013) Microstructural white matter changes in the corpus callosum of young people with bipolar disorder: a diffusion tensor imaging study. PLoS ONE 8:e59108.

Lagopoulos J, Ivanovski B, and Malhi GS (2007) An event-related functional MRI study of working memory in euthymic bipolar disorder. JPN J Psychiat Neur 32(3):174–184.

Lagopoulos J and Malhi GS (2007) A functional magnetic resonance imaging study of emotional Stroop in euthymic bipolar disorder. Neuroreport 18(15):1583–1587.

Lawrence NS, Williams AM, Surguladze S, et al. (2004) Subcortical and ventral prefrontal cortical neural responses to facial expressions distinguish patients with bipolar disorder and major depression. Biol Psychiat 55(6):578–587.

Lisy ME, Jarvis KB, DelBello MP, et al. (2011) Progressive neurostructural changes in adolescent and adult patients with bipolar disorder. Bipolar Disord 13(4):396–405.

Lyoo IK, Dager SR, Kim JE, et al. (2010) Lithium-induced gray matter volume increase as a neural correlate of treatment response in bipolar disorder: a longitudinal brain imaging study. Neuropsychopharmacology 35(8):1743–1750.

Macritchie KAN, Lloyd AJ, Bastin ME, et al. (2010) White matter microstructural abnormalities in euthymic bipolar disorder. Brit J Psychiat 196(1):52–58.

Maes M, Smith R, and Scharpe S (1995) The monocyte-T-lymphocyte hypothesis of major depression. Psychoneuroendocrinology 20(2):111–116.

Mahon K, Burdick KE, and Szeszko PR (2010) A role for white matter abnormalities in the pathophysiology of bipolar disorder. Neurosci Biobehav R 34(4):533–554.

Malhi GS, Lagopoulos J, Sachdev PS, et al. (2004) Cognitive generation of affect in hypomania: an fMRI study. Bipolar Disord 6(4):271–285.

Malhi GS, Lagopoulos J, Sachdev PS, et al. (2005) An emotional Stroop functional MRI study of euthymic bipolar disorder. Bipolar Disord 7(Suppl 5):58–69.

Malhi GS, Lagopoulos J, Sachdev PS, et al. (2007) Is a lack of disgust something to fear? A functional magnetic resonance imaging facial emotion recognition study in euthymic bipolar disorder patients. Bipolar Disord 9(4):345–357.

Manolio TA, Kronmal RA, Burke GL, et al. (1994) Magnetic resonance abnormalities and cardiovascular disease in older adults. The Cardiovascular Health Study. Stroke 25(2):318–327.

Marchand WR, Lee JN, Thatcher GW, et al. (2007a) A functional MRI study of a paced motor activation task to evaluate frontal-subcortical circuit function in bipolar depression. Psychiat Res 155(3):221–230.

Marchand WR, Lee JN, Thatcher J, et al. (2007b) A preliminary longitudinal fMRI study of frontal-subcortical circuits in bipolar disorder using a paced motor activation paradigm. J Affect Disorders 103(1–3):237–241.

Matsuo K, Kopecek M, Nicoletti MA, et al. (2012) New structural brain imaging endophenotype in bipolar disorder. Mol Psychiatr 17:412–420.

Mazzola-Pomietto P, Kaladjian A, Azorin J-M, et al. (2009) Bilateral decrease in ventrolateral prefrontal cortex activation during motor response inhibition in mania. J Psychiat Res 43(4):432–441.

McDonald WM, Tupler LA, Marsteller FA, et al. (1999) Hyperintense lesions on magnetic resonance images in bipolar disorder. Biol Psychiat 45(8):965–971.

McIntyre RS, Alsuwaidan M, Goldstein BI, et al. (2012) The Canadian Network for Mood and Anxiety Treatments (CANMAT) task force recommendations for the management of patients with mood disorders and comorbid metabolic disorders. Ann Clin Psychiat 24:69–81.

Meda SA, Gill A, Stevens MC, et al. (2012) Differences in resting-state functional magnetic resonance imaging functional network connectivity between schizophrenia and psychotic bipolar probands and their unaffected first-degree relatives. Biol Psychiat 71(10):881–889.

Mesman E, Nolen WA Reichart CG, et al. (2013) The Dutch bipolar offspring study: 12-year follow-up. Am J Psychiat 170(5):542–549.

Minzenberg MJ, Laird AR, Thelen S, et al. (2009) Meta-analysis of 41 functional neuroimaging studies of executive function in schizophrenia. Arch Gen Psychiat 66(8):811–822.

Modabbernia A, Taslimi S, Brietzke E, et al. (2013) Cytokine alterations in bipolar disorder: a meta-analysis of 30 studies. Biol Psychiat 74(1):15–25.

Monks PJ, Thompson JM, Bullmore ET, et al. (2004) A functional MRI study of working memory task in euthymic bipolar disorder: evidence for task-specific dysfunction. Bipolar Disord 6(6):550–564.

Moore PB, Shepherd DJ, Eccleston D, et al. (2001) Cerebral white matter lesions in bipolar affective disorder: relationship to outcome. Brit J Psychiat 178:172–176.

Moorhead TW, McKirdy J, Sussmann JE, et al. (2007) Progressive gray matter loss in patients with bipolar disorder. Biol Psychiat 62(8):894–900.

Moreno C, Laje G, Blanco C, et al. (2007) National trends in the outpatient diagnosis and treatment of bipolar disorder in youth. Arch Gen Psychiat 64:1032–1039.

Myint AM, Kim Y-K, Verkerk R, et al. (2007) Tryptophan breakdown pathway in bipolar mania. J Affect Disorders 102(1–3):65–72.

Nery FG, Monkul ES, and Lafer B (2013) Gray matter abnormalities as brain structural vulnerability factors for bipolar disorder: a review of neuroimaging studies of individuals at high genetic risk for bipolar disorder. Aust NZ J Psychiat 47(12):1124–1135.

Nimmerjahn A, Kirchhoff F, and Helmchen F (2005) Resting microglial cells are highly dynamic surveillance of brain parenchyma in vivo. Science 308(5726):1314–1318.

Nortje G, Stein DJ, Radua J, et al. (2013) Systematic review and voxel-based meta-analysis of diffusion tensor imaging studies in bipolar disorder. J Affect Disorders 150(2):192–200.

Olsavsky AK, Brotman MA, Rutenberg JG, et al. (2012) Amygdala hyperactivation during face emotion processing in unaffected youth at risk for bipolar disorder. J Am Acad Child Adolesc Psy 51:294–303.

Ongur D, Lundy M, Greenhouse I, et al. (2010) Default mode network abnormalities in bipolar disorder and schizophrenia. Psychiat Res 183(1):59–68.

Padmos RC, Hillegers MHJ, Knijff EM, et al. (2008) A discriminating messenger RNA signature for bipolar disorder formed by an aberrant expression of inflammatory genes in monocytes. Arch Gen Psychiat 65(4):395–407.

Persaud R, Russow H, Harvey I, et al. (1997) Focal signal hyperintensities in schizophrenia. Schizophr Res 27(1):55–64.

Pfeifer JC, Welge J, Strakowski SM, et al. (2008) Meta-analysis of amygdala volumes in children and adolescents with bipolar disorder. J Am Acad Child Adolesc Psy 47(11):1289–1298.

Pompili M, Ehrlich S, De Pisa E, et al. (2007) White matter hyperintensities and their associations with suicidality in patients with major affective disorders. Eur Arch Psy Clin N 257(8):494–499.

Rao JS, Harry GJ, Rapopor SI, et al. (2010) Increased excitotoxicity and neuroinflammatory markers in postmortem frontal cortex from bipolar disorder patients. Mol Psychiatr 15(4):384–392.

Rasic D, Hajek T, Alda M, et al. (2013) Risk of mental illness in offspring of parents with schizophrenia, bipolar disorder, and major depressive disorder: a meta-analysis of family high-risk studies. Schizophr Bull 40:28–38.

Rich BA, Grimley ME, Schmajuk M, et al. (2008) Face emotion labeling deficits in children with bipolar disorder and severe mood dysregulation. Dev Psychopathol 20:529–546.

Rich BA, Vinton DT, Roberson-Nay R, et al. (2006) Limbic hyperactivation during processing of neutral facial expressions in children with bipolar disorder. Proc Natl Acad Sci USA 103(23):8900–8905.

Roberts G, Green MJ, Breakspear M, et al. (2013) Reduced inferior frontal gyrus activation during response inhibition to emotional stimuli in youth at high risk of bipolar disorder. Biol Psychiat 74(1):55–61.

Robinson JL, Monkul ES, Tordesillas-Gutiérrez D, et al. (2008) Fronto-limbic circuitry in euthymic bipolar disorder: evidence for prefrontal hyperactivation. Psychiat Res 164(2):106–113.

Rubinsztein JS, Fletcher PC, Rogers RD, et al. (2001) Decision-making in mania: a PET study. Brain 124(Pt 12):2550–2563.

Sachdev P, Wen W, Chen X, et al. (2007) Progression of white matter hyperintensities in elderly individuals over 3 years. Neurology 68(3):214–222.

Savitz J, Frank MB, Victor T, et al. (2013) Inflammation and neurological disease-related genes are differentially expressed in depressed patients with mood disorders and correlate with morphometric and functional imaging abnormalities. Brain Behav Immun 31:161–171.

Saxena K, Tamm L, Walley A, et al. (2012) A preliminary investigation of corpus callosum and anterior commissure aberrations in aggressive youth with bipolar disorders. J Child Adol Psychop 22:112–119.

Schafer DP, Lehrman EK, Kautzman AG, et al. (2012) Microglia sculpt postnatal neural circuits in an activity and complement-dependent manner. Neuron 74(4):691–705.

Schneider MR, Delbello MP, McNamara RK, et al. (2012) Neuroprogression in bipolar disorder. Bipolar Disord 14:356–374.

Sierra A, Encinas JM, Deudero JJP, et al. (2010) Microglia shape adult hippocampal neurogenesis through apoptosis-coupled phagocytosis. Cell Stem Cell 7(4):483–495.

Silverstone T, McPherson H, Li Q, et al. (2003) Deep white matter hyperintensities in patients with bipolar depression, unipolar depression and age-matched control subjects. Bipolar Disord 5(1):53–57.

Söderlund J, Olsson SK, Samuelsson M, et al. (2011) Elevation of cerebrospinal fluid interleukin-1ß in bipolar disorder. J Psychiatr Neurosci 36(2):114–118.

Sprooten E, Sussmann JE, Clugston A, et al. (2011) White matter integrity in individuals at high genetic risk of bipolar disorder. Biol Psychiat 70:350–356.

Stertz L, Magalhães PVS, and Kapczinski F (2013) Is bipolar disorder an inflammatory condition? The relevance of microglial activation. Curr Opin Psychiatr 26(1):19–26.

Strakowski SM, Adler CM, Cerullo MA, et al. (2008) Magnetic resonance imaging brain activation in first-episode bipolar mania during a response inhibition task. Early Interv Psychiatry 2(4):225–233.

Strakowski SM, Adler CM, Holland SK, et al. (2004) A preliminary FMRI study of sustained attention in euthymic, unmedicated bipolar disorder. Neuropsychopharmacology 29(9):1734–1740.

Strakowski SM, Adler CM, Holland SK, et al. (2005) Abnormal FMRI brain activation in euthymic bipolar disorder patients during a counting Stroop interference task. Am J Psychiat 162(9):1697–1705.

Strakowski SM, Eliassen JC, Lamy M, et al. (2011) Functional magnetic resonance imaging brain activation in bipolar mania: evidence for disruption of the ventrolateral prefrontal-amygdala emotional pathway. Biol Psychiat 69(4):381–388.

Strakowski SM, Wilson DR, Tohen M, et al. (1993) Structural brain abnormalities in first-episode mania. Biol Psychiat 33(8–9):602–609.

Surguladze SA, Marshall N, Schulze K, et al. (2010) Exaggerated neural response to emotional faces in patients with bipolar disorder and their first-degree relatives. Neuroimage 53(1):58–64.

Thomas AJ, O'Brien JT, Barber R, et al. (2003) A neuropathological study of periventricular white matter hyperintensities in major depression. J Affect Disorders 76(1–3):49–54.

Thomas AJ, Perry R, Barber R, et al. (2002) Pathologies and pathological mechanisms for white matter hyperintensities in depression. Ann N Y Acad Sci **977**:333–339.

Thomas LA, Brotman MA, Bones BL, et al. (2014) Neural circuitry of masked emotional face processing in youth with bipolar disorder, severe mood dysregulation, and healthy volunteers. Dev Cogn Neurosci **8**:110–120.

Thomas LA, Kim P, Bones BL, et al. (2013b) Elevated amygdala responses to emotional faces in youths with chronic irritability or bipolar disorder. Neuroimage Clin **2**:637–645.

Townsend J, Bookheimer SY, Foland-Ross LC, et al. (2010) fMRI abnormalities in dorsolateral prefrontal cortex during a working memory task in manic, euthymic and depressed bipolar subjects. Psychiat Res **182**(1):22–29.

Turkeltaub PE, Eden GF, Jones KM, et al. (2002) Meta-analysis of the functional neuroanatomy of single-word reading: method and validation. Neuroimage **16**(3 Pt 1):765–780.

Van Berckel BN, Bossong MG, Boellaard R, et al. (2008) Microglia activation in recent-onset schizophrenia: a quantitative (R)-[11C]PK11195 positron emission tomography study. Biol Psychiatry **64**(9):820–822.

van Swieten JC, van den Hout JH, van Ketel BA, et al. (1991) Periventricular lesions in the white matter on magnetic resonance imaging in the elderly. A morphometric correlation with arteriolosclerosis and dilated perivascular spaces. Brain **114**(Pt 2):761–774.

Vederine F-E, Wessa M, Leboyer M, et al. (2011) A meta-analysis of whole-brain diffusion tensor imaging studies in bipolar disorder. Prog Neuro-Psychoph **35**(8):1820–1826.

Versace A, Almeida JC, Hassel S, et al. (2008) Elevated left and reduced right orbitomedial prefrontal fractional anisotropy in adults with bipolar disorder revealed by tract-based spatial statistics. Arch Gen Psychiat **65**(9):1041–1052.

Versace A, Ladouceur CD, Romero S, et al. (2010) Altered development of white matter in youth at high familial risk for bipolar disorder: a diffusion tensor imaging study. J Am Acad Child Adolesc Psy **49**:1249–1259, 1259.e1241.

Videbech P (1997) MRI findings in patients with affective disorder: a meta-analysis. Acta Psychiat Scand **96**(3):157–168.

Wang F, Jackowski M, Kalmar JH, et al. (2008a) Abnormal anterior cingulum integrity in bipolar disorder determined through diffusion tensor imaging. Brit J Psychiat **193**(2):126–129.

Wang F, Kalmar JH, Edmiston E, et al. (2008b) Abnormal corpus callosum integrity in bipolar disorder: a diffusion tensor imaging study. Biol Psychiat **64**(8):730–733.

Wen W, Sachdev PS, Li JJ, et al. (2009) White matter hyperintensities in the forties: their prevalence and topography in an epidemiological sample aged 44–48. Hum Brain Mapp **30**(4):1155–1167.

Xekardaki A, Giannakopoulos P, and Haller S (2011) White matter changes in bipolar disorder, Alzheimer disease, and mild cognitive impairment: new insights from DTI. J Aging Res **2011**(6):286564–286510.

Yucel K, McKinnon MC, Taylor VH, et al. (2007) Bilateral hippocampal volume increases after long-term lithium treatment in patients with bipolar disorder: a longitudinal MRI study. Psychopharmacology (Berl) 195(3):357–367.

Yurgelun-Todd DA, Gruber SA, Kanayama G, et al. (2000) fMRI during affect discrimination in bipolar affective disorder. Bipolar Disorders 2(3 Pt 2):237–248.

Yurgelun-Todd DA, Silveri MM, Gruber SA, et al. (2007) White matter abnormalities observed in bipolar disorder: a diffusion tensor imaging study. Bipolar Disord 9(5):504–512.

Zanetti MV, Jackowski MP, Versace A, et al. (2009) State-dependent microstructural white matter changes in bipolar I depression. Eur Arch Psychiat Clin N 259(6):316–328.

Chapter 10

Biomarkers of illness progression in bipolar disorder

Aroldo A. Dargél and Marion Leboyer

Introduction

A biomarker is an indicator of normal biological processes, pathogenic processes, or pharmacological responses to a therapeutic intervention, which can be measured accurately and reproducibly (Biomarkers Definitions Working Group 2001). In medicine, biomarkers are used to support the presence of a specific disease (diagnostic biomarker), to monitor illness progression (prognostic biomarkers), to measure therapeutic interventions (treatment biomarkers), and to predict the onset of future disease (predictive biomarkers) (Biomarkers Definitions Working Group 2001). Biomarker development is a multistep process, in which improvements in clinical care are evaluated at later stages. In oncology, for example, these phases have been outlined as: (1) preclinical; (2) assay validation in independent populations; (3) capacity of the biomarker to detect preclinical disease; (4) assessment of effects on patient management and outcomes; (5) biomarker cost-effectiveness (Pepe et al. 2001). In psychiatry, however, biomarkers with established clinical utility for mental illnesses such as bipolar disorder (BD) are still lacking.

Currently, BD diagnosis is essentially based on patient interviews and self-report questionnaires, which lack objectivity and biological validation (Frey et al. 2013). With an estimated worldwide prevalence of 2.4% (Merikangas et al. 2011), BD is associated with a wide range of detrimental effects on the patient's health and functioning, and is among the top 20 causes of disability worldwide (WHO 2008). Growing evidence has shown the frequency of symptomatic recurrence (i.e. mood episodes) has a negative impact on the illness progression, with marked cognitive and functional impairments, lower pharmacological and psychological treatment responsiveness, and higher rates of medical comorbidities, such as cardiometabolic and neurological diseases (Post et al. 2012). Furthermore, epigenetic mechanisms that are environmentally mediated could interact with genetic mechanisms, which each mediates earlier onset and/or a more severe course of illness (Schmitt et al. 2014).

Neuroprogression has been defined as a pathological brain rewiring process that takes with illness progression in BD (Berk et al. 2011). The end point of such neuroprogressive changes would be tissue injury, structural changes, and functional sequelae that are the neural substrate of mood regulation; these have the potential to increase the risk of further recurrence and reduce the potential of treatment response (Kapczinski et al. 2008; Berk et al. 2011). The neuroprogression is a multifactorial, dynamic process, including biological pathways implicated in inflammation, oxidative stress, and neuroprotection (Fries et al. 2012).

Previous reviews provide a detailed perspective regarding the current state of biomarkers in BD (Frey et al. 2013; Pfaffenseller et al. 2013). Therefore, the aim of this chapter is to summarize the extant literature regarding the relevance of peripheral biomarkers such as neurotrophins, oxidative stress, and proinflammatory markers in illness progression in BD. In addition, we outline some future perspectives through which peripheral biomarkers may contribute to better understanding the pathophysiology of BD and to design novel therapeutic strategies.

Peripheral biomarkers in bipolar disorder

Neurotrophic factors

Neurotrophins are proteins with a crucial role in neuronal development, plasticity, and connectivity (Lang et al. 2007; Klein et al. 2011). Growing evidence has demonstrated that patients with BD have abnormal blood levels of neurotrophic factors, such as brain-derived neurotrophic factor (BDNF) (Post 2007; Lin 2009), neurotrophin-3 (NT-3), neurotrophin-4/5 (NT-4/5), glial cell-derived neurotrophic factor (GDNF), and nerve growth factor (NGF) (Berk et al. 2011; Post et al. 2012).

BDNF is a neurotrophin widely distributed in the nervous system, acting as a key regulator of neuronal growth and synaptic activity/

plasticity (Lang et al. 2007; Klein et al. 2011). Preclinical studies reported correlations between serum BDNF levels and BDNF expression in cortical and hippocampal areas (Lang et al. 2007; Schmidt and Duman 2010), which are implicated in regulation of mood and emotion (Post 2007; Lin 2009; Schmidt and Duman 2010). Peripherally, BDNF is expressed at relatively high levels in vascular endothelial cells, lymphocytes, and smooth muscle (Schmidt and Duman 2010). The BDNF val66met polymorphism, associated with low BDNF function, has been linked to prefrontal cortical morphometric and metabolic alterations in BD (Frey et al. 2007; Matsuo et al. 2009) as well as with early onset of the disease (Geller et al. 2004; Tang et al. 2008).

Several studies have shown that circulating levels of BDNF were significantly decreased during mania or depression (Cunha et al. 2006; Vieira et al. 2007; Oliveira et al. 2009; Grande et al. 2010). Pandey et al. (2008) found decreased levels of mRNA lymphocyte-derived BDNF as well as of BDNF protein in platelets of drug-free manic children and adolescents compared to controls. Recently, two meta-analyses have shown that BD patients had decreased plasmatic/serum levels of BDNF compared to healthy subjects, particularly during manic or depressive episodes (Lin 2009; Fernandes et al. 2011). Fernandes et al. (2011) in a meta-regression analysis ($n = 548$ BD patients; $n = 565$ controls) have found decreased BDNF, with large effect sizes (ES) for depression (ES −0.97) and mania (ES −0.81) versus controls (Fernandes et al. 2011). However, BDNF levels among euthymic BD patients compared to controls subjects were not significant, with a small magnitude (ES −0.20). There was a substantial variability in the results in euthymic phase, and both age and illness duration significantly influenced this variability (Fernandes et al. 2011). Of note, decreased BDNF levels have been reported in euthymic patients at late stages of BD (Kauer-Sant'Anna et al. 2009; Barbosa et al. 2012). Indeed, associations of lower levels of peripheral BDNF with age, illness duration (Yatham et al. 2009), and late stage of BD (Kauer-Sant'Anna et al. 2009) contribute to the hypothesis of BD as a neuroprogressive illness (Berk et al. 2011; Fries et al. 2012).

Other neurotrophic factors have also been studied in BD. NGF was the first neurotrophin to be discovered, by Rita Levi-Montalcini in 1951.

Recently, one study in BD reported a negative correlation between the severity of manic episodes and NGF levels (Barbosa et al. 2011). Increased levels of NT-3, which shares signal transduction pathways with BDNF, have been found in BD patients during mania and depression compared to euthymic patients and healthy controls (Walz et al. 2007; Fernandes et al. 2010; Kapczinski et al. 2011). One study found increased circulating levels of NT-4/5 in BD, but no difference across mood phases (Walz et al. 2009). Under stress, astrocytes/microglial cells increase production of GDNF to avoid neuronal loss (Miller 2011). Abnormal levels of GDNF have been found across the different BD mood phases (Rosa et al. 2006; Takebayashi et al. 2006; Zhang et al. 2010). Additionally, increased plasma levels of vascular endothelial growth factor (VEGF) were found during major depressive or manic episodes in patients with mood disorders (Lee and Kim 2012). Other studies have indicated that VEGF could be one of the modulators for the therapeutic effect of mood stabilizers (Sugawara et al. 2010; Gupta et al. 2012). Taken together, these findings reinforce the possibility that alteration in neurotrophin levels may be a compensatory response to restore neurogenesis in turn to the potential toxicity of mood episodes. Although further studies are needed to investigate the applicability of the neurotrophic factors as markers of illness progression in BD, in particular to identify individuals in the earlier stages of the disease, facilitating early intervention and potentially reducing the allostatic load in the early phase (Kapczinski et al. 2008).

Inflammatory biomarkers

Growing evidence has shown that inflammatory mechanisms may exert a crucial role in BD pathophysiology (Leboyer et al. 2012), in particular via their regulation of synaptic transmission/plasticity and neuronal survival (Dantzer et al. 2008; Yirmiya and Goshen 2011).

In BD patients, immune dysfunctions have been related to the severity and number of mood episodes (Tsai et al. 2001; Ortiz-Dominguez et al. 2007; Brietzke et al. 2009;Goldstein et al. 2009), high prevalence of comorbidities (Goldstein et al. 2009; Magalhães et al. 2012a), medication effects (Boufidou et al. 2004; Knijff et al. 2007), and illness progression (Berk et al. 2011; Pfaffenseller et al. 2013).

Several studies have reported increased peripheral levels of proinflammatory cytokines, including interleukins (IL-2, IL-4, IL-6, and IL-1) and tumour necrosis factor-α (TNF-α) during mania (O'Brien et al. 2006; Kim et al. 2007; Ortiz-Dominguez et al. 2007; Brietzke et al. 2009; Barbosa et al. 2011, 2012; Hope et al. 2011) and depression (O'Brien et al. 2006; Ortiz-Dominguez et al. 2007). Compelling evidence has demonstrated increased levels of soluble receptors of TNF (sTNF-R1 and sTNF-R2) and IL-2 (sIL-2) in manic patients compared to euthymic and control patients (Barbosa et al. 2011, 2012; Hope et al. 2011; Cetin et al. 2012; Tsai et al. 2012). Additionally, increased levels of sTNF-R1 and sTNF-R2 were positively correlated with patients' age and illness duration of BD (Barbosa et al. 2011, 2012), and BD patients with increased levels of TNFR1 had poor functioning in late adulthood (Hope et al. 2013). Pre-existing increased levels of IL-1β and IL-1Ra might predict vulnerability for future mood episodes (Ortiz-Dominguez et al. 2007). Furthermore, a recent study has demonstrated that markers of neuroinflammation are significantly increased in postmortem frontal cortex from BD patients (Rao et al. 2010). In particular, this study found an important activation of the IL-1 receptor cascade (Rao et al. 2010),which is involved in several regulatory process of inflammation (Buttner et al. 2007). IL-10 exerts a central role in immune response through down-regulation of proinflammatory cytokines, including TNF-α, IL-1β, and IL-6. Elevated levels of IL-10 have been demonstrated in BD patients in remission after manic (Boufidou et al. 2004; Remlinger-Molenda et al. 2012) or depressive episodes (Barbosa et al. 2012), while other reports did not find any significant difference in IL-10 levels (Remlinger-Molenda et al. 2012). Levels of IL-10 seem to reduce significantly from early to late stages of BD (Kauer-Sant'Anna et al. 2009). Therefore, a cumulative effect of successive mood episodes, as well as illness duration, appears to influence levels of proinflammatory cytokines, which act as key mediators in both central and peripheral inflammation, and may contribute to neuroprogression in BD.

It is worth mentioning that TNF-α, IL-1β, and particularly IL-6 are the chief inducers of acute-phase proteins, including C-reactive protein (CRP) (Gabay and Kushner 1999). CRP is a marker of systemic, low-grade inflammation as well as an established risk factor for cardiovascular disease (CVD). In a recent meta-analysis (including 11 studies; 1,618 individuals) to estimate the size of the association between CRP levels and BD, we found a significant elevation in CRP levels in BD patients compared to control subjects, with a moderate effect size (ES = 0.39) (95% CI, 0.24–0.55; $P < 0.0001$) (Dargél et al. 2014). In the subgroup analysis by mood phases, we found that manic BD patients had levels of CRP significantly higher than control subjects with a large ES (0.74) (95% CI, 0.44–1.02; $P < 0.001$) (Dargél et al. 2014). A 2-year follow-up study demonstrated that increased levels of CRP were an important risk factor for the onset of manic symptoms in depressed men (Becking et al. 2013). Another study reported an association between severity of manic symptoms and high-sensitivity CRP as well as a negative association between serum IL-6 and BDNF protein levels in adolescents with BD (Goldstein et al. 2011). A proinflammatory state seems to be related with manic symptoms. That adds to the notion that CRP could be a state marker in BD. Although explanatory mechanisms to this relationship are still unclear, one possible mechanism might be linked to sleep dysfunction, which is often in manic (Harvey 2008). BD patients are known to be associated to elevated cytokines and CRP levels (Mullington et al. 2009). In the same meta-analysis, differences in CRP levels among euthymic patients versus controls were significantly higher albeit with a slight magnitude (Dargél et al. 2014), suggesting that there may be an inflammatory component in non-acutely ill BD patients. These meta-analytic results reinforce evidence showing that activation of the inflammatory response persists after remission (Mullington et al. 2009), suggesting CRP as a potential marker of trait in BD (Dargél et al. 2014). However, it is important to bear in mind that many studies included in this subgroup analysis used different criteria to characterize the different mood phases of BD, raising the idea that some BD patients categorized as euthymic had residual symptoms (subsyndromal), which could also influence CRP levels (Dargél et al. 2014). The burden of acute episodes appears to contribute to CVD mortality among individuals with BD (Fiedorowicz et al. 2009). Compelling evidence has shown that CRP is an independent predictor of CVD (Emerging Risk Factors Collaboration et al. 2010), which is the leading cause of excess mortality in BD patients (Kupfer 2005). Measurement of CRP levels associated with other parameters commonly used in clinical practice such as blood pressure, waist circumference, lipid, and glucose levels may be a useful biomarker in BD patients at risk of CVD as well as in individuals who are otherwise healthy, but suffer from BD.

Hypothalamic-pituitary-adrenal (HPA) axis

The HPA is the main system implicated in the response to physical or psychological stress (Teixera et al. 2013). Various parameters of HPA function such as cortisol levels, dexamethasone suppression test (DST), and DEX/CHR have been related to severity of mood symptoms. In depression, for example, serum cortisol levels measured after the overnight 1 mg DST were related to severity of illness and were thought to discriminate severity of depression (Maes et al. 1986). Studies have demonstrated increased activity of the HPA axis and basal cortisol levels during depressive or manic episodes in BD patients (Maes et al. 1986; Schmider et al. 1995; Watson et al. 2004), as well as a trend to increased levels of cortisol in response to the DEX/CRH test during euthymia (Maes et al. 1986; Watson et al. 2004). Measurements of HPA function, reflecting the severity of a particular disease state, might be putative biomarkers of illness progression in BD.

Oxidative stress biomarkers

The brain is susceptible to oxidative stress damage, due to high oxygen consumption and hence the generation of free radicals, and its low antioxidant capacity (Olmez and Ozyurt 2012). An imbalance between oxidant/antioxidant mechanisms contributes to accumulation of oxidative species, which react with cell components, such as proteins, lipids, mitochondria, and nucleic acid, contributing to neuronal degradation and dysfunctional neurogenesis (Andreazza et al. 2007; Zhang and Yao 2013). The mechanisms of oxidative injury have been reported in various conditions, including ageing (Poulose and Raju 2014), cancer, cardiovascular, and neurodegenerative diseases (Friese et al. 2014). In BD, significant alterations in antioxidant enzymes, lipid peroxidation, and nitric oxide (NO) levels have been reported (Andreazza et al. 2008).

Altered oxidative stress parameters and activated antioxidant defences have been associated with the different mood phases in BD and/or the number of the manic episodes (Savas et al. 2006).

It has been shown that NO levels increase during acute episodes of mania (Savaş et al. 2002) and depression (Selek et al. 2008), as well as in euthymic BD patients (Savas et al. 2006). Altered activity of erythrocyte superoxide dismutase (SOD), an antioxidant enzyme, is another important finding in BD patients. Many studies have demonstrated a significant elevation in SOD concentration in manic and depressed BD patients compared to euthymic patients or controls (Andreazza et al. 2007; Kunz et al. 2008). In contrast, other studies have reported reduced levels of SOD across all mood phases of BD (Ranjekar et al. 2003; Gegerlioglu et al. 2007; Selek et al. et al. 2008) as well as no significant difference in the SOD activity between BD patients and controls (Raffa et al. 2012). Despite NO levels have reduced after treatment of BD patients, SOD activity remained high (Selek et al. 2008). SOD increasing activity may be a defence-antioxidant mechanism against increased NO levels in BD. Additionally, high SOD activity in mood episodes may reflect a preceding cellular oxidative stress or serve as a compensatory mechanism, suggesting that SOD may be involved in neuroprogression in BD. Increased activity of serum catalase (CAT), another antioxidant enzyme, was found in manic patients (Andreazza et al. 2007) including those medication-free (Vieira et al. 2007), with a reduced activity during euthymia (Ranjekar et al. 2003; Andreazza et al. 2007). Despite normal levels of glutathione peroxidase observed during mania (Andreazza et al. 2007), an increased oxidant/antioxidant ratio (SOD/GPx + catalase) was found in manic and depressive BD patients compared to euthymic patients and controls (Andreazza et al. 2007). Several conditions related with ageing (e.g. higher visceral adiposity, inflammation, abnormal glucose/lipid levels) have been linked to oxidative damage to lipids (Poulose and Raju 2014), which could be assessed by measuring serum/plasma levels of thiobarbituric acid reactive substances (TBARS). Elevated levels of TBARS have been reported across all mood phases of BD (Andreazza et al. 2007; Kunz et al. 2008). Although Kunz et al. (2008) demonstrated that only manic patients had significantly increased levels of TBARS in comparison to other patient's groups (depressed, euthymic, or schizo-phrenic) (Kunz et al. 2008). Magalhães et al. (2012) have found an asso-ciation between current manic episode and abnormal concentrations of protein carbonyl content (PCC), which is a measure of oxidative dam-age to protein (Magalhães et al. 2012b). Higher PCC levels have been associated to apoptosis and necrosis cellular as well as to adverse clinical outcomes (e.g. colorectal cancer) (Poulose and Raju 2014). Moreover, oxidative stress may also lead to DNA damage in BD patients mainly in those with severe mood episodes (Andreazza et al. 2007, 2008). Oxidative damage therefore occurs during acute mood episodes, supporting the idea that mood episodes (mania in particular) might be toxic to patients with BD. However, the lipid and protein damage could be a consequence of dysfunction in different pathways and further studies are needed to elucidate oxidative stress biomarkers in BD illness progression.

Peripheral biomarkers associated with the treatment of BD neurotrophins

Studies reported that manic patients had significant increase in BDNF levels following treatment with mood stabilizers, in particular with lith-ium (Tramontina et al. 2009; Fernandes et al. 2011; Sousa et al. 2011). In addition, BD patients non-responders to lithium had lower plasmatic levels of BDNF than those with a good response to lithium (Rybakowski and Suwalska 2010). Another study that examined changes in BDNF lev-els among BD patients, initially unmedicated, found increased levels of BDNF in depressed patients but a reduced level in patients during manic/mixed episodes after treatment with extended-release quetiapine (Grande et al. 2012). Given these findings, peripheral levels of BDNF may also be a potential marker of treatment response in BD. Longitudinal studies are needed to measure BDNF levels in the same patients experiencing dif-ferent mood episodes as well as in those receiving multiple treatments.

Oxidative stress and antioxidant defence markers

It is important to highlight that the therapeutic effects of mood stabiliz-ers may be related to their regulatory effect on oxidative stress pathways (Andreazza et al. 2008). BD patients medication-free treated with lithium during manic episodes exhibit reduced levels of SOD, CAT, and TBARS (Vieira et al. 2007). Similarly, first-episode psychotic patients treated with olanzapine or risperidone had decreased SOD activity and lipid peroxidation (Vieira et al. 2007; Andreazza et al. 2008; Kunz et al. 2008). Oxidative stress therefore might be implicated in illness progression in BD, and use of antioxidants can be a relevant therapeutic strategy on this disorder.

N-acetyl-cysteine (NAC) is the precursor of glutathione (GSH), the most important non-enzymatic cellular antioxidant, and is known to maintain the oxidative balance in the cell. Recent clinical trials have shown that adjunctive treatment with NAC appears to be beneficial in BD (Berk 2008; Magalhães et al. 2011b). Preclinical evidence has demonstrated some antioxidant/neuroprotective properties of the ω-3 polyunsaturated fatty acids (PUFAs) (Wu et al. 2004). Recently, a meta-analysis of clinical trials using ω-3PUFAs associated with standard treatment in BD reported that ω-3 amended BD depressive symptoms (Sarris et al. 2012). Of note, add-on supplementation of vitamin C, vitamin E, the combination of vitamin C and vitamin E, or the mixture of fish oil has been shown to reduce oxidative stress markers and improve clinical symptoms in schizophrenic patients (Pandya et al. 2013). Given these data, development of novel therapeutic approaches to reduce oxidative stress and repair membrane impairments may be useful in early intervention to prevent neuroprogression in BD.

Inflammatory biomarkers

Conventional mood stabilizers seem to down-regulate the production of proinflammatory mRNA and protein gene expression (Harman et al. 2014).

Given that inflammatory pathways seem to be involved in illness progression of BD, adjunctive therapies to modulate inflammatory response seem to be another relevant therapeutic strategy to more accurate interventions in BD. In keeping with this view, a randomized, double-blind, placebo-controlled study reported substantial antidepressant effects following adjunctive treatment with celecoxib (cyclooxygenase-2 inhibitor) in BD patients during depressive or mixed episodes (Nery et al. 2008) beneficial effects of aspirin as an adjunctive treatment in BD (Savitz et al. 2012). Interestingly, alterations in the arachidonic acid metabolism cascade were found in the postmortem brain of BD (Rao et al. 2010).

Disturbances in inflammatory response, however, can be prominent only in a subset of individuals with BD. Recently, a study has evaluated the effect of a TNF-α antagonist (infliximab) in patients with treatment-resistant depression. Infliximab was superior to placebo in mitigating depressive symptoms only in individuals who exhibited elevated inflammation (hsCRP >5 mg/L) at baseline (Raison et al. 2013). This preliminary result supports the idea that measurements of CRP levels may be useful to stratify BD patients who respond to a specific immune or anti-inflammatory treatment, suggesting that CRP may be a potential marker for enhancing treatment matching in BD.

To date, several biomarkers that display potential information about treatment response overlap with prognostic markers that could predict risk or progression of illness. Moreover, non-pharmacologic therapeutic approaches, such as psychotherapy and healthy behaviour, may modulate peripheral biomarkers of neuroprogression, including neurotrophins, inflammation, and oxidative markers (see Fig. 10.1) (Conus et al. 2008; Brietzke et al 2011).

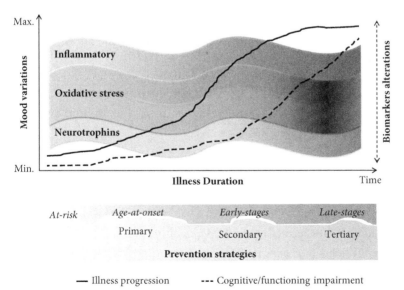

Fig. 10.1 Peripheral biomarkers in illness progression in bipolar disorder.

Evidences have shown that physical exercise (Eyre et al. 2013) and good dietary habits (King et al. 2003) are associated to significant reduction in CRP levels as well as to improvement in depression-like behaviour and depressive symptoms (Eyre et al. 2013; Sanchez-Villegas and Martinez-Gonzalez 2013). In paediatrics, poor sleep and unhealthy diet habits have been linked to unhealthy growth by modifying the architecture of the plastic brain (Garner and Shonkoff 2012). Moreover, smoking increases the risk of mood disorders, and appears to affect similar biological pathways (Moylan et al. 2013).

Future perspectives

As discussed in this chapter, a number of neurotrophic, inflammatory, and oxidative stress biomarkers are associated with BD (Pfaffenseller et al. 2013). However, a question remains about how to implement these putative biomarkers in the clinical practice to identify individuals at risk or earlier stages of BD and to prevent illness progression.

BD is a heterogeneous disorder, where different peripheral biomarker profiles have been linked to particular characteristics of patients, specific mood phases, length of illness, or even different stages of disease, thereby making generalized conclusions difficult. Heterogeneous populations used in most of the studies are also another critical point. Examining well-defined groups may enhance accuracy of peripheral biomarkers of illness progression in BD. Moreover, it may be necessary to shift focus away from a one-size-fits-all approach and instead generate biomarkers profiles, highlighting core domains of dysfunction or strengths for each patient towards tailored interventions.

Although BD is associated with several inflammatory or oxidative stress biomarkers, confounding/moderator variables need to be accounted for. For example, despite CRP being commonly used as a marker of inflammation (Gabay and Kushner 1999) as well as a risk factor for CVD (Emerging Risk Factors Collaboration et al. 2010), its levels may be influenced by gender, BMI, medical comorbidities, alcohol/drug abuse, smoking, and stressors (O'Connor et al. 2009), with an impact on the results. Further studies including within-subject comparisons and subgroup analyses (e.g. BD subtype, sex, and family history of BD) are required to identify useful biomarkers of illness progression in BD. Moreover, it would be interesting to examine whether these peripheral biomarkers can inform our understanding, treatment, and prevention of crucial non-mood conditions in BD as cardiometabolic disorders and cognitive-functioning impairment (Barbosa et al. 2012).

The effect of treating BD on biomarkers has primarily focused on pharmacological treatments. Research into other treatments such as psychological therapies and lifestyle interventions (sleep, diet, and exercise) are still scarce. The influence of more targeted anti-inflammatory treatments and antioxidant therapies on mood symptoms and biomarkers levels is also required. Finally, while a selection of more commonly assessed biomarkers in BD research, specifically targeting inflammation, oxidative stress, and neurotrophins, has been covered in this chapter, there remains an array of other potential options. Other potential biomarkers would include measurements of amino acid levels which are the precursors to neurotransmitters (Miller et al. 2008); growth factors such as insulin-like growth factor-1 (Kim et al. 2013), markers of associated with tryptophan pathways (e.g. kynurenic acid, quinolic acid) (Olsson et al. 2012) genetic polymorphisms associated with dopamine and serotonin transporters and receptors as well as with P450 metabolic pathways (Patel et al. 2010; Singh et al. 2012).

Conclusion

BD is complex, and a multidimensional approach is germane to guide disease diagnosis and therapeutic interventions. Advances in research have identified promising biomarkers of illness progression, including neurotrophins, oxidative stress, and inflammatory markers. However, more work is needed to elucidate the clinical utility of these biomarkers. Future studies combining different approaches, such as integrative omics (e.g. proteomics, epi/genomics, and metabolomics), computational models, as well as pooling various biomarkers, may contribute to the development of useful biomarkers in BD. Ultimately, more consistent nosology and accurate classification of biomarkers will be crucial to determine how these tests could help us to better understand pathophysiological mechanisms and to identify biological targets, providing individualized treatment and preventing illness progression in BD.

References

Andreazza AC, Cassini C, Rosa AR, et al. (2007) Serum S100B and antioxidant enzymes in bipolar patients. J Psychiat Res **41**(6):523–529.

Andreazza AC, Kauer-Sant'anna M, Frey BN, et al. (2008) Oxidative stress markers in bipolar disorder: a meta-analysis. J Affect Disorders **111**(2–3):135–144.

Barbosa IG, Huguet RB, Sousa LP, et al. (2011) Circulating levels of GDNF in bipolar disorder. Neurosci Lett **502**(2):103–106.

Barbosa IG, Rocha NP, de Miranda AS, et al. (2012) Increased levels of adipokines in bipolar disorder. J Psychiat Res **46**(3):389–393.

Barbosa IG, Rocha NP, Huguet RB, et al. (2012) Executive dysfunction in euthymic bipolar disorder patients and its association with plasma biomarkers. J Affect Disorders **137**(1–3):151–155.

Becking K, Boschloo L, Vogelzangs N, et al. (2013) The association between immune activation and manic symptoms in patients with a depressive disorder. Transl Psychiatry. **3**(10):e314.

Berk M (2008) Neuroprogression: pathways to progressive brain changes in bipolar disorder. Int J Neuropsychoph **12**(4):441–445.

Berk M, Kapczinski F, Andreazza AC, et al. (2011) Pathways underlying neuroprogression in bipolar disorder: focus on inflammation, oxidative stress and neurotrophic factors. Neurosci Biobehav R **35**(3):804–817.

Biomarkers Definitions Working Group (2001) Biomarkers and surrogate endpoints: preferred definitions and conceptual framework. Clin Pharmacol Ther **69**(3):89–95.

Boufidou F, Nikolaou C, Alevizos B, et al. (2004) Cytokine production in bipolar affective disorder patients under lithium treatment. J Affect Disorders **82**(2):309–313.

Brietzke E, Kapczinski F, Grassi-Oliveira R, et al. (2011) Insulin dysfunction and allostatic load in bipolar disorder. Exp Rev Neurother **11**(7):1017–1028.

Brietzke E, Stertz L, Fernandes BS, et al. (2009) Comparison of cytokine levels in depressed, manic and euthymic patients with bipolar disorder. J Affect Disorders **116**(3):214–217.

Buttner N, Bhattacharyya S, Walsh J, et al. (2007) DNA fragmentation is increased in non-GABAergic neurons in bipolar disorder but not in schizophrenia. Schizophr Res **93**(1–3):33–41.

Cetin T, Guloksuz S, Cetin EA, et al. (2012) Plasma concentrations of soluble cytokine receptors in euthymic bipolar patients with and without subsyndromal symptoms. BMC Psychiat **12**:158.

Conus P, Ward J, Hallam KT, et al. (2008) The proximal prodrome to first episode mania a new target for early intervention. Bipolar Disord 10(5):555–565.

Cunha ABM, Frey BN, Andreazza AC, et al. (2006) Serum brain-derived neurotrophic factor is decreased in bipolar disorder during depressive and manic episodes. Neurosci Lett 398(3):215–219.

Dantzer R, O'Connor JC, Freund GG, et al. (2008) From inflammation to sickness and depression: when the immune system subjugates the brain. Nat Rev Neurosci 9(1):46–56.

Dargél AA, Godin O, Kapczinski F, et al. (2015) C-reactive protein alterations in bipolar disorder: a and meta-analysis. J Clin Psychiat 76:142–150.

Emerging Risk Factors Collaboration, Kaptoge S, Di Angelantonio E, Lowe G, et al. (2010) C-reactive protein concentration and risk of coronary heart disease, stroke, and mortality: an individual participant meta-analysis. Lancet 375(9709): 132–140.

Eyre HA, Papps E, and Baune BT (2013) Treating depression and depression-like behavior with physical activity: an immune perspective. Front Psychiatry [Internet]. Available from <http://www.frontiersin.org/Journal/10.3389/fpsyt.2013.00003/full> (accessed 21 November 2014).

Fernandes BS, Gama CS, Cereśer KM, et al. (2011) Brain-derived neurotrophic factor as a state-marker of mood episodes in bipolar disorders: a systematic review and meta-regression analysis. J Psychiat Res 45(8):995–1004.

Fernandes BS, Gama CS, Walz JC, et al. (2010) Increased neurotrophin-3 in drug-free subjects with bipolar disorder during manic and depressive episodes. J Psychiat Res 44(9):561–565.

Fiedorowicz JG, Solomon DA, Endicott J, et al. (2009) Manic/hypomanic symptom burden and cardiovascular mortality in bipolar disorder. Psychosom Med 71(6):598–606.

Frey BN, Andreazza AC, Houenou J, et al. (2013) Biomarkers in bipolar disorder: a positional paper from the International Society for Bipolar Disorders Biomarkers Task Force. Aust NZ J Psychiat 47(4):321–332.

Frey BN, Walss-Bass C, Stanley JA, et al. (2007) Brain-derived neurotrophic factor val66met polymorphism affects prefrontal energy metabolism in bipolar disorder. Neuroreport 18(15):1567–1570.

Fries GR, Pfaffenseller B, Stertz L, et al. (2012) Staging and neuroprogression in bipolar disorder. Curr Psychiatry Rep 14(6):667–675.

Friese MA, Schattling B, and Fugger L (2014) Mechanisms of neurodegeneration and axonal dysfunction in multiple sclerosis. Nat Rev Neurol 10(4):225–238.

Gabay C and Kushner I (1999) Acute-phase proteins and other systemic responses to inflammation. N Engl J Med 340(6):448–454

Garner AS and Shonkoff JP, Committee on Psychosocial Aspects of Child and Family Health, Committee on Early Childhood, Adoption, and Dependent Care, Section on Developmental and Behavioral Pediatrics (2012) Early childhood adversity, toxic stress, and the role of the pediatrician: translating developmental science into lifelong health. Pediatrics 129(1):e224–231.

Geller B, Badner JA, Tillman R, et al. (2004) Linkage disequilibrium of the brain-derived neurotrophic factor Val66Met polymorphism in children with a prepubertal and early adolescent bipolar disorder phenotype. Am J Psychiat 161(9):1698–1700.

Gergerlioglu HS, Savas HA, Bulbul F, et al. (2007) Changes in nitric oxide level and superoxide dismutase activity during antimanic treatment. Prog Neuro-Psychoph 31(3):697–702.

Goldstein BI, Collinger KA, Lotrich F, et al. (2011) Preliminary findings regarding proinflammatory markers and brain-derived neurotrophic factor among adolescents with bipolar spectrum disorders. J Child Adol Psychop 21(5):479–484.

Goldstein BI, Kemp DE, Soczynska JK, et al. (2009) Inflammation and the phenomenology, pathophysiology, comorbidity, and treatment of bipolar disorder: a systematic review of the literature. J Clin Psychiat 70(8):1078–1090.

Grande I, Fries GR, Kunz M, et al. (2010) The role of BDNF as a mediator of neuroplasticity in bipolar disorder. Psychiat Invest 7(4):243–250.

Grande I, Kapczinski F, Stertz L, et al. (2012) Peripheral brain-derived neurotrophic factor changes along treatment with extended release quetiapine during acute mood episodes: an open-label trial in drug-free patients with bipolar disorder. J Psychiat Res 46(11):1511–1514.

Guloksuz S, Altinbas K, Aktas Cetin E, et al. (2012) Evidence for an association between tumor necrosis factor-alpha levels and lithium response. J Affect Disorders 143(1–3):148–152.

Gupta A, Schulze TG, Nagarajan V, et al. (2012) Interaction networks of lithium and valproate molecular targets reveal a striking enrichment of apoptosis functional clusters and neurotrophin signaling. Pharmacogenomics J 12(4):328–341.

Haarman BBC, Riemersma-Van der Lek RF, Burger H, et al. (2014) Relationship between clinical features and inflammation-related monocyte gene expression in bipolar disorder—towards a better understanding of psychoimmunological interactions. Bipolar Disord 16(2):137–150.

Harvey AG (2008) Sleep and circadian rhythms in bipolar disorder: seeking synchrony, harmony, and regulation. Am J Psychiat 165(7):820–829.

Hope S, Dieset I, Agartz I, et al. (2011) Affective symptoms are associated with markers of inflammation and immune activation in bipolar disorders but not in schizophrenia. J Psychiat Res 45(12):1608–1616.

Hope S, Ueland T, Steen NE, et al. (2013) Interleukin 1 receptor antagonist and soluble tumor necrosis factor receptor 1 are associated with general severity and psychotic symptoms in schizophrenia and bipolar disorder. Schizophr Res 145 (1–3):36–42. 56.

Kapczinski F, Dal-Pizzol F, Teixeira AL, et al. (2011) Peripheral biomarkers and illness activity in bipolar disorder. J Psychiat Res 45(2):156–161.

Kapczinski F, Vieta E, Andreazza AC, et al. (2008) Allostatic load in bipolar disorder: implications for pathophysiology and treatment. Neurosci Biobehav R 32(4):675–692.

Kauer-Sant'Anna M, Kapczinski F, Andreazza AC, et al. (2009) Brain-derived neurotrophic factor and inflammatory markers in patients with early- vs. late-stage bipolar disorder. Int J Neuropsychoph 12(4):447–458.

Kim Y-K, Jung H-G, Myint A-M, et al. (2007) Imbalance between pro-inflammatory and anti-inflammatory cytokines in bipolar disorder. J Affect Disorders 104(1–3):91–95.

Kim Y-K, Na K-S, Hwang J-A, et al. (2013) High insulin-like growth factor-1 in patients with bipolar I disorder: A trait marker? J Affect Disorders 151(2):738–743.

King DE, Egan BM, and Geesey ME (2003) Relation of dietary fat and fiber to elevation of C-reactive protein. Am J Cardiol 92(11):1335–1339.

Klein AB, Williamson R, Santini MA, et al. (2011) Blood BDNF concentrations reflect brain-tissue BDNF levels across species. Int J Neuropsychoph 14(3):347–353.

Knijff EM, Breunis MN, Kupka RW, et al. (2007) An imbalance in the production of IL-1beta and IL-6 by monocytes of bipolar patients: restoration by lithium treatment. Bipolar Disord 9(7):743–753.

Kunz M, Gama CS, Andreazza AC, et al. (2008) Elevated serum superoxide dismutase and thiobarbituric acid reactive substances in different phases of bipolar disorder and in schizophrenia. Prog Neuro-Psychoph 32(7):1677–1681.

Kupfer DJ (2005) The increasing medical burden in bipolar disorder. JAMA 293(20):2528.

Lang UE, Hellweg R, Seifert F, et al. (2007) Correlation between serum brain-derived neurotrophic factor level and an in vivo marker of cortical integrity. Biol Psychiat 62(5):530–535.

Leboyer M, Soreca I, Scott J, et al. (2012) Can bipolar disorder be viewed as a multisystem inflammatory disease? J Affect Disorders 141(1):1–10.

Lee B-H and Kim Y-K (2012) Increased plasma VEGF levels in major depressive or manic episodes in patients with mood disorders. J Affect Disorders 136(1–2):181–184.

Lin P-Y (2009) State-dependent decrease in levels of brain-derived neurotrophic factor in bipolar disorder: a meta-analytic study. Neurosci Lett 466(3):139–143.

Liu H-C, Yang Y-Y, Chou Y-M, et al. (2004) Immunologic variables in acute mania of bipolar disorder. J Neuroimmunol 150(1–2): 116–122.

Maes M, De Ruyter M, Hobin P, et al. (1986) Repeated dexamethasone suppression test in depressed patients. J Affect Disorders 11(2):165–172.

Magalhães PV, Dean OM, Bush AI, et al. (2011a) N-acetylcysteine for major depressive episodes in bipolar disorder. Rev Bras Psiquiatr 33(4):374–378.

Magalhães PV, Dean OM, Bush AI, et al. (2011b) N-acetyl cysteine add-on treatment for bipolar II disorder: a subgroup analysis of a randomized placebo-controlled trial. J Affect Disorders 129(1–3):317–320.

Magalhães PV, Jansen K, Pinheiro RT, et al. (2012b) Peripheral oxidative damage in early-stage mood disorders: a nested population-based case-control study. Int J Neuropsychoph 15:1043–1050.

Magalhães PV, Kapczinski F, Nierenberg AA, et al. (2012a) Illness burden and medical comorbidity in the Systematic Treatment Enhancement Program for Bipolar Disorder. Acta Psychiat Scand 125(4):303–308.

Matsuo K, Walss-Bass C, Nery FG, et al. (2009) Neuronal correlates of brain-derived neurotrophic factor Val66Met polymorphism and morphometric abnormalities in bipolar disorder. Neuropsychopharmacology 34(8):1904–1913.

Merikangas KR, Jin R, He JP, et al. (2011) Prevalence and correlates of bipolar spectrum disorder in the World Mental Health Survey Initiative. Arch Gen Psychiat 68(3):241–251.

Miller CA (2011) Stressed and depressed? Check your GDNF for epigenetic repression. Neuron 69(2):188–190.

Miller CL, Llenos IC, Cwik M, et al. (2008) Alterations in kynurenine precursor and product levels in schizophrenia and bipolar disorder. Neurochem Int 52(6):1297–1303.

Moylan S, Eyre HA, Maes M, et al. (2013) Exercising the worry away: how inflammation, oxidative and nitrogen stress mediates the beneficial effect of physical activity on anxiety disorder symptoms and behaviours. Neurosci Biobehav R 37(4):573–584.

Mullington JM, Haack M, Toth M, et al. (2009) Cardiovascular, inflammatory, and metabolic consequences of sleep deprivation. Prog Cardiovasc Dis 51(4):294–302.

Nery FG, Monkul ES, Hatch JP, et al. (2008) Celecoxib as an adjunct in the treatment of depressive or mixed episodes of bipolar disorder: a double-blind, randomized, placebo-controlled study. Hum Psychopharmacol 23(2):87–94.

O'Brien SM, Scully P, Scott LV, et al. (2006) Cytokine profiles in bipolar affective disorder: focus on acutely ill patients. J Affect Disorders 90(2–3):263–267.

O'Connor M-F, Bower JE, Cho HJ, et al. (2009) To assess, to control, to exclude: effects of biobehavioral factors on circulating inflammatory markers. Brain Behav Immun 23(7):887–897.

Oliveira GS, Ceresér KM, Fernandes BS, et al. (2009) Decreased brain-derived neurotrophic factor in medicated and drug-free bipolar patients. J Psychiat Res 43(14):1171–1174.

Olmez I and Ozyurt H (2012) Reactive oxygen species and ischemic cerebrovascular disease. Neurochem Int 60(2):208–212.

Olsson SK, Sellgren C, Engberg G, et al. (2012) Cerebrospinal fluid kynurenic acid is associated with manic and psychotic features in patients with bipolar I disorder: KYNA correlates to mania and psychosis. Bipolar Disord 14(7):719–726.

Ortiz-Domínguez A, Hernández ME, Berlanga C, et al. (2007) Immune variations in bipolar disorder: phasic differences. Bipolar Disord 9(6):596–602.

Pandey GN, Rizavi HS, Dwivedi Y, et al. (2008) Brain-derived neurotrophic factor gene expression in pediatric bipolar disorder: effects of treatment and clinical response. J Am Acad Child Adolesc Psy 47(9):1077–1085.

Pandya CD, Howell KR, and Pillai A (2013) Antioxidants as potential therapeutics for neuropsychiatric disorders. Prog Neuro-Psychoph 46:214–223.

Patel SD, Le-Niculescu H, Koller DL, et al. (2010) Coming to grips with complex disorders: genetic risk prediction in bipolar disorder using panels of genes identified through convergent functional genomics. Am J Med Genet Part B Neuropsychiat Genet 153B(4):850–877.

Pepe MS, Etzioni R, Feng Z, et al. (2001) Phases of biomarker development for early detection of cancer. J Natl Cancer Inst 93(14):1054–1061.

Pfaffenseller B, Fries GR, Wollenhaupt-Aguiar B, et al. (2013) Neurotrophins, inflammation and oxidative stress as illness activity biomarkers in bipolar disorder. Expert Rev Neurother 13(7):827–842.

Post RM (2007) Role of BDNF in bipolar and unipolar disorder: clinical and theoretical implications. J Psychiat Res 41(12):979–990.

Post RM, Fleming J, and Kapczinski F (2012) Neurobiological correlates of illness progression in the recurrent affective disorders. J Psychiat Res 46(5):561–573.

Potvin S, Stip E, Sepehry AA, et al. (2008) Inflammatory cytokine alterations in schizophrenia: a systematic quantitative review. Biol Psychiat 63(8):801–808.

Poulose N and Raju R (2014) Aging and injury: alterations in cellular energetics and organ function. Aging Dis 5(2):101–108.

Raffa M, Barhoumi S, Atig F, et al. (2012) Reduced antioxidant defense systems in schizophrenia and bipolar I disorder. Prog Neuro-Psychoph 39(2):371–375.

Raison CL, Rutherford RE, Woolwine BJ, et al. (2013) A randomized controlled trial of the tumor necrosis factor antagonist infliximab for treatment-resistant depression: the role of baseline inflammatory biomarkers. JAMA Psychiat 70(1):31–41.

Ranjekar PK, Hinge A, Hegde MV, et al. (2003) Decreased antioxidant enzymes and membrane essential polyunsaturated fatty acids in schizophrenic and bipolar mood disorder patients. Psychiat Res 121(2):109–122.

Rao JS, Harry GJ, Rapoport SI, et al. (2010) Increased excitotoxicity and neuroinflammatory markers in postmortem frontal cortex from bipolar disorder patients. Mol Psychiatr 15(4):384–392.

Remlinger-Molenda A, Wojciak P, Michalak M, et al. (2012) Selected cytokine profiles during remission in bipolar patients. Neuropsychobiology 66(3):193–198.

Rosa AR, Frey BN, Andreazza AC, et al. (2006) Increased serum glial cell line-derived neurotrophic factor immunocontent during manic and depressive episodes in individuals with bipolar disorder. Neurosci Lett 407(2):146–150.

Rybakowski JK and Suwalska A (2010) Excellent lithium responders have normal cognitive functions and plasma BDNF levels. Int J Neuropsychoph 13(5):617–622.

Sanchez-Villegas A and Martínez-González MA (2013) Diet, a new target to prevent depression? BMC Med 11(1):3.

Sarris J, Mischoulon D, and Schweitzer I (2011) Adjunctive nutraceuticals with standard pharmacotherapies in bipolar disorder: a systematic review of clinical trials. Bipolar Disord 13(5–6):454–465.

Sarris J, Mischoulon D, and Schweitzer I (2012) Omega-3 for bipolar disorder: meta-analyses of use in mania and bipolar depression. J Clin Psychiat 73(1):81–86.

Savas HA, Gergerlioglu HS, Armutcu F, et al. (2006) Elevated serum nitric oxide and superoxide dismutase in euthymic bipolar patients: impact of past episodes. World J Biol Psychiat 7(1):51–55.

Savaş HA, Herken H, Yürekli M, et al. (2002) Possible role of nitric oxide and adrenomedullin in bipolar affective disorder. Neuropsychobiology 45(2):57–61.

Savitz J, Preskorn S, Teague TK, et al. (2012) Minocycline and aspirin in the treatment of bipolar depression: a protocol for a proof-of-concept, randomised, double-blind, placebo-controlled, 2x2 clinical trial. BMJ Open 2(1):e000643.

Schmider J, Lammers CH, Gotthardt U, et al. (1995) Combined dexamethasone/corticotropin-releasing hormone test in acute and remitted manic patients, in acute depression, and in normal controls: I. Biol Psychiat 38(12):797–802.

Schmidt HD and Duman RS (2010) Peripheral BDNF produces antidepressant-like effects in cellular and behavioral models. Neuropsychopharmacology 35(12):2378–2391.

Schmitt A, Malchow B, Hasan A, et al. (2014) The impact of environmental factors in severe psychiatric disorders. Front Neurosci 8:19.

Selek S, Savas HA, Gergerlioglu HS, et al. (2008) The course of nitric oxide and superoxide dismutase during treatment of bipolar depressive episode. J Affect Disorders 107(1–3):89–94.

Singh AB, Bousman CA, Ng CH, et al. (2012) ABCB1 polymorphism predicts escitalopram dose needed for remission in major depression. Transl Psychiatry 2:e198.

Sousa RT, van de Bilt MT, Diniz BS, et al. (2011) Lithium increases plasma brain-derived neurotrophic factor in acute bipolar mania: a preliminary 4-week study. Neurosci Lett 494(1):54–56.

Sugawara H, Iwamoto K, Bundo M, et al. (2010) Effect of mood stabilizers on gene expression in lymphoblastoid cells. J Neural Transm 117(2):155–164.

Takebayashi M, Hisaoka K, Nishida A, et al. (2006) Decreased levels of whole blood glial cell line-derived neurotrophic factor (GDNF) in remitted patients with mood disorders. Int J Neuropsychoph 9(5):607–612.

Tang J, Xiao L, Shu C, et al. (2008) Association of the brain-derived neurotrophic factor gene and bipolar disorder with early age of onset in mainland China. Neurosci Lett 433(2):98–102.

Teixeira AL, Barbosa IG, Machado-Vieira R, et al. (2013) Novel biomarkers for bipolar disorder. Exp Opin Med Diagn 7(2):147–159.

Tramontina JF, Andreazza AC, Kauer-Sant'anna M, et al. (2009) Brain-derived neurotrophic factor serum levels before and after treatment for acute mania. Neurosci Lett 452(2):111–113.

Tsai S-Y, Chung K-H, Wu J-Y, et al. (2012) Inflammatory markers and their relationships with leptin and insulin from acute mania to full remission in bipolar disorder. J Affect Disorders 136(1–2):110–116.

Tsai SY, Yang YY, Kuo CJ, et al. (2001) Effects of symptomatic severity on elevation of plasma soluble interleukin-2 receptor in bipolar mania. J Affect Disorders 64(2–3):185–193.

Vieira RM, Andreazza AC, Viale CI, et al. (2007) Oxidative stress parameters in unmedicated and treated bipolar subjects during initial manic episode: a possible role for lithium antioxidant effects. Neurosci Lett 421(1):33–36.

Vieira RM, Dietrich MO, Leke R, et al. (2007) Decreased plasma brain derived neurotrophic factor levels in unmedicated bipolar patients during manic episode. Biol Psychiat 61(2):142–144.

Walz JC, Andreazza AC, Frey BN, et al. (2007) Serum neurotrophin-3 is increased during manic and depressive episodes in bipolar disorder. Neurosci Lett 415(1):87–89.

Walz JC, Magalhães PV, Giglio LM, et al. (2009) Increased serum neurotrophin-4/5 levels in bipolar disorder. J Psychiat Res 43(7):721–723.

Watson S, Gallagher P, Ritchie JC, et al. (2004) Hypothalamic-pituitary-adrenal axis function in patients with bipolar disorder. Brit J Psychiat 184:496–502.

World Health Organization (2008) The Global Burden of Disease: 2004 Update. Geneva: WHO.

Wu A, Ying Z, and Gomez-Pinilla F (2004) Dietary omega-3 fatty acids normalize BDNF levels, reduce oxidative damage, and counteract learning disability after traumatic brain injury in rats. J Neurotrauma 21(10):1457–1467.

Yatham LN, Kapczinski F, Andreazza AC, et al. (2009) Accelerated age-related decrease in brain-derived neurotrophic factor levels in bipolar disorder. Int J Neuropsychoph 12(1):137–139.

Yirmiya R and Goshen I (2011) Immune modulation of learning, memory, neural plasticity and neurogenesis. Brain Behav Immun 25(2):181–213.

Zhang X, Zhang Z, Sha W, et al. (2010) Effect of treatment on serum glial cell line-derived neurotrophic factor in bipolar patients. J Affect Disorders 126(1–2):326–329.

Zhang XY and Yao JK (2013) Oxidative stress and therapeutic implications in psychiatric disorders. Prog Neuro-Psychoph 46:197–199.

Chapter 11

Childhood adversity and illness progression in bipolar disorder

Joana Bücker, Marcia Kauer-Sant'Anna, and Lakshmi N. Yatham

Relatively little is understood regarding the aetiology of bipolar disorder (BD); however, it is generally agreed that psychiatric disorders are multifactorial as no single variable whether biological, psychological, or social can adequately account for the complexity of clinical features (Rutter et al. 2006). While genetic factors play a significant role, psychosocial factors also contribute significantly to BD and a complex gene–environment interaction seems to account for the development of the condition (Leverich and Post 2006; Fowke et al. 2012). Studies suggest that not only do stressful life events tend to precede mood episodes in BD, but also patients report higher rates of negative life events, even before BD onset, which could exert a cumulative effect to worse outcomes (Liu 2010). In this chapter, we review the association of childhood adversity with neurobiological and clinical features of BD.

Childhood trauma (CT) is a complex experience that can include emotional, physical, and sexual abuse, as well as emotional and physical neglect (Dannlowski et al. 2012). CT is considered to be the most severe environmental stress and probably the most important event for investigation (Etain et al. 2008). The incidence of CT in the general population is high, and in North America has been estimated to be around 35% (Gorey and Leslie 1997) with an estimated annual cost exceeding $100 billion (Wang and Holton 2007). Studies suggest that up to 82% of patients with severe mental disease report a history of CT (Larsson et al. 2013b) and majority of patients with mood disorders receiving care in the public mental health system report experiencing childhood stress

(Lu et al. 2008). CT has been found to be associated with poor physical and poor mental health, impaired functioning, and increased substance abuse in the general adult population (Dube et al. 2001, 2002) and in adults with severe mood disorders (Lu et al. 2008). A study by Sugaya et al. (2012) showed that the risk of psychiatric disorders in adults is related to the frequency of child physical abuse, suggesting a clear dose–response relationship between these two variables. Patients with mood disorders report, in general, more physical and sexual abuse, overall life-time trauma, and post-traumatic stress symptoms than those with other psychiatric illness, such as schizophrenia (O'Hare et al. 2013). It can be inferred that there are different developmental windows of vulnerability in which early negative experience may induce greater susceptibility to future psychopathology (Goldberg and Garno 2005). CT can occur before the development of BD and trigger the first episode, which is often associated with psychosocial stressors (Vieira and Gauer 2003).

Childhood adversity and clinical outcomes in bipolar disorder

BD patients with a history of CT reported more stressful events before the onset of the first and the most recent mood episode compared to patients without CT (Leverich et al. 2002). These data suggest that an increased occurrence and accumulation of serious adverse experiences may contribute to the triggering of a pathological response mechanism and may be reactivated in the future by even less stressful events, or predispose to a high number of adverse life events (Leverich et al. 2002; Hoersch and Iancu 2010). There is a growing evidence suggesting that exposure to serious adverse experiences in childhood may have a negative impact on response to treatment in bipolar patients (Marchand et al. 2005).

The association between CT and the development of psychiatric disease, such as BD, have been reported in several studies (Etain et al. 2010; Hoersch and Iancu 2010; Larsson et al. 2013a). CT is considered a risk factor for psychosis and poor course in severe BD (Neria et al. 2005; Daruy-Filho et al. 2011; Schäfer and Fisher 2011). The incidence of CT is more frequent and severe in bipolar patients compared to healthy controls, with a high frequency of childhood emotional abuse and neglect in this patient group (Leboyer et al. 2007; Etain et al. 2010; Fowke et al. 2012). Besides predisposing subjects to BD, CT may also modulate the clinical expression and course of the disease, increasing the vulnerability to symptoms during its development (Hammersley et al. 2003; Etain et al. 2008; Daruy-Filho et al. 2001). However, one caveat is that most of these studies evaluated adverse life events retrospectively, thus limiting the conclusions about the cause and effect of CT in BD illness (Daruy-Filho et al. 2001). The risk of potential memory recall bias cannot be underestimated (Daruy-Filho et al. 2001). An alternative hypothesis suggests that children with hereditary or environmental vulnerability to BD might be more exposed to traumatic events (Daruy-Filho et al. 2001).

CT in BD seems to be related to rapid illness progression, accelerating the evolution of the disease, and also is considered a strong risk factor for the chronicity of the illness, impacting its pathophysiology (Daruy-Filho et al. 2001; Angst et al. 2011). There is evidence to suggest that BD patients exposed to CT are more symptomatic (Neria et al. 2005), have more psychiatric hospitalizations (Carballo et al. 2008), earlier onset of disease (Garno et al. 2005; Larsson et al. 2013a; Bücker et al. 2013), greater frequency and severity of psychotic features and hallucinations (Hammersley et al. 2003), substance abuse disorder (Garno et al. 2005; Leverich and Post 2006; Brown et al. 2005), and internalized shame (Fowke et al. 2012). CT in BD patients is also associated with recurrent depressive symptoms in adulthood, along with lower premorbid functioning levels, poorer adherence to treatment, higher rates of forensic history, and lesser likelihood of living with family members during the treatment (Conus et al. 2010). CT is considered a risk factor for suicidality in BD and these patients report higher incidence of suicide attempts compared with those without trauma (Brown et al. 2005; Garno et al. 2005; Leverich and Post 2006; Dilsaver et al. 2007; Carballo et al. 2008; Halfon et al. 2013). BD patients with a history of childhood adversity also seem to report comorbidity with numerous medical conditions, including allergies, arthritis, asthma, chronic fatigue syndrome, chronic menstrual irregularities, fibromyalgia, head injury, hypotension, irritable bowel syndrome, and migraine headaches (Post et al. 2013).

The course of BD in patients reporting CT also includes a rapid cycling course (Garno et al. 2005; Leverich and Post 2006), higher prevalence of affective disorders in first-degree relatives (Carballo et al. 2008), a pattern of increasing severity of mania (Leverich et al. 2002), especially in patients with childhood physical abuse (Levitan et al. 1998), along with aggression and impulsivity (Daruy-Filho et al. 2001), and less time well than those without early trauma (Leverich et al. 2002). BD patients with CT had a significantly longer delay to treatment compared to patients without early abuse (Leverich et al. 2002), and this delay might also contribute to the increased incidence of alcohol and substance abuse in these patients, in part as an attempt at self-medication (Leverich and Post 2006). Post-traumatic stress disorder (PTSD) is one of the most frequent consequences of CT (Brown et al. 2005) and is strongly, and perhaps directly, associated with BD, and vice versa (Maniglio 2013). Rates of current PTSD in individuals with BD range from 11% to 24% (Goldberg and Garno 2005; Quarantini et al. 2010), while in the general population the rates range from 3% to 5% (Kessler et al. 2005). About a third of BD patients with history of trauma, particularly sexual abuse, develop PTSD (Goldberg and Garno 2005).

Given that CT has significant adverse effects on progression of BD, it is important to investigate the history of childhood abuse and neglect in BD and identify treatments that might benefit these patients (Daruy-Filho et al. 2001; Schäfer and Fisher 2011); thus potentially preventing the development of psychiatric comorbidities and substance abuse (Leverich and Post 2006). Preliminary studies have shown that interventions focusing on trauma experience might be more effective and more beneficial for patients with psychosis than for other psychiatric patients (Trappler and Newville 2007; Mueser et al. 2008) and for patients who had the longest period without a specific treatment for bipolar illness (Leverich and Post 2006).

Exposure to adverse events may be common as well among paediatric bipolar patients and has a negative impact on prognosis. A study evaluating a BD youth sample showed that 53% of these patients had experienced maltreatment and that childhood stress was associated with delay of diagnosis, psychiatric hospitalization, and a decreased response to treatment (Marchand et al. 2005). Children with BD are likely to have a greater number of family members that experience alcohol abuse, which is related to parental disorganization, and a greater risk of CT (Etain et al. 2008). History of abuse was correlated with lifetime history of PTSD, psychosis, conduct disorder, and a positive family history of mood disorder in youths with BD (Romero et al. 2009).

CT also has been reported in as many as half of the adults with BD in several studies (Goldberg and Garno 2005; Garno et al. 2005; Etain et al. 2010), showing the importance of exploring this point during the treatment of such patients (Conus et al. 2010). However, the prevalence of trauma measured by self-report questionnaires is higher than the prevalence measured by case notes reports, probably because clinicians do not enquire frequently about trauma during the treatment (Shannon et al. 2011). Garno et al. (2005) evaluated BD patients with CT and showed that emotional abuse was the most frequent type of trauma reported by 37% of the patients; 24% reported physical abuse, 24% emotional neglect, 21% sexual abuse, and 12% physical neglect. In addition, one-third of those patients presented a combination of different types of trauma and showed increased risk for suicide attempts and rapid cycling. Another study of this kind also reported a higher frequency of childhood emotional abuse and neglect in BD patients compared with another types of trauma (Fowke et al. 2012).

However, there seems to be a difference between types of trauma and course of illness in BD, associated with different clinical characteristics of the disorder (Larsson et al. 2013a). In a study by Etain et al. (2010), only emotional abuse was associated with BD, with a suggestive dose-effect. In another studies, emotional abuse also was associated with lifetime substance misuse comorbidity and past-year rapid cycling, and sexual abuse was associated with lifetime suicide attempts (Garno et al. 2005) and increased number of mood episodes (Larsson et al. 2013a). Childhood maltreatment predicted worsening clinical course of BD (Daruy-Filho et al. 2011), and can be strongly associated with poor functioning, increased number of mood episodes, and self-harm in patients with BD (Larsson et al. 2013a). In a BD youth sample, physical abuse was associated with longer duration of BP illness, non-intact family, PTSD, psychosis, and first-degree family history of mood disorder, while sexual abuse was associated with PTSD (Romero et al. 2009).

The frequency of the CT appears to be important, as well, to the course of the illness. Leverich et al. (2002 and 2003) showed that patients who reported single or rare incidence of physical abuse had a smaller impact on suicidality than individuals who reported experiencing these traumas more frequently. In contrast, childhood sexual abuse, even occurring only once, is associated with increased incidence of subsequent medically serious suicide attempts.

Many studies of CT, in general, focus on female samples and BD women patients reported significantly higher rates of lifetime sexual or physical abuse (Meade et al. 2009; Conus et al. 2010; Mauritz et al. 2013). On the other hand, in a study that evaluated predominantly male military veteran patients showed that CT was reported by 47.3% of the men. Male patients reported more frequency of physical abuse compared to female patients (20.7% vs. 6.7%) (Brown et al. 2005) and are more often exposed to sexual and physical abuse than men with major depressive disorder (Hyun et al. 2000).

Taken together, these data suggest that early traumatic experiences in those with genetic vulnerability might result in earlier onset and poor outcomes in BD (Leverich et al. 2002) and it is important to explore this issue during the treatment of these patients (Larsson et al. 2013b). In order to diminish the prevalence of CT, it would be important to investigate the context in which such traumas can occur and develop early intervention strategies (Conus et al. 2010).

The impact of childhood trauma on cognition in patients with bipolar disorder

Cognitive functions are sensitive to the timing of the environmental experience (Knudsen 2004), and higher intelligence scores (IQ) are associated with a decreased risk of exposure to traumatic events (Breslau et al. 2006). From a developmental perspective, CT has potentially the highest odds for a pervasive deleterious effect on cognitive function and neurobiology.

It is well known that patients with BD have cognitive impairment compared to healthy subjects, especially in sustained attention, verbal and visual memory, executive function, processing speed and verbal fluency, even during euthymic periods (Robinson et al. 2006; Bora et al. 2009; Torres et al. 2007). CT is also associated with decline in cognitive function in children without a diagnosis of psychiatric disorder (Bücker et al. 2012) and in healthy adults, especially in short-term and nonverbal memory (Bremner et al. 1995; Navalta et al. 2006; Majer et al. 2010), perceptual abilities (Aas et al. 2011), and executive function (Spann et al. 2012).

A possible association of CT with a more severe cognitive impairment in BD patients also has been reported. CT and BD have been associated with adverse effects on cognitive functions such as verbal and visual recall, verbal fluency, and cognitive flexibility (Savitz et al. 2008). Physical abuse in BD patients has been reported to be associated with reductions in working memory, executive function, perception, visuospatial abilities, and verbal abilities while sexual abuse is associated with impairment in executive function, perception, visuospatial, and verbal abilities (Aas et al. 2012). BD patients that reported higher rates of adverse life events showed poor memory performance (Savitz et al. 2007).

Furthermore, the cognitive impairment can be detectable even early in the course of illness, after a first episode of mania. A previous study (Aas et al. 2011) showed that BD patients with CT and recently recovered from a first episode of mania had poorer performance in language, visuoconstruction, and perceptual domains compared to patients without trauma. Furthermore, a more recent study that evaluated BD patients early in the course of their illness, with a larger sample size, also showed diminished cognitive functioning associated with trauma (Bücker et al. 2013). This study showed that trauma in patients was especially associated with decreased IQ, auditory attention, verbal memory, and working memory. These data thus suggest that the CT-related changes observed in patients may be due to cognitive impairment in domains of known vulnerability in BD (Bücker et al. 2013).

These results suggest that CT has an independent adverse effect on cognition, and, therefore, it is not surprising that cognitive impairment is more severe in BD patients with a history of CT. Therefore, it is important to evaluate the presence of CT BD samples in neuropsychological studies, especially if these patients have been exposed to high rates of stressful events (Savitz et al. 2008).

Childhood trauma and biological markers in bipolar disorder

The involvement of cortisol and hypothalamic-pituitary-adrenal (HPA) axis dysfunction in persistent stress response alterations after early adverse experiences is well documented, although not always consistent (Lu et al. 2013). Nevertheless, hyperactivation of the HPA axis has been reported in those with early life stress independent of the diagnosis of psychosis. It is conceivable that these alterations in stress response are key in mediating other changes in neurobiology, such as inflammatory response, neurotrophic changes (given brain-derived neurotrophic factor (BDNF) would counteract stress effects in hippocampus), and brain volume; this would be cumulative, with changes associated with mood episodes (Kapczinski et al. 2008).

In fact, CT may contribute to chronic inflammation in psychotic disorders (Suvisaari and Mantere 2013), as it is associated with elevated serum proinflammatory cytokines in adulthood (Danese et al. 2009). A potential neurobiological candidate for the interaction between CT and an adverse course of BD may be BDNF. BDNF is a member of the neurotrophins and is also important for brain development, plasticity, and maintenance of neurons in adult life (Lewin and Barde 1996) and can be critical for the control of cognition (Ernfors et al. 1990).

Alterations in BDNF levels and genes have been implicated in stress (Rattiner et al. 2005), during manic and depressive episodes (Fernandes et al. 2011), and in first episode of psychosis (Mondelli et al. 2011). A history of CT also partially induces the down-regulation of BDNF expression in first-episode psychosis patients through a pathway that may involve increased inflammation (Mondelli et al. 2011). Kauer-Sant'Anna et al. (2007) examined the impact of CT on BDNF levels in BD patients and found that a history of childhood abuse was associated with lower levels of serum BDNF in BD patients, and it may account for increased psychiatric comorbidity. Among traumatic events, sexual abuse showed the strongest association with a reduction in BDNF levels. These data suggest that a sexual component of CT has the greatest impact on psychopathology and BDNF levels. Conversely, the genetic predisposition to reduced levels of BDNF also could contribute to higher vulnerability to BD and the neurobiological effects of traumatic events (Kauer-Sant'Anna et al. 2007).

BDNF gene has at least one functional variant, resulting in a low active methionine (met) variant being related to reduced BDNF levels (Egan et al. 2003). Individuals with low activity in the *Met* allele of the BDNF gene (val66met) might be at increased risk for BD when exposed to childhood abuse (Liu et al. 2010). Family-based association studies have shown that the BDNF gene polymorphism val66met is associated with BD (Skibinska et al. 2004) and rapid cycling (Green et al. 2006). Miller et al. (2013) also showed that among patients with BD, those with a history of childhood sexual abuse and BDNF *met* allele carriers showed greater severity and chronicity of the illness and earlier BD onset age. From these results, it can be inferred that BD patients who are carriers of the BDNF val66met are more susceptible to the negative effects of CT on BD illness severity (Miller et al. 2013).

A growing body of evidence indicates that in those with history of CT (Savitz et al. 2007; Shaltiel et al. 2007; Kurnianingsih et al. 2011) lower levels of the BDNF Val66 allele are associated with cognitive decline, especially memory. Similarly, patients with psychosis (BD and schizophrenia) who are *met* carriers of the BDNF val66met, with a history of exposer to high levels of CT, especially physical abuse and emotional abuse, demonstrated significantly poorer cognitive functioning compared to homozygotic valine (*val/val*) carriers (Aas et al. 2013). In this study, the cognitive impairment was prominent in executive function/ verbal fluency, working memory, and verbal abilities. These results demonstrate that BDNF val66met modulates the association between childhood abuse and cognition abnormalities in psychoses and that both environment and genetic factors are important to evaluate cognitive impairment in psychosis (Aas et al. 2013) and BD.

A functional polymorphism in the promoter region of the serotonin transporter (5-HTT) gene is also considered a relevant candidate gene in BD in view of the role of serotonin in this disease. The short allele of the *5-HTTLPR* polymorphism of the 5-HTT gene may be considered a risk factor for psychotic symptoms in BD (DePradier et al. 2010). An interaction between serotonin transporter gene variants and CT in BD also has been suggested. Leboyer et al. (2007) showed that earlier age at illness onset and higher rates of CT were correlated only in *5-HTTLPR* 'ss' homozygous bipolar patients, and emotional neglect was identified as the potentially most important subtype of trauma in these samples. Childhood sexual abuse is also associated with cannabis abuse or dependence in BD patients, especially in those carrying the s allele (DePradier et al. 2010).

In summary, the existing research indicates that CT has an independent and interactive effect in the aetiology of BD, and the understanding of these mechanisms on the development of the illness is helpful to designing effective prevention and treatment strategies (Liu et al. 2010).

Influence of childhood trauma on brain structures in bipolar disorder

Childhood is a period of great vulnerability, and the most important phase of brain maturation occur during early childhood (Toga et al. 2006). Thus, environmental factors such as CT can cause important changes in the maturation of the central nervous system (Etain et al. 2008). The neurobiological consequences of early stress may have an important role in the emergence of psychiatric disorders during the course of brain development, which could make some individuals vulnerable to certain types of psychopathology (Teicher et al. 2003, 2004). Therefore, BD may be partly determined by early changes in brain structures (Murray et al. 2004).

The long-term negative consequences of childhood traumatic experiences in adults with mental illness comprise changes in brain morphology, particularly in the hippocampus (Woon and Hedges 2008), amygdala (Vermetten et al. 2006), prefrontal cortex (Treadway et al. 2009), and corpus callosum (Villarreal et al. 2004; Bucker et al. 2014).

Different forms of child maltreatment may affect the central nervous system differently, depending on the severity and chronicity of the events (Etain et al. 2008; Sugaya et al. 2012).

A relationship between CT and volume reduction in amygdala and hippocampus has been recently observed in a sample of patients in first-episode psychosis (Hoy et al. 2012). The results showed that the experience of CT was a significant predictor of small left hippocampal volume and small right and total amygdalar volumes. In other relevant study about first-episode psychosis (Aas et al. 2012b), the CT was associated with poor cognitive function (executive function, language, and verbal intelligence) and smaller amygdala volume and it seems to mediate the relationship between trauma history and cognitive dysfunction.

A potentially causal relationship between early trauma and corpus callosum volume has been suggested due to the fact that the most consistent finding in children and adolescents who experienced psychological trauma seems to be structural abnormalities of the corpus callosum (Rinne-Albers et al. 2013). Nonetheless, the literature about the effects of CT in the corpus callosum is scarce in BD. Preliminary results suggested a significant reduction of the corpus callosum in first-episode mania patients with trauma compared with those without trauma. However, there is no significant difference in the CC volume of patients with/without trauma compared to the healthy subjects. It is possible that callosal abnormalities might be more related to childhood maltreatment than bipolar illness early in its course, and reductions in CC volume may occur late in the course of BD. It might mean that there may be two sources of CC volume reduction in these patients: the reduction due to trauma and the further reduction due to the illness (Bücker et al. 2014). Fig. 11.1 shows the volume reduction associated with trauma in patients with BD, even after a first manic episode.

BDNF is most strongly expressed in the hippocampus (Yan et al. 1997), and damage in this brain structure results in reduced BDNF mRNA expression in other areas of the brain (Rybakowski et al. 2003). Lower BDNF expression predicted a smaller left hippocampal volume in a sample of first-episode psychosis, demonstrating that stress may activate biological changes that represent a significant factor that may

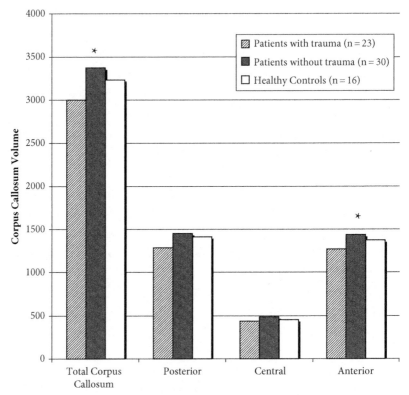

Fig. 11.1 Brain morphometry in first-episode BD with and without childhood trauma. Reprinted from J Psychiatr Res, 48(1), Bücker J, Muralidharan K, Torres IJ, Su W, Kozicky J, Silveira LE, Bond DJ, Honer WG, Kauer-Santanna M, Lam RW, Yatham LN, Childhood maltreatment and corpus callosum volume in recently diagnosed patients with bipolar I disorder: data from the Systematic Treatment Optimization Program for Early Mania (STOP-EM), 65–72, Copyright (2014), with permission from Elsevier.

influence brain structures in first-episode psychosis through BDNF (Mondelli et al. 2011).

The BDNF val66met functional polymorphism may lead to global changes in brain structure, specifically in patients with early trauma (Aas et al. 2013). Reduced hippocampal volume in met carriers has been found independent of the effect of CT (Hajek et al. 2012). In patients with psychosis (BD and schizophrenia), met carriers with higher levels of childhood sexual abuse showed reduced right hippocampal volume and larger right and left lateral ventricles (Aas et al. 2013).

Conclusion

Patients with BD have high rates of CT, and there is mounting evidence that CT is associated with adverse effects on clinical outcomes, cognitive functions, neurobiology, and brain structures. However, to the best of our knowledge, no study has demonstrated a strong causal relationship between CT and BD (Etain et al. 2008). To clarify the role of CT in the expression of BD is important to consider the fact that adverse experiences might be related to a toxic effect to the development of the illness. Children who were born in an environment with higher rates of stress will have to modify their psychological and neurological structures to deal with the toxic effects of the trauma. However, in the early stages of the development such modifications and rearrangements might be potentially harmful, especially in a traumatic environment (Grassi-Oliveira et al. 2008) (Fig. 11.2).

On the other hand, animal model studies showed that genetic factors, and not only the environment, might modulate the response to early traumatic events (Claessens et al. 2011). A growing body of evidence also suggests that stress and traumatic events may have effects on BDNF expression through the modulation of epigenetic mechanisms, including DNA methylation and histone modifications (Roth et al. 2009; Bennett

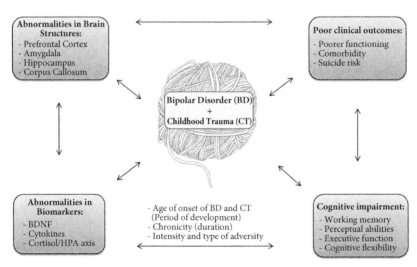

Fig. 11.2 The impact of childhood trauma on bipolar disorder.

and Lagopoulos 2014). Recent studies have also suggested that different genotypes may differentially interact with epigenetic mechanisms in determining the expression levels of some proteins (Klengel et al. 2013). Then, genetic studies may help to clarify the fact that traumatic events during childhood may predispose only some people to morbidity, since it does not happen in all cases.

It is important that future studies, through a follow-up design, try to focus on the influence of the neurobiological sequelae of childhood abuse in the aetiology of BD in order to clarify the role of CT in the evolution of the illness. Evaluation of the epigenetic alterations on the genes involved or the associated histone modifications would be useful in future studies, particularly in light of the association of poor outcomes in patients with a history of CT. Recognizing CT as an adverse event with negative consequences also may be important to design effective prevention and treatment strategies so as to avoid the occurrence of childhood adverse experiences, and minimize their impact.

References

Aas M, Dazzan P, Fisher HL, et al. (2011) Childhood trauma and cognitive function in first-episode affective and non-affective psychosis. Schizophr Res **129**(1):12–19.

Aas M, Haukvik UK, Djurovic S, et al. (2013) BDNF val66met modulates the association between childhood trauma, cognitive and brain abnormalities in psychoses. Prog Neuro-Psychoph **46**:181–188.

Aas M, Navari S, Gibbs A, et al. (2012b) Is there a link between childhood trauma, cognition, and amygdala and hippocampus volume in first-episode psychosis? Schizophr Res **137**(1–3):73–79.

Aas M, Steen NE, Agartz I, et al. (2012a) Is cognitive impairment following early life stress in severe mental disorders based on specific or general cognitive functioning? Psychiat Res **15**(198):495–500.

Angst J, Gamma A, Rössler W, et al. (2011) Childhood adversity and chronicity of mood disorders. Eur Arch Psy Clin N **261**(1):21–27.

Bennett MR and Lagopoulos J (2014) Stress and trauma: BDNF control of dendritic-spine formation and regression. Prog Neurobiol **112**:80–99.

Bora E, Yucel M, and Pantelis C (2009) Cognitive endophenotypes of bipolar disorder: a meta-analysis of neuropsychological deficits in euthymic patients and their first-degree relatives. J Affect Disorders **113**(1–2):1–20.

Bremner JD, Randall P, Scott TM, et al. (1995) Deficits in short-term memory in adult survivors of childhood abuse. Psychiat Res **59**(1–2):97–107.

Breslau N, Lucia VC, and Alvarado GF (2006) Intelligence and other predisposing factors in exposure to trauma and posttraumatic stress disorder: a follow-up study at age 17 years. Arch Gen Psychiat 63(11):1238–1245.

Brown GR, McBride L, Bauer MS, et al. (2005) Impact of childhood abuse on the course of bipolar disorder: a replication study in US veterans. J Affect Disorders 89:57–67.

Bücker J, Kapczinski F, Post R, et al. (2012) Cognitive impairment in school-aged children with early trauma. Compr Psychiat 53(6):758–764.

Bücker J, Kozicky J, Torres IJ, et al. (2013) The impact of childhood trauma on cognitive functioning in patients recently recovered from a first manic episode: data from the Systematic Treatment Optimization Program for Early Mania (STOP-EM). J Affect Disorders 148(2–3):424–430.

Bücker J, Muralidharan K, Torres IJ, et al. (2014) Childhood maltreatment and corpus callosum volume in recently diagnosed patients with bipolar I disorder: data from the Systematic Treatment Optimization Program for Early Mania (STOP-EM). J Psychiat Res 48(1):65–72.

Carballo JJ, Harkavy-Friedman J, Burke AK, et al. (2008) Family history of suicidal behavior and early traumatic experiences: additive effect on suicidality and course of bipolar illness? J Affect Disorders 109(1–2):57–63.

Claessens SE, Daskalakis NP, van der Veen R, et al. (2011) Development of individual differences in stress responsiveness: an overview of factors mediating the outcome of early life experiences. Psychopharmacology (Berl) 214(1):141–154.

Conus P, Cotton S, Schimmelmann BG, et al. (2010) Pretreatment and outcome correlates of past sexual and physical trauma in 118 bipolar I disorder patients with a first episode of psychotic mania. Bipolar Disord 12(3):244–252.

Danese A, Moffitt TE, Harrington H, et al. (2009) Adverse childhood experiences and adult risk factors for age-related disease: depression, inflammation, and clustering of metabolic risk markers. Arch Pediat Adol Med 163(12):1135–1143.

Dannlowski U, Stuhrmann A, Beutelmann V, et al. (2012) Limbic scars: long-term consequences of childhood maltreatment revealed by functional and structural magnetic resonance imaging. Biol Psychiat 71(4):286–293.

Daruy-Filho L, Brietzke E, Lafer B, et al. (2011) Childhood maltreatment and clinical outcomes of bipolar disorder. Acta Psychiat Scand 124(6):427–434.

De Pradier M, Gorwood P, Beaufils B, et al. (2010) Influence of the serotonin transporter gene polymorphism, cannabis and childhood sexual abuse on phenotype of bipolar disorder: a preliminary study. Eur Psychiat 25(6):323–327.

Dilsaver SC, Benazzi F, and Akiskal KK (2007) Posttraumatic stress disorder among adolescents with bipolar disorder and its relationship to suicidality. Bipolar Disord 9:649–655.

Dube SR, Anda RF, Felitti VJ, et al. (2001) Childhood abuse, household dysfunction, and the risk of attempted suicide throughout the life span: findings from the Adverse Childhood Experiences study. JAMA 286:3089–3096.

Dube SR, Anda RF, Felitti VJ, et al. (2002) Adverse childhood experiences and personal alcohol abuse as an adult. Addict Behav 27:713–725.

Egan MF, Kojima M, Callicott JH, et al. (2003) The BDNF val66met polymorphism affects activity-dependent secretion of BDNF and human memory and hippocampal function. Cell 112:257–269.

Ernfors P, Wetmore C, Olson L, et al. (1990) Identification of cells in rat brain and peripheral tissues expressing mRNA for members of the nerve growth factor family. Neuron 5(4):511–526.

Etain B, Henry C, Bellivier F, et al. (2008) Beyond genetics: childhood affective trauma in bipolar disorder. Bipolar Disord 10(8):867–876.

Etain B, Mathieu F, Henry C, et al. (2010) Preferential association between childhood emotional abuse and bipolar disorder. J Trauma Stress 23(3):376–383.

Fernandes BS, Gama CS, Ceresér KM, et al. (2011) Brain-derived neurotrophic factor as a state-marker of mood episodes in bipolar disorders: a systematic review and meta-regression analysis. J Psychiat Res 45(8):995–1004.

Fowke A, Ross S, and Ashcroft K (2012) Childhood maltreatment and internalized shame in adults with a diagnosis of bipolar disorder. Clin Psychol Psychother 19(5):450–457.

Garno JL, Goldberg JF, Ramirez PM, et al. (2005) Impact of childhood abuse on the clinical course of bipolar disorder. Brit J Psychiat 186:121–125.

Goldberg JF and Garno JL (2005) Development of posttraumatic stress disorder in adult bipolar patients with histories of severe childhood abuse. J Psychiat Res 39:595–601.

Gorey KM and Leslie DR (1997) The prevalence of child sexual abuse: integrative review adjustment for potential response and measurement biases. Child Abuse Neglect 21:391–398.

Grassi-Oliveira R, Ashy M, and Stein LM (2008) Psychobiology of childhood maltreatment: effects of allostatic load? Rev Bras Psiquiatr 30:60–68.

Green EK, Raybould R, Macgregor S, et al. (2006) Genetic variation of brain-derived neurotrophic factor (BDNF) in bipolar disorder: case-control study of over 3000 individuals from the UK. Brit J Psychiat 188:21–25.

Hajek T, Kopecek M, and Hoschl C (2012) Reduced hippocampal volumes in healthy carriers of brain-derived neurotrophic factor Val66Met polymorphism: meta-analysis. World J Biol Psychiat 13:178–187.

Halfon N, Labelle R, Cohen D, et al. (2013) Juvenile bipolar disorder and suicidality: a review of the last 10 years of literature. Eur Child Adoles Psy 22(3):139–151.

Hammersley P, Dias A, Todd G, et al. (2003) Childhood trauma and hallucinations in bipolar affective disorder: preliminary investigation. Brit J Psychiat 182:543–547.

Horesh N and Iancu I (2010) A comparison of life events in patients with unipolar disorder or bipolar disorder and controls. Compr Psychiat 51(2):157–164.

Hoy K, Barrett S, Shannon C, et al. (2012) Childhood trauma and hippocampal and amygdalar volumes in first-episode psychosis. Schizophr Bull 38(6):1162–1169.

Hyun M, Friedman SD, and Dunner DL (2000) Relationship of childhood physical and sexual abuse to adult bipolar disorder. Bipolar Disord 2(2):131–135.

Kapczinski F, Vieta E, Andreazza AC, et al. (2008) Allostatic load in bipolar disorder: implications for pathophysiology and treatment. Neurosci Biobehav R 32(4):675–692.

Kauer-SantAnna M, Tramontina J, Andreazza AC, et al. (2007) Traumatic life events in bipolar disorder: impact on BDNF levels and psychopathology. Bipolar Disord 9(1):128–135.

Kessler RC, Chiu WT, Demler O, et al. (2005) Prevalence, severity, and comorbidity of 12-month DSM-IV disorders in the National Comorbidity Survey Replication. Arch Gen Psychiat 62:617–627.

Klengel T, Mehta D, Anacker C, et al. (2013) Allele-specific FKBP5 DNA demethylation mediates gene-childhood trauma interactions. Nat Neurosci 16:33–41.

Knudsen EI (2004) Sensitive periods in the development of the brain and behavior. J Cognitive Neurosci 16(8):1412–1425.

Kurnianingsih YA, Kuswanto CN, McIntyre RS, et al. (2011) Neurocognitive-genetic and neuroimaging-genetic research paradigms in schizophrenia and bipolar disorder. J Neural Transm 118(11):1621–1639.

Larsson S, Aas M, Klungsøyr O, et al. (2013a) Patterns of childhood adverse events are associated with clinical characteristics of bipolar disorder. BMC Psychiat 22(13):97.

Larsson S, Andreassen OA, Aas M, et al. (2013b) High prevalence of childhood trauma in patients with schizophrenia spectrum and affective disorder. Compr Psychiat 54(2):123–127.

Leboyer M, Etain B, Mathieu F, et al. (2007) Childhood affective trauma in bipolar affective disorder. Bipolar Disord 9(1):9.

Leverich GS, Altshuler LL, Frye MA, et al. (2003) Factors associated with suicide attempts in 648 patients with bipolar disorder in the Stanley Foundation Bipolar Network. Clin Psychiat 64:506–515.

Leverich GS, McElroy SL, Suppes T, et al. (2002) Early physical and sexual abuse associated with an adverse course of bipolar illness. Biol Psychiat 51:288–297.

Leverich GS and Post RM (2006) Course of bipolar illness after history of childhood trauma. Lancet 367:1040–1042.

Levitan RD, Parikh SV, Lesage AD, et al. (1998) Major depression in individuals with a history of childhood physical or sexual abuse: relationship to neurovegetative features, mania, and gender. Am J Psychiat 155(12):1746–1752.

Lewin GR and Barde YA (1996) Physiology of the neurotrophins. Annu Rev Neurosci 19:289–317.

Liu RT (2010) Early life stressors and genetic influences on the development of bipolar disorder: The roles of childhood abuse and brain-derived neurotrophic factor. Child Abuse Neglect 34:516–522.

Lu S, Gao W, Wei Z, et al. (2013) Reduced cingulate gyrus volume associated with enhanced cortisol awakening response in young healthy adults reporting childhood trauma. PLoS One 8(7):e69350.

Lu W, Mueser KT, Rosenberg SD, et al. (2008) Correlates of adverse childhood experiences among adults with severe mood disorders. Psychiatr Serv 59(9):1018–1026.

Majer M, Nater UM, Lin JM, et al. (2010) Association of childhood trauma with cognitive function in healthy adults: a pilot study. BMC Neurol 14:10–61.

Maniglio R (2013) The impact of child sexual abuse on the course of bipolar disorder: a systematic review. Bipolar Disord 15(4):341–358.

Marchand WR, Wirth L, and Simon C (2005) Adverse life events and pediatric bipolar disorder in a community mental health setting. Community Ment Hlt J 41(1):67–75.

Mauritz MW, Goossens PJ, Draijer N, van Achterberg T (2013) Prevalence of interpersonal trauma exposure and trauma-related disorders in severe mental illness. Eur J Psychotraumatol 4. doi: 10.3402/ejpt.v4i0.19985.

Meade CS1, McDonald LJ, Graff FS, et al. (2009). A prospective study examining the effects of gender and sexual/physical abuse on mood outcomes in patients with co-occurring bipolar I and substance use disorders. Bipolar Disord 11(4):425–433.

Miller S, Hallmayer J, Wang PW, et al. (2013) Brain-derived neurotrophic factor val66met genotype and early life stress effects upon bipolar course. J Psychiat Res 47(2):252–258.

Mondelli V, Cattaneo A, Belvederi Murri M, et al. (2011) Stress and inflammation reduce brain-derived neurotrophic factor expression in first-episode psychosis: a pathway to smaller hippocampal volume. J Clin Psychiat 72(12):1677–1684.

Mueser KT, Rosenberg SD, Xie H, et al. (2008) A randomized controlled trial of cognitive-behavioral treatment for posttraumatic stress disorder in severe mental illness. J Consult Clin Psych 76:259–271.

Murray RM, Sham P, Van Os J, et al. (2004) A developmental model for similarities and dissimilarities between schizophrenia and bipolar disorder. Schizophr Res 71:405–416.

Navalta CP, Polcari A, Webster DM, et al. (2006) Effects of childhood sexual abuse on neuropsychological and cognitive function in college women. J Neuropsych Clin N 18(1):45–53.

Neria Y, Bromet EJ, Carlson GA, et al. (2005) Assaultive trauma and illness course in psychotic bipolar disorder: findings from the Suffolk county mental health project. Acta Psychiat Scand 111(5):380–383.

OHare T, Shen C, and Sherrer M (2013) Differences in trauma and posttraumatic stress symptoms in clients with schizophrenia spectrum and major mood disorders. Psychiat Res 30;205(1–2):85–89.

Post RM, Altshuler LL, Leverich GS, et al. (2013) Role of childhood adversity in the development of medical co-morbidities associated with bipolar disorder. J Affect Disorders 147(1–3):288–294.

Post RM and Leverich GS (2006) The role of psychosocial stress in the onset and progression of bipolar disorder and its comorbidities: the need for earlier and alternative modes of therapeutic intervention. Dev Psychopathol 18(4):1181–1211.

Quarantini LC, Miranda-Scippa A, Nery-Fernandes F, et al. (2010) The impact of comorbid posttraumatic stress disorder on bipolar disorder patients. J Affect Disorders 123:71–76.

Rattiner LM, Davis M, and Ressler KJ (2005) Brain-derived neurotrophic factor in amygdala-dependent learning. Neuroscientist 11:323–333.

Rinne-Albers MA, van der Wee NJ, Lamers-Winkelman F, et al. (2013) Neuroimaging in children, adolescents and young adults with psychological trauma. Eur Child Adoles Psy 22(12):745–755.

Robinson LJ, Thompson JM, Gallagher P, et al. (2006) A meta-analysis of cognitive deficits in euthymic patients with bipolar disorder. J Affect Disorders 93:105–115.

Romero S, Birmaher B, Axelson D, et al. (2009) Prevalence and correlates of physical and sexual abuse in children and adolescents with bipolar disorder. J Affect Disorders 112(1–3):144–150.

Roth TL, Lubin FD, Funk AJ, et al. (2009) Lasting epigenetic influence of early-life adversity on the BDNF gene. Biol Psychiat 65:760–769.

Rutter M, Moffitt TE, and Caspi A (2006) Gene-environment interplay and psychopathology: multiple varieties but real effects. J Child Psychol Psyc 47(3–4):226–261.

Rybakowski JK, Borkowska A, Czerski PM, et al. (2003) Polymorphism of the brain-derived neurotrophic factor gene and performance on a cognitive prefrontal test in bipolar patients. Bipolar Disord 5:468–472.

Savitz J, van der Merwe L, Stein DJ, et al. (2007) Genotype and childhood sexual trauma moderate neurocognitive performance: a possible role for brain-derived neurotrophic factor and apolipoprotein E variants. Biol Psychiat 1(62):391–399.

Savitz JB, van der Merwe L, Stein DJ, et al. (2008) Neuropsychological task performance in bipolar spectrum illness: genetics, alcohol abuse, medication and childhood trauma. Bipolar Disord 10(4):479–494.

Schäfer I and Fisher HL (2011) Childhood trauma and psychosis—what is the evidence? Dialogues Clin Neurosci 13(3):360–365.

Shaltiel G, Chen G, and Manji HK (2007) Neurotrophic signaling cascades in the pathophysiology and treatment of bipolar disorder. Curr Opin Pharmacol 7:22–26.

Shannon C, Maguire C, Anderson J, et al. (2011) Enquiring about traumatic experiences in bipolar disorder: a case note and self-report comparison. J Affect Disorders 133(1–2):352–355.

Skibinska M, Hauser J, Czerski PM, et al. (2004) Association analysis of brain-derived neurotrophic factor (BDNF) gene Val66Met polymorphism in schizophrenia and bipolar affective disorder. World J Biol Psychiat 5:215–220.

Spann MN, Mayes LC, Kalmar JH, et al. (2012) Childhood abuse and neglect and cognitive flexibility in adolescents. Child Neuropsychol 18(2):182–189.

Sugaya L, Hasin DS, Olfson M, et al. (2012) Child physical abuse and adult mental health: a national study. J Trauma Stress 25(4):384–392.

Suvisaari J and Mantere O (2013) Inflammation theories in psychotic disorders: a critical review. Infect Disord Drug Targets 13(1):59–70.

Teicher MH, Andersen SL, Polcari A, et al. (2003) The neurobiological consequences of early stress and childhood maltreatment. Neurosci Biobehav R **27**:33–44.

Teicher MH, Dumont NL, Ito Y, et al. (2004) Childhood neglect is associated with reduced corpus callosum area. Biol Psychiat **56**(2):80–85.

Toga AW, Thompson PM, and Sowell ER (2006) Mapping brain maturation. Trends Neurosci **29**:148–159.

Torres IJ, Boudreau VG, and Yatham LN (2007) Neuropsychological functioning in euthymic bipolar disorder: a meta-analysis. Acta Psychiat Scand Suppl (**434**):17–26.

Torres IJ, DeFreitas VG, DeFreitas CM, et al. (2010) Neurocognitive functioning in patients with bipolar I disorder recently recovered from a first manic episode. J Clin Psychiat **71**(9):1234–1242.

Trappler B and Newville H (2007) Trauma healing via cognitive behavior therapy in chronically hospitalized patients. Psychiatr Q **78**:317–325.

Treadway MT, Grant MM, Ding Z, et al. (2009) Early adverse events, HPA activity and rostral anterior cingulate volume in MDD. PLoS One **4**:e4887.

Vermetten E, Schmahl C, Lindner S, et al. (2006) Hippocampal and amygdalar volumes in dissociative identity disorder. Am J Psychiat **163**:630–636.

Vieira RM and Gauer GJ (2003) Posttraumatic stress disorder and bipolar mood disorder. Rev Bras Psiquiatr **25**(1):55–61.

Villarreal G, Hamilton DA, Graham DP, et al. (2004) Reduced area of the corpus callosum in posttraumatic stress disorder. Psychiat Res **131**:227–235.

Wang C and Holton J (2007) Total estimated cost of child abuse and neglect in the United States. Chicago: Prevent Child Abuse America.

Woon FL and Hedges DW (2008) Hippocampal and amygdala volumes in children and adults with childhood maltreatment-related posttraumatic stress disorder: a meta-analysis. Hippocampus **18**:729–736.

Yan Q, Rosenfeld RD, Matheson CR, et al. (1997) Expression of brain-derived neurotrophic factor protein in the adult rat central nervous system. Neuroscience **78**:431–448.

Chapter 12

Vascular and metabolic medical comorbidities and neuroprogression in bipolar disorder

Anusha Baskaran, Benjamin I. Goldstein, and Roger McIntyre

Introduction

Bipolar disorder (BD) is a prevalent, lifelong disorder associated with high rates of non-recovery and interepisodic dysfunction (Judd et al. 1996). A recent report from the Global Alliance for Chronic Diseases identifies BD as a leading cause of disability amongst all mental, neurological, and substance use disorders (Collins et al. 2011). In addition to the mood symptoms that define the illness, patients with BD more frequently suffer from medical conditions with the most common medical comorbidities being endocrine/metabolic disease (23%) and vascular disease (21%) (Maina et al. 2013). Mortality studies indicate that individuals with BD have excess and premature mortality from multiple causes with the highest rate of premature mortality due to cardiovascular disease (CVD) (Taylor and Macqueen 2006). Fully one-third of patients with BD also meet criteria for metabolic syndrome, a group of risk factors associated with the development of heart disease, stroke, and type II diabetes (Fagiolini et al. 2005). Furthermore, general medical conditions are associated with delay of treatment in patients with BD (Maina et al. 2013).

Clinical characterization of bipolar disorder and medical comorbidity

Several clinical characteristics of BD have been reported to be associated with the frequency of medical comorbidity. Magalhães and colleagues (2012) reported on associations between variables reflecting illness chr-onicity and burden with comorbid medical conditions in patients enrolled in the Systematic Treatment Enhancement Program for Bipolar Disorder (STEP-BD). Having more than 10 previous mood episodes, childhood onset, smoking, lifetime comorbidity with anxiety, and substance use disorders were independently associated with having a medical comorbidity (Magalhães et al. 2012). Strong associations between variables related to illness chronicity and medical burden in BD lend support to multidimensional models incorporating medical morbidity as a core feature of BD.

Medical comorbidity has also been associated with more complex illness presentations and greater severity of mood symptoms in BD. Kemp et al. (2013) demonstrated that the burden of comorbid medical illnesses appears to be associated with worsened course of illness in the BD population. Patients with high medical burden were more likely to present in a major depressive episode, meet criteria for obsessive–compulsive disorder, and experience a greater number of lifetime mood episodes. They were also more likely to be prescribed a greater number of psychotropic medications (Kemp et al. 2013). However, there is incongruity as to the role comorbid medical conditions play in moderating or predicting treatment response. Some authors have found significant associations between the absolute number of comorbid medical illnesses and worsened BD outcomes (Beyer et al. 2005; McIntyre et al. 2006), whereas others have identified no such relationships (Pirraglia et al. 2009). Thompson and colleagues (2006), studying patients with bipolar I or schizoaffective disorder, found the presence of a high number of baseline medical comorbidities to be associated with depressive episodes of greater severity and longer duration. Moreover, patients with greater baseline medical burden in that study improved more slowly throughout the course of treatment. Hence, medical comorbidity in BD may not only represent a consequence of the illness but may also be an epiphenomenon of the underlying disease process and also accelerate illness progression.

The staging model of bipolar disorder and medical comorbidity

The 'staging' model of BD proposes that, in some cases, illness may progress through successive steps. Initially, individuals at risk of being declared as having BD demonstrate an asymptomatic latency period, which is closely followed by a set of early, often non-specific, symptoms called the prodromal stage. In the majority of cases, the first episode of BD is usually depressive in nature with a gradual transition to hypo/mania (Berk et al. 2007). The course of BD then generally worsens over time, in terms of both increasing severity and frequency of mood episodes (Kessing et al. 2004). These changes in clinical presentation that take place over time have been conceptualized as 'neuroprogression' (Grande et al. 2012).

As BD progresses, physical comorbidities, along with residual symptoms, often worsen, resulting in additional physical health burden and low quality of life (Young and Grunze 2013). The accumulation of medical burden in BD has previously been described as 'somatoprogression' (Goldstein et al. 2009a). Moreover, the early onset of BD has been correlated with an earlier onset of comorbid medical conditions such as ischaemic heart disease, stroke, hypertension, and diabetes, compared with the general population (Kilbourne et al. 2004). Patients who develop BD during childhood or adolescence are the ones who wait the longest for the correct diagnosis (Berk et al. 2007). It can take up to 10–12 years between the time of initial onset of BD symptom(s), and correct diagnosis, significantly delaying the initiation of treatment (Berk et al. 2007; Macneil 2012). The problems with delayed diagnosis and lack of timely treatment include increased morbidity, increased severity of depression, decreased quality of life, and greater likelihood of suicide (Howes and Falkenberg 2011; Taylor et al. 2011).

In a large national cohort study, the association between BD and mortality from chronic diseases (ischaemic heart disease, diabetes, chronic obstructive pulmonary disease, or cancer) was shown to be weaker amongst persons with a prior diagnosis of these conditions than amongst those without a prior diagnosis (Crump et al. 2013). Hence, chronic disease mortality amongst those with more timely medical diagnosis approached that of the general population, suggesting that better provision of primary medical care may effectively reduce premature mortality amongst persons with BD (Crump et al. 2013).

Theoretical links between medical comorbidities and illness progression in bipolar disorder

Several models have emerged as useful paradigms to provide an explanation for the illness progression in BD. One such model involves the concept of allostatic load. According to the model of allostatic load, chronic stress plays an important role in how one ages and his disease trajectory (Grande et al. 2012). Chronic stress activates mechanisms in the body that are normally activated in order to deal with stress, but the repetitive activation of such compensatory systems leaves the body physically worn down, giving way to allostatic load (Grande et al. 2012). The pathophysiology underlying BD may foster the development of a variety of medical disorders that occur comorbid to BD (Soreca et al. 2009).

Although allostatic load provides a framework for our understanding, several mediators have been postulated as theoretical links between medical comorbidities and illness progression in BD. These include hypothalamic-pituitary-adrenal (HPA) axis disturbances, mitochondrial dysfunction, oxidative stress, and inflammation (Fries et al 2012; Grande et al. 2012; Lopresti and Drummond 2013). BD and many of the medical comorbidities observed in BD share several of these common dysregulated biological pathways, as discussed in subsequent sections. It is evident that BD is characterized by HPA dysfunction, including increased level of basal cortisol, lack of suppression of cortisol levels by dexamethasone, and abnormal responses of the HPA system to various physical and psychological stressors. The stress that underlies elevated noradrenergic tone and activation of the HPA axis results in hypercortisolaemia (Fitzgerald 2009).

BD is further accompanied by changes in the mitrochondrial electron transport chain (ETC). Converging evidence consistently demonstrates down-regulation of many mitochondrial ETC-related genes in BD patients (Andreazza and Young 2013). This lends way to increased levels of reactive oxidative species (Budni et al. 2013). Oxidative stress, conversely, can inhibit mitochondrial ETC complexes, leading to reduced ATP production and cellular dysfunction. Moreover, oxidative stress is a mediator of the inflammatory process (Budni et al. 2013). Available evidence indicates that BD and inflammation are linked through shared genetic polymorphisms and gene expression as well as altered cytokine levels during symptomatic (i.e. mania and depression) and asymptomatic intervals (Goldstein et al. 2009a). A recent meta-analysis of 30 studies reported elevated concentrations of interleukin (IL)-4, IL-6, IL-10, soluble IL-2 receptor (sIL-2R), sIL-6R, tumour necrosis factor (TNF)-α, soluble TNF receptor-1 (sTNFR1), and IL-1 receptor antagonist in patients compared with healthy controls (Modabbernia et al. 2013). Moreover, IL-1β and IL-6 tended to show higher values in BD patients. Moreover, it has been suggested that inflammation may be associated with cognitive deficits that are observed in BD (Berk et al. 2011).

Diabetes

Epidemiology

BD patients have up to three times increased risk of type 2 diabetes mellitus (T2DM) compared to the general population (Calkin et al. 2013). This is a major contributing factor to the elevated risk of CVD mortality, the leading cause of death in BD patients. In a review of epidemiological studies, the prevalence of T2DM in patients with BD was reported to be 8–17% (Newcomer 2006). The first 10-year nationwide population-based prospective matched control cohort study showed increased risks of initiation of antidiabetic and antihyperlipidaemia medications amongst patients with BD and schizophrenia (Bai et al. 2013). Patients with BD and T2DM have a more severe course of illness and are more refractory to treatment. Moreover, control of their diabetes is poorer when compared to diabetics without BD.

Clinical correlates

Patients with BD and comorbid T2DM suffer from greater psychiatric symptom severity including a more chronic course, with increased rapid cycling, increased number of psychiatric admissions to hospital, and increased mortality (30% shortened life expectancy) (Ruzickova et al. 2003; Colton et al. 2006). These patients also have an overall poor quality of life and functioning, compared to their counterparts without diabetes. Several factors likely play an underlying role towards the increased prevalence of T2DM in BD. There may be shared pathophysiology linking BD and diabetes, including HPA and mitochondrial dysfunction, common genetic links, and epigenetic interactions (Calkin et al. 2013). Life-style factors, phenomenology of BD symptoms, and adverse effects of pharmacotherapy may also be contributing factors (Calkin et al. 2013).

The stress that underlies elevated noradrenergic tone and activation of the HPA axis leading to hypercortisolaemia in BD can also lead to a decrease in insulin secretion and increase in gluconeogenesis, resulting in hyperglycaemia with progression to diabetes (Fitzgerald 2009). This in turn promotes the deposition of body fat as well as the formation of atherosclerotic plaques in the coronary arteries (Brindley and Rolland 1989), contributing to abdominal obesity and CVD, respectively.

Mitochondrial dysfunction has been implicated in the pathogenesis of both BD and diabetes (Kato and Kato 2000). Patients with BD have reduced pH, phosphocreatine, and ATP in the brain, all hallmarks of decreased aerobic metabolism. Bipolar patients also have increased brain lactate levels, indicating an increase in anaerobic metabolism. Similarly, patients with diabetes have reduced muscle mitochondrial capacity to produce ATP (Szendroedi et al. 2007). BD patients and diabetic patients also share mitochondrial DNA deletions, mutations, and polymorphisms (Kato 2006). Glucose abnormalities in BD patients need to be screened for and treated. Metformin appears to have the best benefit/risk ratio, and the dipeptidyl peptidase-4 inhibitors and glucagon-like peptide-1 receptor agonists and analogues also appear promising, although they have not been specifically investigated in mood disorder populations (Calkin et al. 2013). Physicians should be mindful of the increased risk for T2DM in BD patients, and appropriate prevention, screening, case finding, and treatment are recommended.

Obesity

Epidemiology

Clinical and epidemiological studies reveal that more than half of the BD patients are either overweight or obese, a finding that appears independent of treatment with weight-promoting psychotropic medications (Kemp et al. 2010). While overweight/obesity is highly prevalent amongst adults with BD and has been associated with illness severity, the prevalence of overweight/obesity amongst youth with BD may be modestly greater than in the general population (Goldstein et al. 2008). Moreover, similar to adults, overweight/obesity amongst youth with BD may be associated with increased psychiatric burden.

Clinical correlates

Obesity in BD appears to be associated with greater psychiatric symptom severity and progression of illness. Retrospective studies have found that obese BD patients report an increased frequency of depressive and manic episodes compared to non-obese patients, as well as positive correlations between body mass index (BMI) and markers of illness severity (Fagiolini et al. 2004). Similarly, poorer treatment outcomes are more likely in BD patients with generalized obesity (Fagiolini et al. 2002). Not only do obese BD patients experience an increased lifetime number of depressive and manic episodes, but they also relapse more quickly following stabilization, primarily into depressive episodes (Fagiolini et al. 2003). Prospective studies have also shown that obese BD patients have shorter euthymic periods, more frequent depressive relapses, and that clinically significant weight gain is associated with functional impairment (Bond et al. 2010). In a 3-year longitudinal study, obesity was shown to independently predict the accumulation of medical conditions amongst adults with BD (Goldstein et al. 2013). Hence, treatment of obesity could potentially mitigate the psychiatric and medical burden of BD.

Furthermore, the neuropathology of BD is exacerbated with elevated BMI. Elevated BMI in BD is associated with reduced brain volume in regions of known vulnerability in BD (Bond et al. 2011). Bond et al. (2013) reported that BD patients with higher BMI, at recovery from their first manic episode, have both grey matter and white matter reductions in emotion-generating and -regulating regions of the brain. These results suggest a possible neurobiological mechanism to explain the well-validated association between obesity and the course of illness severity in BD.

Obese BD patients also demonstrate poorer response to lithium-based treatment (Fagiolini et al. 2003). Calkin and colleagues (2009) found an inverse correlation between BMI and response to lithium, the gold standard treatment for BD. Subjects achieving complete remission of symptoms on lithium showed significantly lower BMI (in the healthy range) compared to those in the obese range who had no clinical response to lithium (Calkin et al. 2009). Kemp et al. (2010) reported that for every 1-unit increase in BMI, the likelihood of response to any bipolar treatment decreased by 7.5%, and the likelihood of remission decreased by 7.3%. Therefore, BD patients with comorbid obesity may suffer from treatment refractoriness.

Many different hypotheses have been used to explain the association between obesity and BD. BD and obesity share core phenomenological features, such as overeating, reduced physical activity, sleep disturbance, and impulsivity, that adversely affect the balance between energy intake and expenditure (McElroy and Keck 2012). However, BD and obesity also share neurobiological abnormalities, such as HPA dysfunction, neurotransmitter system imbalance, and brain-derived neurotrophic factor dysfunction (McElroy and Keck 2012).

Abnormalities in metabolic-inflammatory networks suggest that inflammation as observed in BD is also common to metabolic disorders such as obesity. For instance, women with BD store a greater proportion of fat in visceral or abdominal regions than obese controls (Fleet-Michaliszyn et al. 2008). Visceral fat is metabolically active, secreting proinflammatory cytokines and other acute-phase reactants that have been correlated with increased severity of depressive symptoms (McIntyre et al. 2007).

Cardiovascular disease

Epidemiology

Of the disproportionate burden of medical conditions faced by BD patients, CVD is notable, due to both impaired functioning and premature mortality. Goldstein and colleagues (2009b) reported that the mean age of BD subjects with CVD and hypertension was 14 and 13 years younger, respectively, than controls with CVD and hypertension. Persons with BD die of CVD approximately 10 years earlier than the general population (Westman et al. 2013). In a population-based cohort study in Sweden, Westman and colleagues (2013) reported that one-third (38%) of all deaths in persons with BD were caused by CVD and almost half (44%) by other somatic diseases. Excess mortality of both CVD and other somatic diseases was higher than that of suicide and other external causes (Westman et al. 2013). Mortality rate ratios for cerebrovascular disease, coronary heart disease, and acute myocardial infarction were twice as high in individuals with BD compared to the general population.

Clinical correlates

Chronicity of BD symptoms has been shown to contribute to vasculopathy in a dose-dependent fashion. For example, patients with more manic/hypomanic symptoms have been shown to have poorer endothelial function (Fiedorowicz et al. 2012). Exposure to first-generation antipsychotic medications has also been associated with arterial stiffness, higher augmentation pressure, and elevated blood pressure (Fiedorowicz et al. 2012). Vascular phenotyping methods may provide a promising means of elucidating the mechanisms linking mood disorders to vascular disease. Further research is warranted to study whether CVDs affect illness progression in BD.

The excess rate of CVD in BD is due to the clustering of both traditional (e.g. obesity) and emerging (e.g. inflammation) risk factors. A recent report from the Brazilian Research Network in BD demonstrated that variables such as medication use pattern, alcohol use disorder, and physical activity were associated with selected cardiovascular risk factors. Also, of the multiple biological pathways that have been implicated in the pathology of CVD, oxidative stress, and inflammation are the most commonly reported (Stoner et al. 2013).

Some experts have suggested that shared pathophysiological processes may link BD to CVD. Such factors conceptually intrinsic to the proposed disease process of BD may theoretically lead to elevated cardiovascular risk (Murray et al. 2009). Potential links include serum epinephrine levels, decreased heart rate variability, lipid metabolism, and inflammation.

Lipid metabolism may be one particularly important area of research into the link between BD and CVD. Individuals with BD have lower cholesterol and higher triglycerides, both of which may influence the course of illness (Fiedorowicz et al. 2010). Patients with BD and lower cholesterol levels have a higher burden of manic symptoms, suggesting a possible relationship between low cholesterol and manic morbidity without an expected increased risk for vascular disease (Fiedorowicz et al. 2010). Low levels of cholesterol and triglycerides have also been associated with a higher rate of suicide attempts in individuals with BD (Vuksan-Cusa et al. 2009).

On the contrary, high triglycerides and the metabolic syndrome may predispose individuals to vascular disease.

BD is characterized by a dysregulated or overactive inflammatory response. C-reactive protein, a circulating inflammatory marker, has been previously linked to coronary heart disease (Lowe 2005). Recent work has demonstrated elevated levels of C-reactive protein in acutely ill and non-acutely ill patients with BD but not in patients with severe depression (Lowe 2005; Huang and Lin 2007). Furthermore, individuals with BD who are free from vascular disease were found to have elevated serum proapoptotic activity, perhaps triggered by an exaggerated proinflammatory state, which could lead to endothelial dysfunction and vascular disease (Politi et al. 2008).

The increased cardiovascular mortality in persons with BD calls for renewed efforts to prevent and treat somatic diseases in this group (Gomes et al. 2013). It would also be critical to ensure that individuals with BD receive the same quality care for CVD as those without BD.

Conclusions and future directions

It is unclear why comorbid medical conditions are associated with more severe course of illness in BD. It is possible that various comorbid conditions such as obesity represent a more severe variant of BD. It is also plausible to say that comorbid physical conditions can exert a toxic effect on the brain, impairing cognition, and ultimately leading to worsened course of illness. Neuroimaging techniques may also help explain why comorbid medical conditions in BD accelerate and/or worsen illness progression.

Patients with BD more frequently suffer from medical conditions, more commonly endocrine/metabolic disease (e.g. T2DM, obesity), and CVD. Mortality studies also indicate that individuals with BD have excess and premature mortality. Medical comorbidity may represent a core feature of BD, rather than an incidental event or side effect of treatment due to strong associations between variables related to illness chronicity and medical burden in BD. Moreover, medical comorbidity in BD may not only represent a consequence of the illness but may also be an epiphenomenon of the underlying disease process and as well accelerate illness progression.

The pathophysiology underlying BD may foster the development of a variety of medical disorders that occur comorbid to BD. Several mediators have been postulated as theoretical links between medical comorbidities and illness progression in BD. These include HPA axis disturbances, mitochondrial dysfunction, oxidative stress, and inflammation. These mediators also provide a link to the theory of allostatic load in BD and the resulting 'wear and tear' of the body. Taken together, findings to date suggest the importance of approaching BD, both scientifically and clinically, as a systemic disorder with both physical and psychiatric manifestations.

References

Andreazza AC and Young LT (2013) The neurobiology of bipolar disorder: identifying targets for specific agents and synergies for combination treatment. Int J Neuropsychoph 1:1–14.

Bai YM, Su TP, Chen MH, et al. (2013) Risk of developing diabetes mellitus and hyperlipidemia among patients with bipolar disorder, major depressive disorder, and schizophrenia: a 10-year nationwide population-based prospective cohort study. J Affect Disorders 150(1):57–62.

Berk M, Dodd S, Callaly P, et al. (2007). History of illness prior to diagnosis of bipolar disorder or shizoaffective disorder. J Affect Disorders **103**:181–186.

Berk M, Kapczinski F, Andreazza AC, et al. (2011) Pathways underlying neuroprogression in bipolar disorder: focus on inflammation, oxidative stress and neurotrophic factors. Neurosci Biobehav R **35**(3):804–817.

Beyer J, Kuchibhatla M, Gersing K, et al. (2005) Medical comorbidity in a bipolar outpatient clinical population. Neuropsychopharmacology **30**:401–404.

Bond DJ, Ha TH, Lang DJ, et al. (2013) Body mass index-related regional gray and white matter volume reductions in first-episode mania patients. Biol Psychiat 15;**76**(2):138–145.

Bond DJ, Kunz M, Torres IJ, et al. (2010) The association of weight gain with mood symptoms and functional outcomes following a first manic episode: prospective 12-month data from the Systematic Treatment Optimization Program for Early Mania (STOP-EM). Bipolar Disord **12**:616–626.

Bond DJ, Lang DJ, Noronha MM, et al. (2011) The association of elevated body mass index with reduced brain volumes in first-episode mania. Biol Psychiat **70**(4):381–387.

Brindley DN and Rolland Y (1989) Possible connections between stress, diabetes, obesity, hypertension and altered lipoprotein metabolism that may result in atherosclerosis. Clin Sci (Lond) **77**:453–461.

Budni J, Valvassori SS, and Quevedo J (2013) Biological mechanisms underlying neuroprogression in bipolar disorder. Rev Bras Psiquiatr **35**:1–2.

Calkin CV, Gardner DM, Ransom T, et al. (2013) The relationship between bipolar disorder and type 2 diabetes: more than just co-morbid disorders. Ann Med **45**:171–181.

Calkin C, van de Velde C, Ruzickova M, et al. (2009) Can body mass index help predict outcome in patients with bipolar disorder? Bipolar Disord **11**:650–656.

Collins PY, Patel V, Joestl SS, et al. (2011) Grand challenges in global mental health. Nature **475**(7354):27–30.

Colton CW and Manderscheid RW (2006) Congruencies in increased mortality rates, years of potential life lost, and causes of death among public mental health clients in eight states. Prev Chronic Dis **3**:A42.

Crump C, Sundquist K, Winkleby MA, et al. (2013) Comorbidities and mortality in bipolar disorder: a Swedish national cohort study. AMA Psychiat **70**(9):931–939.

Fagiolini A, Frank E, Houck PR, et al. (2002) Prevalence of obesity and weight change during treatment in patients with bipolar I disorder. J Clin Psychiat **63**:528–533.

Fagiolini A, Frank E, Scott JA, et al. (2005) Metabolic syndrome in bipolar disorder: findings from the Bipolar Disorder Center for Pennsylvanians. Bipolar Disord **7**:424–430.

Fagiolini A, Kupfer DJ, Houck PR, et al. (2003) Obesity as a correlate of outcome in patients with bipolar I disorder. Am J Psychiat **160**:112–117.

Fagiolini A, Kupfer DJ, Rucci P, et al. (2004) Suicide attempts and ideation in patients with bipolar I disorder. J Clin Psychiat 65:509–514.

Fiedorowicz JG, Coryell WH, Rice JP, et al. (2012) Vasculopathy related to manic/hypomanic symptom burden and first-generation antipsychotics in a sub-sample from the collaborative depression study. Psychother Psychosom 81(4):235–243.

Fiedorowicz JG, Palagummi NM, Behrendtsen O, et al. (2010) Cholesterol and affective morbidity. Psychiat Res 175(1–2):78–81.

Fitzgerald PJ (2009) Is elevated noradrenaline an aetiological factor in a number of diseases? Auton Autacoid Pharmacol 29:143–156.

Fleet-Michaliszyn SB, Soreca I, Otto AD, et al. (2008) A prospective observational study of obesity, body composition, and insulin resistance in 18 women with bipolar disorder and 17 matched control subjects. J Clin Psychiat 69:1892–1900.

Fries GR, Pfaffenseller B, Stertz L, et al. (2012) Staging and neuroprogression in bipolar disorder. Curr Psychiat Rep 14:667–675.

Goldstein BI, Birmaher B, Axelson DA, et al. (2008) Preliminary findings regarding overweight and obesity in pediatric bipolar disorder. J Clin Psychiat 69(12):1953–1959.

Goldstein BI, Fagiolini A, Houck P, et al. (2009b) Cardiovascular disease and hypertension among adults with bipolar I disorder in the United States. Bipolar Disord 11(6):657–662.

Goldstein BI, Kemp DE, Soczynska JK, et al. (2009a) Inflammation and the phenomenology, pathophysiology, comorbidity, and treatment of bipolar disorder: a systematic review of the literature. J Clin Psychiat 70(8):1078–1090.

Goldstein BI, Liu SM, Schaffer A, Sala R, and Blanco C (2013) Obesity and the three-year longitudinal course of bipolar disorder. Bipolar Disord 15(3):284–293.

Gomes FA, Almeida KM, Magalhaes PV, et al. (2013) Cardiovascular risk factors in outpatients with bipolar disorder: a report from the Brazilian Research Network in Bipolar Disorder. Rev Bras Psiquiatr 35(2):126–130.

Grande I, Magalhaes PV, Kunz M, et al. (2012) Mediators of allostasis and systemic toxicity in bipolar disorder. Physiol Behav 106:46–50.

Howes OD and Falkenberg I (2011) Early detection and intervention in bipolar affective disorder: targeting the development of the disorder. Curr Psychiat Rep 13:493–499.

Huang TL and Lin FC (2007) High-sensitivity C-reactive protein levels in patients with major depressive disorder and bipolar mania. Prog Neuro-Psychoph 31:370–372.

Judd LL, Paulus MP, Wells KB, et al. (1996) Socioeconomic burden of subsyndromal depressive symptoms and major depression in a sample of the general population. Am J Psychiat 153(11):1411–1417.

Kato T (2006) The role of mitochondrial dysfunction in bipolar disorder. Drug News Perspect 19:597–602.

Kato T and Kato N (2000) Mitochondrial dysfunction in bipolar disorder. Bipolar Disord **2**(3 Pt 1):180–90.

Kemp DE, Gao K, Chan PK, et al. (2010) Medical comorbidity in bipolar disorder: relationship between illnesses of the endocrine/metabolic system and treatment outcome. Bipolar Disord **12**:404–413.

Kemp DE, Sylvia LG, Calabrese JR, et al., The LiTMUS Study Group (2013) General medical burden in bipolar disorder: findings from the LiTMUS comparative effectiveness trial. Acta Psychiat Scand **129**(1):24–34.

Kessing LV, Hansen MG, Andersen PK, et al. (2004) The predictive effect of episodes on the risk of recurrence in depressive and bipolar disorders—a life-long perspective. Acta Psychiat Scand **109**(5):339–344.

Kilbourne AM, Cornelius JR, Han X, et al. (2004) Burden of general medical conditions among individuals with bipolar disorder. Bipolar Disord **6**:368–373.

Lopresti AL and Drummond PD (2013) Obesity and psychiatric disorders: Commonalities in dysregulated biological pathways and their implications for treatment. Prog Neuro-Psychoph **45**:92–99.

Lowe GD (2005) Circulating inflammatory markers and risks of cardiovascular and non-cardiovascular disease. J Thromb Haemost **3**:1618–1627.

Macneil CA (2012) Are we missing opportunities for early intervention in bipolar disorder? Expert Rev Neurother **12**(1):5–7.

Magalhães PV, Kapczinski F, Nierenberg AA, et al. (2012) Illness burden and medical comorbidity in the Systematic Treatment Enhancement Program for Bipolar Disorder. Acta Psychiat Scand **125**(4):303–308.

Maina G, Bechon E, Rigardetto S, et al. (2013) General medical conditions are associated with delay to treatment in patients with bipolar disorder. Psychosomatics **54**(5):437–442.

McElroy SL and Keck PE Jr (2012) Obesity in bipolar disorder: an overview. Curr Psychiat Rep **14**(6):650–658.

McIntyre RS, Konarski JZ, Soczynska JK, et al. (2006) Medical comorbidity in bipolar disorder: implications for functional outcomes and health service utilization. Psychiatr Serv **57**:1140–1144.

McIntyre RS, Soczynska JK, Konarski JZ, et al. (2007) Should depressive syndromes be reclassified as 'metabolic syndrome type II?' Ann Clin Psychiat **19**:257–264.

Modabbernia A, Taslimi S, Brietzke E, et al. (2013) Cytokine alterations in bipolar disorder: a meta-analysis of 30 studies. Biol Psychiat **74**(1):15–25.

Murray DP, Weiner M, Prabhakar M, et al. (2009) Mania and mortality: why the excess cardiovascular risk in bipolar disorder? Curr Psychiat Rep **11**:475–480.

Newcomer JW (2006) Medical risk in patients with bipolar disorder and schizophrenia. J Clin Psychiat **67**(Suppl 9):25–30.

Pirraglia PA, Biswas K, Kilbourne AM, et al. (2009) A prospective study of the impact of comorbid medical disease on bipolar disorder outcomes. J Affect Disorders **115**:355–359.

Politi P, Brondino N, and Emanuele E (2008) Increased proapoptotic serum activity in patients with chronic mood disorders. Arch Med Res **39**:242–245.

Ruzickova M, Slaney C, Garnham J, et al. (2003) Clinical features of bipolar disorder with and without comorbid diabetes mellitus. Can J Psychiat **48**:458–461.

Soreca I, Frank E, and Kupfer DJ (2009) The phenomenology of bipolar disorder: what drives the high rate of medical burden and determines long-term prognosis. Depress Anxiety **26**:73–82.

Stoner L, Lucero AA, Palmer BR, et al. (2013) Inflammatory biomarkers for predicting cardiovascular disease. Clin Biochem **46**(15):1353–1371.

Szendroedi J, Schmid AI, Chmelik M, et al. (2007) Muscle mitochondrial ATP synthesis and glucose transport/phosphorylation in type 2 diabetes. PLoS Med **4**:e154.

Taylor M, Bressan RA, Pan Neto P, et al. (2011) Early intervention for bipolar disorder: current imperatives, future directions. Rev Bras Psiquiatr **33**(Suppl 2): s197–212.

Taylor V and Macqueen G (2006) Associations between bipolar disorder and metabolic syndrome: A review. J Clin Psychiat **67**(7):1034–1041.

Thompson WK, Kupfer DJ, Fagiolini A, et al. (2006) Prevalence and clinical correlates of medical comorbidities in patients with bipolar I disorder: analysis of acutephase data from a randomized controlled trial. J Clin Psychiat **67**:783–788.

Vuksan-Cusa B, Marcinko D, Nad S, et al. (2009) Differences in cholesterol and metabolic syndrome between bipolar disorder men with and without suicide attempts. Prog Neuro-Psychoph **33**:109–112.

Westman J, Hällgren J, Wahlbeck K, et al. (2013) Cardiovascular mortality in bipolar disorder: a population-based cohort study in Sweden. BMJ Open **3**(4):pii: e002373.

Young AH and Grunze H (2013) Physical health of patients with bipolar disorder. Acta Psychiat Scand Suppl **442**:3–10.

Chapter 13

Substance misuse in staging bipolar affective disorder

Romain Icick and Frank Bellivier

Introduction

The association between substance misuse and bipolar disorder (BD) has long been recognized as a major source of burden for both patients and clinicians, and data from the past 20 years have highlighted the preoccupying extent of that association. Thus, substance misuse has been integrated among factors involved in the progression of bipolar illness, as described by staging models recently established by several authors (see Scott et al. 2013 for a digest). However, we believed there were several reasons to go further and we propose in this chapter a much larger implication of substance misuse in the staging model described throughout this book. To support this view, we will first gather epidemiological, clinical, and biological evidence that bridge substance use disorders (SUD) and current staging models for BD. Second, we will briefly describe how the definition of SUD itself could be used when enlarging their implication in staging models in light with recent changes in *Diagnostic and Statistical Manual of Mental Disorders* (DSM) criteria. However, several limitations still prevent the full integration of SUD as a modelling factor in BD staging, as discussed in our final section.

Throughout this chapter, we will indifferently use the terms 'substance misuse' or SUD to refer to substance abuse or dependence.

Substance use disorders should be included in the definition of staging

Data from separate fields of research clearly show that SUD have a potential role at multiple levels in the allostatic load involved in bipolar illness progression (Kapczinski et al. 2008).

Substance use disorders are very prevalent among individuals with bipolar disorder

The association between SUD and BD has now been established based on results from national (Regier et al. 1990) and cross-national (Merikangas et al. 2011) epidemiological studies, such as the National Epidemiological Study on Alcohol and Related Conditions (NESARC) (Grant et al. 2005) conducted in the United States. In this national sample of 43,000+ subjects assessed with the Alcohol Use Disorders and Associated Disabilities Interview Schedule, DSM-IV version (AUDADIS-IV) (Grant et al. 2003), BD was highly associated with alcohol use disorders (adjusted odds ratio (OR) 3.5, CI 95% 3.0–4.1 for lifetime prevalence) and with drug use disorders (adjusted OR 4.8, CI 95% 4.1–5.6 for lifetime prevalence). One-year prospective data from NESARC's wave 2 (n = 34,653) are in line with these results, yielding an increased risk of drug abuse of 2.9 (CI 95% 1.01–7.92) found among bipolar type I (BD-I) subjects with no such comorbidity at baseline. Of note, the overall incidence for psychiatric disorders was relatively low in that sample. Ten-year prospective results from another US national survey (National Comorbidity Survey—Replication (NCS-R)) (Swensden et al. 2010) reported stronger links between baseline BD and further incidence of nicotine, alcohol, and drug dependence than the NESARC study. The ORs were all significant ($p < 0.05$), but the adjustments were made only with sociodemographic characteristics, whereas comorbid psychiatric disorders were included in the final regression model of NESARC's wave 2 study.

In the clinical population, SUDs are also highly associated with BD. McElroy et al. (2001) found that 42% of 288 outpatients with BD also had a lifetime SUD, nicotine excluded. The main misused substance was alcohol for 32% of patients, stimulants—including cocaine—for 18%, and marijuana for 16%.

Eventually, nicotine dependence might be almost as prevalent among bipolar patients as with schizophrenia, with lifetime prevalence between 44% and 69% in the general population (Lasser et al. 2000; Grant et al. 2005), similar to that found in outpatient settings (Vanable et al. 2003). The adjusted odds of having lifetime nicotine dependence in case of BD compared to unaffected subjects are 3.4 (CI 95% 2.9–4.0) in the general population (Grant et al. 2005).

Of note, these results are to be interpreted in light of the diagnostic issues related to complex comorbid conditions, especially when applied to the general population in a lifetime basis, and the variability of SUD prevalence according to current mood symptoms (Nery-Fernandes et al. 2009) and the samples' origin. Thus, studies on the most severe patients, tending to exhibit higher rates of addictive comorbidity, and studies focusing on primarily substance-dependent patients tend to report relatively low rates of BD (Rounsaville et al. 1991; Savant et al. 2013).

Impact of SUD on BD outcome

SUD have a major negative impact on the course of BD. Several key features associated with that impact are part of the elements defining staging BD, and thus warrant further description.

First, comorbid SUD increase the odds of relapse with a major mood episode. For example, prospective clinical studies have shown indeed that an increase in alcohol intake was associated with further depression (Jaffee et al. 2009), whereas marijuana use was associated with later manic episodes (Strakowski et al. 2007). Moreover, remission is often incomplete in comorbid patients, with higher rates of residual symptoms (Ostacher et al. 2010). All these factors may contribute to the lower rates of functional remission described with comorbid patients (Weiss et al. 2005). Eventually, suicidal behaviour is more frequent among bipolar patients with SUDs (Pompili et al. 2013).

Shared biomarkers of SUD and BD

Addictive disorders have been associated with a wide range of biological and neuroanatomical disturbances, some of which are common to those observed in BD. These biomarkers are usually more prominent in the later stages of BD progression, which implies that their early occurrence linked to substance use may accelerate illness progression. Moreover, biomarkers associated with comorbid addiction and bipolar disorder (BIPADD) condition are highly susceptible to vary with substance type, duration of use, and mood state. Therefore, we focus on state markers that have been associated with both bipolar and addictive disorders, although separately to date.

Inflammatory chemokines

Interleukin-6 and interleukin-10 levels have been found elevated in subjects with alcohol dependence (Laso et al. 2007; Nicolaou et al. 2004). Interleukin-10 levels were also increased among subjects with opiate (Azarang et al. 2007), and cocaine (Narvaez et al. 2013) dependence.

Brain-derived neurotrophic factor (BDNF)

Peripheral concentrations of BDNF have shown opposite results with regard to studied substances. Compared to control subjects, they were found higher in case of crack cocaine use (Narvaez et al. 2013) and lower in alcohol-dependent subjects, although higher during acute withdrawal (Köhler et al. 2013). This result is supported by the fact that BDNF levels return to normal with protracted abstinence of alcohol (Costa et al. 2011).

Neuroimaging

SUD have also been associated with alterations of brain structure in several key areas involved in memory, decision-making, and in the limbic system. Alteration of brain white matter (WM), responsible for between-areas connectivity, might be even more pronounced. Loss of WM volume has been associated with misuse of cocaine (Moreno-López et al. 2012), alcohol (Monnig et al. 2013), and ecstasy (De Win et al. 2008).

As for grey matter (GM) alterations, case–control studies have shown reduced hippocampal volume in subjects with ecstasy (Den Hollander et al. 2012), cocaine (Moreno-López et al. 2012), and alcohol use disorders (Durazzo et al. 2011). More specifically, higher GM volume in reward circuitry may predict relapse/abstinence of alcohol dependence (Cardenas et al. 2011). Conversely, reduced cortical thickness has been correlated with both current and lifetime drinking status (Cardenas et al. 2011) among alcohol abusers. As for marijuana, a reduction of global GM volume has been suggested in bipolar adolescents with cannabis use disorders (Jarvis et al. 2008), whereas cannabidiol, when given separately, may have neuroprotective effects (Demirakca et al. 2011). Eventually, lifetime tobacco smoking considering subjects at age 64+ has been associated with heterogeneous effects on striatal volume (Das et al. 2012) and thus warrants further investigation.

Overall, it seems that drugs such as psychostimulants have widespread toxic effects on both GM and WM, while alcohol rather impairs GM structure. The effect of marijuana and tobacco might be age-dependent. Of note, these changes in brain structures are in line with more functional results of neuropsychological studies.

Hypothalamic-pituitary-adrenal axis (HPA) dysregulation

HPA axis dysregulation has been extensively studied in psychiatric disorders, with interesting, yet varied results in the field of addiction psychiatry (Friedman and Eisenstein 2004). This hormonal system is highly important because of its mediating role between stress and neurotoxicity, mainly through the effects of cortisol (de Kloet et al. 2005). In SUD, peripheral cortisol has exhibited blunted response to Adrenocorticotropic hormone (ACTH), higher mean plasma levels, and lower circadian reactivity (Lovallo 2006). Of note, the reactivity of the HPA axis can be mediated by stressful life events, especially childhood trauma (Van Leeuwen et al. 2011; Perroud et al. 2013).

Neuropsychological abnormalities

During the last two decades, there has been a paradigm shift in the concept of addiction from an initial 'intoxication/withdrawal' sequence to considerably long-lasting impairment, involving alteration of decision-making underlain by impairment in attention and memory (Hyman 2005; Heyman 2013). Similar disturbances have been described among euthymic bipolar patients (Bellivier 2012), and one can expect additive effects in case of concurrent substance use and addiction, with regard to some specificity described further. Moreover, preliminary evidence has shown that bipolar patients with SUD seem to perform worse than those without on several tasks of attention and learning in the case of comorbid alcohol dependence (Levy et al. 2008). Of note, executive functions such as decision-making seem to predict relapse of stimulant dependence whether patients were bipolar or not (Nejtek et al. 2013), suggesting similar mechanisms (De Wilde et al. 2013; Wang et al. 2013).

Regarding dimensional profiles, impulsivity is frequently associated with SUDs among bipolar patients, and with an overall higher severity of such patients (Etain et al. 2013).

It is noteworthy that most of these studies on biomarkers used a cross-sectional design, which prevents concluding any formal causal effect of these drugs on brain structure. Such causal link is still supported by the fact that remitted subjects with SUD tend to show intermediate levels of alteration between active users and controls.

Environmental

Current staging models highlight the impact of bipolar illness on the subjects' environment and social life, especially in later stages. These could be split into early consequences, such as the slowing of academic achievement due to early depressive or manic episodes, and later consequences, with divorce or separation due to episode repetition, or even cognitive dysfunction for even later stages. These consequences favour the subjects' isolation, which can in turn increase bipolar illness symptomatology. SUDs are known providers of such environmental alterations, depending on their legal status, but also because of impaired decision-making abilities (Volkow et al. 2011) or increased harm to others (Witt et al. 2013). They should thus be considered more largely for staging in that domain.

From this narrow and selective review, it seems clear that SUDs warrant larger involvement in the criteria used for staging BD, which could benefit from a much broader endorsement of criteria linked to substance misuse. Several pathophysiological alterations that could be useful in staging BD can be drawn from these results, with two main pathways: one involving BDNF, cognition, episode repetition, and neuronal loss, and another involving the HPA axis, emotional dysregulation, and early trauma. Inflammatory states, WM abnormalities, and repetition of major mood episodes probably participate equally to both.

Despite this evidence, the phenomenology of SUDs is complex and warrants further description to be integrated into staging models.

How to incorporate SUDs into staging models for BD?

DSM-V criteria

Substance misuse has long been referring to abuse and dependence, despite some historical variations in existing classifications. Briefly, diagnosis of abuse mainly relies on isolated but relatively severe negative consequences of drug use for an individual, whereas diagnosis of dependence rather refers to fixed pattern of use leading to relapse and aggravating problems in different areas of one's functioning, all reflecting a loss of control of substance use (Goodman 1990). Given the lack of specificity associated with the diagnosis of abuse, and the relatively high severity implied by dependence diagnosis, researchers have validated a semi-dimensional classification now called 'Substance Use and Addictive Disorders' in the recent 5th edition of the DSM (American Psychiatric Association 2013). These changes resulted in a continuous score with three levels of severity. Such a pattern of classification has intriguing similarities with staging models, although it does not imply progression from one symptom cluster to another across illness duration.

Specifiers for substance misuse to be used in staging definitions

Substance use and relapse of BD

The first step for a course specifier of any substance use within the staging definition of BD would be to its association with relapse or not. Thus, individuals with BD exhibit variable mood sensitivity to substance use, which also depends on the type of substance used and its modalities. Of note, a workgroup on co-occurring mental illness and SUD recently proposed that any pattern of substance use inducing or worsening symptoms of an associated psychiatric disorder should be integrated when scoring SUD. We definitely support such a view and would include such a criterion in our staging model.

Substance use because of mood symptoms

Apart from controversial theories of self-medication processes, in which individuals with psychiatric disorders are thought to use psychotropic substances in order to alleviate their illness symptoms, several situations in BD may lead to an increase or initiation of substance use.

First, manic episodes are often associated with disinhibition and sensation-seeking, leading to substance intake that is sometimes not even present at baseline. This is better considered as core symptoms rather than secondary consequences of manic states, although some patients also report using sedatives or alcohol to calm down during such moments.

Second, patients frequently report the use of alcohol in depressive states, in an attempt to improve sleep and anxiety.

Third, between-episode alterations such as emotional hyperreactivity (M'bailara et al. 2009) could also lead to substance intake.

With that regard, a very interesting clinical study had a close look into bipolar patients' motivations for drinking alcohol (Meyer et al. 2012). Using a structured questionnaire, the Drinking Motives Questionnaire (DMQ), patients reported that they were drinking for social enhancement when manic, whereas they were prone to use alcohol to alleviate symptoms when depressed. Of note, such effects are often held as positive and can delay treatment-seeking.

Polysubstance use

Polysubstance use and misuse are rather the rule than the exception in SUDs, and BD might even play a catalytic role in multiplying substance use for a given individual. Such patterns should be specified separately if used in a staging model of BD, since they are a major provider of clinical and environmental instability (Hoblyn et al. 2009; Icick and Bellivier 2013), although correlates of polysubstance use in BD have yet not been specifically assessed to our knowledge.

Transnosographic dimensions

As mentioned earlier, SUDs are highly associated with dimensions such as impulsivity among bipolar patients, to the extent that it may partly mediate their impact on the course of bipolar illness (Icick and Bellivier 2013). This may justify supplementary specifiers aside from SUD, given that individuals with higher impulsivity levels are expected to present with a worse course of bipolar illness, including comorbid SUDs and suicidal behaviour (Etain et al. 2013).

Overall, we believe that these minimum specifiers should be used to weight the importance of substance use for a given individual with BD so as to be relevant for illness staging. However, despite the evidence gathered so far and the refinement of SUD patterns brought by DSM-V definitions, several limitations impede from building staging models of BD with a larger involvement of SUDs.

Barriers against an operational definition of staging that would include SUD as a key factor

The phenomenology of addictive disorders implies personal and environmental instability that may influence BD outcomes and symptoms, with additional impact on treatment-seeking and adherence, all with between-subject and within-subject variability. Thus, we will briefly explain how such complexity still stands against operationalizing staging, with more implication of SUDs.

First of all, substance use itself is a complex, heterogeneous, and time-varying phenomenon. A closer look to marijuana use provides a good illustration of that complexity.

- *Routes of administration.* Marijuana is usually smoked, which can be done pure or associated with tobacco in cigarettes or 'bongs', and eaten in oil form. These routes have different onset and duration of effect, and thus might not affect mood states in the same way. A major effect of administration route is also seen in cocaine use (Nichols 2013).

- *Drug composition.* First, marijuana is a complex composite of more than 60 cannabinoids, the two major ones, tetrahydrocannabinol and cannabidiol, exhibiting almost opposite psychotropic effects (Demirakca et al. 2011). Their respective proportions usually vary according to the final drug sample that is sold, and can hardly be anticipated. Second, the almost constant use of tobacco when marijuana is smoked may not only have an impact on its pharmacokinetics, but also directly on the brain, since tobacco smoke has monoamine oxidase inhibitor (MAOI) effects that add to the stimulant effect of nicotine. There is indeed some preliminary work, which suggested either worse (Cahil et al. 2006) or better (Braga et al. 2012) cognitive functioning among bipolar patients with chronic cannabis use, although these studies did not control for the effect of tobacco smoking. This further highlights the issue of polysubstance use, with known additive effects of several substances of abuse on their addictive properties or their toxic effects, as seen with biochemical interactions between cocaine and alcohol, for example (Natakar et al. 2012).

- *Between-subject and within-subject variability.* Individual and time-related variables are also a main factor of variability when assessing the effects of substance intake on mood symptoms. The age at onset (AAO) of substance use might be of importance, and adolescents' brain seems a highly vulnerable target for both psychotropic (i.e. their ability to accelerate BD onset) and neurotoxic (i.e. cognitive) effects of substances, the use of which are very common at that age (Heffner et al. 2008, 2012; Meier et al. 2012). Psychological, but also inflammatory, states (Hamdani et al. 2013) linked to BD or other associated conditions (Krishnan 2005) could also confer very different vulnerability to the reinforcing (i.e. addictive) or neurotoxic effects of substance intake.

- *Propensity to induce relapse.* Of note, substances of abuse have effects on mood that do not induce the same type of symptoms and relapse polarity (Icick et al. 2012), but also given to various amounts or duration of use.

- *Craving.* This subjective and unpleasant urge to use a given substance of abuse is highly drug- and subject-dependent. It is particularly seen among stimulant-dependent subjects, but also in the case of alcohol dependence. It is highly associated with relapse, and one could wonder if bipolar individuals experience craving just as unaffected subjects, but also if craving itself could bring enough discomfort and anxiety to induce major mood episodes. Its repetition may also have stress-mediated neurotoxicity.

◆ *Duration and sequences of use.* Chronic exposure to a given substance probably has different effects on the brain compared to multiple withdrawals and/or relapses after long-term abstinence. Brutal withdrawal of most substances of abuse has thus been associated with glutamate release (Quntero 2013), which may have additive effects to those of chronic drug exposure on selected domains such as neurotoxicity. For example, ecstasy use has been linked with WM abnormalities and manic symptoms in early stages of use (De Win et al. 2008), whereas tobacco smoking might rather be associated with higher suicidal risk and neurovascular complications after many years of use (Das et al. 2012).

All these factors associated with SUD have to be taken into account before enlarging their involvement into staging models of BD, and still prevent from immediately building an operational 'bipolar-addiction' staging model.

Conclusion

Throughout this chapter, we have tried to argue for a much larger inclusion of substance use and misuse into future models of staging BD, starting from evidence of shared impairment and dysregulation (Swann 2010). We believe that their role has to be better highlighted at multiple levels of illness progression: this should be highlighted from first tobacco use reinforcing emotional instability among high-risk subjects (BD stage 0) to later cognitive impairment linked to multiple episodes and direct neurotoxicity due to stimulant or polysubstance dependence (BD stages 3–4). The complex phenomenology of SUD still prevents their operationalized inclusion into staging models. However, it could be used as a powerful igniter for future research in the area of comorbidity, and might bring new insights into the pathophysiology of addictive and BD.

References

American Psychiatric Association (2013) Diagnostic and Statistical Manual of Mental Disorders, 5th edn. Arlington, VA: American Psychiatric Publishing.

Azarang A, Mahmoodi M, Rajabalian S, et al. (2007) T-helper 1 and 2 serum cytokine assay in chronic opioid addicts. Eur Cytokine Netw **18**(4):210–214.

Bellivier F (2012) [Cognitions and functioning in euthymic bipolar patients: screening and treatment]. Encephale **38**(Suppl 4):S151–154.

Braga RJ, Burdick KE, Derosse P, et al. (2012) Cognitive and clinical outcomes associated with cannabis use in patients with bipolar I disorder. Psychiat Res **200**(2–3):242–245.

Cahill CM, Malhi GS, Ivanovski B, et al. (2006) Cognitive compromise in bipolar disorder with chronic cannabis use: cause or consequence? Expert Rev Neurother **6**(4):591–598.

Cardenas VA, Durazzo TC, Gazdzinski S, et al. (2011) Brain morphology at entry into treatment for alcohol dependence is related to relapse propensity. Biol Psychiat **70**(6):561–567.

Costa M-A, Girard M, Dalmay F, et al. (2011) Brain-derived neurotrophic factor serum levels in alcohol-dependent subjects 6 months after alcohol withdrawal. Alcohol Clin Exp Res **35**(11):1966–1973.

Das D, Cherbuin N, Anstey KJ, et al. (2012) Lifetime cigarette smoking is associated with striatal volume measures. Addict Biol **17**(4):817–825.

Demirakca T, Sartorius A, Ende G, et al. (2011) Diminished gray matter in the hippocampus of cannabis users: possible protective effects of cannabidiol. Drug Alcohol Depend **114**(2–3):242–245.

Den Hollander B, Schouw M, Groot P, et al. (2012) Preliminary evidence of hippocampal damage in chronic users of ecstasy. J Neurol Neurosurg Psychiatry **83**(1):83–85.

De Wilde B, Verdejo-García A, Sabbe B, et al. (2013) Affective decision-making is predictive of three-month relapse in polysubstance-dependent alcoholics. Eur Addict Res **19**(1):21–28.

De Win MML, Jager G, Booij J, et al. (2008) Sustained effects of ecstasy on the human brain: a prospective neuroimaging study in novel users. Brain J Neurol **131**(Pt 11): 2936–2945.

Durazzo TC, Tosun D, Buckley S, et al. (2011) Cortical thickness, surface area, and volume of the brain reward system in alcohol dependence: relationships to relapse and extended abstinence. Alcohol Clin Exp Res **35**(6):1187–1200.

Etain B, Mathieu F, Liquet S, et al. (2013) Clinical features associated with trait-impulsiveness in euthymic bipolar disorder patients. J Affect Disorders **144**(3): 240–247.

Friedman H and Eisenstein TK (2004) Neurological basis of drug dependence and its effects on the immune system. J Neuroimmunol **147**(1–2):106–108.

Goodman A (1990) Addiction: definition and implications. Brit J Addict **85**(11): 1403–1408.

Grant BF, Dawson DA, Stinson FS, et al. (2003) The Alcohol Use Disorder and Associated Disabilities Interview Schedule-IV (AUDADIS-IV): reliability of alcohol consumption, tobacco use, family history of depression and psychiatric diagnostic modules in a general population sample. Drug Alcohol Depend **71**(1):7–16.

Grant BF, Stinson FS, Hasin DS, et al. (2005) Prevalence, correlates, and comorbidity of bipolar I disorder and axis I and II disorders: results from the National Epidemiologic Survey on Alcohol and Related Conditions. J Clin Psychiat 66(10):1205–1215.

Hamdani N, Doukhan R, Kurtlucan O, et al. (2013) Immunity, inflammation, and bipolar disorder: diagnostic and therapeutic implications. Curr Psychiat Rep 15(9):387.

Heffner JL, DelBello MP, Anthenelli RM, et al. (2012) Cigarette smoking and its relationship to mood disorder symptoms and co-occurring alcohol and cannabis use disorders following first hospitalization for bipolar disorder. Bipolar Disord 14(1):99–108.

Heffner JL, DelBello MP, Fleck DE, et al. (2008) Cigarette smoking in the early course of bipolar disorder: association with ages-at-onset of alcohol and marijuana use. Bipolar Disord 10(7):838–845.

Heyman GM (2013) Addiction and choice: theory and new data. Front Addict Disord Behav Dyscontrol 4:31.

Hoblyn JC, Balt SL, Woodard SA, et al. (2009) Substance use disorders as risk factors for psychiatric hospitalization in bipolar disorder. Psychiatr Serv Wash DC 60(1):50–55.

Hyman SE (2005) Addiction: a disease of learning and memory. Am J Psychiat 162(8): 1414–1422.

Icick R and Bellivier F (2013) Correlates of substance use disorders among bipolar patients from Fondamental Advanced Centers of Expertise-Bipolar Disorder (FACE-BD). Unpublished data, 2013.

Icick R, Desage A, Gard S, et al. (2012) Comorbid addiction in bipolar affective disorder. Neuropsychiatry 2(6): 531–541.

Jaffee WB, Griffin ML, Gallop R, et al. (2009) Depression precipitated by alcohol use in patients with co-occurring bipolar and substance use disorders. J Clin Psychiat 70(2):171–176.

Jarvis K, DelBello MP, Mills N, et al., 2008. Neuroanatomic comparison of bipolar adolescents with and without cannabis use disorders. J Child Adol Psychop 18: 557–563. doi:10.1089/cap.2008.033

Kapczinski F, Vieta E, Andreazza AC, et al. (2008) Allostatic load in bipolar disorder: implications for pathophysiology and treatment. Neurosci Biobehav R 32(4):675–692.

Kloet ER de, Joëls M, and Holsboer F (2005) Stress and the brain: from adaptation to disease. Nat Rev Neurosci 6(6):463–475.

Köhler S, Klimke S, Hellweg R, et al. (2013) Serum brain-derived neurotrophic factor and nerve growth factor concentrations change after alcohol withdrawal: preliminary data of a case-control comparison. Eur Addict Res 19(2):98–104.

Krishnan KRR (2005) Psychiatric and medical comorbidities of bipolar disorder. Psychosom Med 67(1):1–8.

Laso FJ, Vaquero JM, Almeida J, et al. (2007) Chronic alcohol consumption is associated with changes in the distribution, immunophenotype, and the inflammatory cytokine secretion profile of circulating dendritic cells. Alcohol Clin Exp Res 31(5):846–854.

Lasser K, Boyd JW, Woolhandler S, et al. (2000) Smoking and mental illness: a population-based prevalence study. JAMA 284(20):2606–2610.

Levy B, Monzani BA, Stephansky MR, et al. (2008) Neurocognitive impairment in patients with co-occurring bipolar disorder and alcohol dependence upon discharge from inpatient care. Psychiat Res 161(1): 28–35.

Lovallo WR (2006) Cortisol secretion patterns in addiction and addiction risk. Int J Psychophysiol 59(3):195–202.

M'bailara K, Demotes-Mainard J, Swendsen J, et al. (2009) Emotional hyper-reactivity in normothymic bipolar patients. Bipolar Disord 11(1):63–69.

McElroy SL, Altshuler LL, Suppes T, et al. (2001) Axis I psychiatric comorbidity and its relationship to historical illness variables in 288 patients with bipolar disorder. Am J Psychiat 158(3):420–426.

Meier MH, Caspi A, Ambler A, et al. Persistent cannabis users show neuropsychological decline from childhood to midlife. Proc Natl Acad Sci U S A 109(40):E2657–E2664.

Merikangas KR, Jin R, He J, et al. (2011) Prevalence and correlates of bipolar spectrum disorder in the world mental health survey initiative. Arch Gen Psychiat 68(3):241–251.

Meyer TD, McDonald JL, Douglas JL, et al. (2012) Do patients with bipolar disorder drink alcohol for different reasons when depressed, manic or euthymic? J Affect Disorders 136(3):926–932.

Monnig MA, Tonigan JS, Yeo RA, et al. (2013) White matter volume in alcohol use disorders: a meta-analysis. Addict Biol 18(3):581–592.

Moreno-López L, Catena A, Fernández-Serrano MJ, et al. (2012) Trait impulsivity and prefrontal gray matter reductions in cocaine dependent individuals. Drug Alcohol Depend 125(3):208–214.

Narvaez JCM, Magalhães PV, Fries GR, et al. (2013) Peripheral toxicity in crack cocaine use disorders. Neurosci Lett 544:80–84.

Natekar A, Motok I, Walasek P, et al. (2012) Cocaethylene as a biomarker to predict heavy alcohol exposure among cocaine users. J Popul Ther Clin Pharmacol J Thérapeutique Popul Pharmacologie Clin 19(3):e466–472.

Nejtek VA, Kaiser KA, Zhang B, et al. (2013) Iowa Gambling Task scores predict future drug use in bipolar disorder outpatients with stimulant dependence. Psychiat Res 210:871–879.

Nery-Fernandes F, Quarantini LC, Galvão-De-Almeida A, et al. (2009) Lower rates of comorbidities in euthymic bipolar patients. World J Biol Psychiat 10(4 Pt 2): 474–479.

Nichols E (2013) Psychotic Symptoms Induced by Cocaine Use. Poster presented at the International Conference on Dual Disorders (ICDD), Barcelona, Spain, October 2013.

Nicolaou C, Chatzipanagiotou S, Tzivos D, et al. (2004) Serum cytokine concentrations in alcohol-dependent individuals without liver disease. Alcohol Fayettev N 32(3):243–247.

Ostacher MJ, Perlis RH, Nierenberg AA, et al. (2010) Impact of substance use disorders on recovery from episodes of depression in bipolar disorder patients: prospective data from the Systematic Treatment Enhancement Program for Bipolar Disorder (STEP-BD). Am J Psychiat 167(3):289–297.

Perroud N, Dayer A, Piguet C, et al. (2013) Childhood maltreatment and methylation of the glucocorticoid receptor gene NR3C1 in bipolar disorder. Brit J Psychiat 204:30–35.

Pompili M, Gonda X, Serafini G, et al. (2013) Epidemiology of suicide in bipolar disorders: a systematic review of the literature. Bipolar Disord 15(5):457–90.

Quintero G (2013) Role of nucleus accumbens glutamatergic plasticity in drug addiction. Neuropsychiatr Dis Treat 9:1499–1512.

Regier DA, Farmer ME, Rae DS, et al. (1990) Comorbidity of mental disorders with alcohol and other drug abuse. Results from the Epidemiologic Catchment Area (ECA) Study. JAMA 264(19):2511–2518.

Rounsaville BJ, Anton SF, Carroll K, et al. (1991) Psychiatric diagnoses of treatment-seeking cocaine abusers. Arch Gen Psychiat 48(1):43–51.

Savant JD, Barry DT, Cutter CJ, et al. (2013) Prevalence of mood and substance use disorders among patients seeking primary care office-based buprenorphine/naloxone treatment. Drug Alcohol Depend 127(1–3):243–247.

Scott J, Leboyer M, Hickie I, et al. (2013) Clinical staging in psychiatry: a cross-cutting model of diagnosis with heuristic and practical value. Br J Psychiat J Ment Sci 202:243–245.

Strakowski SM, DelBello MP, Fleck DE, et al. (2007) Effects of co-occurring cannabis use disorders on the course of bipolar disorder after a first hospitalization for mania. Arch Gen Psychiat 64(1):57–64.

Swann AC (2010) The strong relationship between bipolar and substance-use disorder. Ann N Y Acad Sci 1187:276–293.

Swendsen J, Conway KP, Degenhardt L, et al. (2010) Mental disorders as risk factors for substance use, abuse and dependence: results from the 10-year follow-up of the National Comorbidity Survey. Addict Abingdon Engl 105(6):1117–1128.

Vanable PA, Carey MP, Carey KB, et al. (2003) Smoking among psychiatric outpatients: relationship to substance use, diagnosis, and illness severity. Psychol Addict Behav J Soc Psychol Addict Behav 17(4):259–265.

Van Leeuwen AP, Creemers HE, Greaves-Lord K, et al. (2011) Hypothalamic-pituitary-adrenal axis reactivity to social stress and adolescent cannabis use: the TRAILS study. Addict Abingdon Engl 106(8):1484–1492.

Volkow ND, Baler RD, and Goldstein RZ (2011) Addiction: pulling at the neural threads of social behaviors. Neuron **69**(4): 599–602.

Wang G, Shi J, Chen N, et al. (2013) Effects of length of abstinence on decision-making and craving in methamphetamine abusers. PloS One **8**(7):e68791.

Weiss RD, Ostacher MJ, Otto MW, et al. (2005) Does recovery from substance use disorder matter in patients with bipolar disorder? J Clin Psychiat **66**(6):730–735; quiz 808–809.

Witt K, van Dorn R, and Fazel S (2013) Risk factors for violence in psychosis: systematic review and meta-regression analysis of 110 studies. PLoS One **8**:e55942. doi:10.1371/journal.pone.0055942

Chapter 14

Excellent lithium responders, resilience, and staging in bipolar disorder

Janusz K. Rybakowski

Staging in bipolar disorder

In a significant proportion of patients with bipolar disorder (BD), the course of illness can be described in terms of 'staging'. The staging model of psychiatric disorder assumes a progression from prodromal (at risk) to more severe and treatment-refractory conditions. An original proposal of staging for various psychiatric illnesses was made by Fava and Kellner (1993) 20 years ago. Four different staging models have been proposed for BD. The earliest concept of Robert Post (1992) is based on the phenomenon of kindling and neurosensitization, assuming a role of stressors in triggering the first episode of illness, with subsequent persistent changes in the activity of neurons, greater vulnerability to relapse, and worse response to treatment. The model of Michael Berk (2009) was conceived in parallel to therapeutic algorithms. Berk's model classifies the stages of illness based on clinical features, prognosis, and response to treatment. It also identifies high-risk individuals, highlights the need for early intervention, and is proposed as a course specifier for BD. The model of Flavio Kapczinski (2009a) is based on the assessment of patients in the interepisodic period according to functioning and cognition. In this model, the possible use of biomarkers in the future is also highlighted. Finally, the concept of Anne Duffy (2010) should be mentioned. This is based on the research of high-risk bipolar offspring and describes the early development of the illness as successive stages: i.e. non-mood disorders, minor mood disorders, and acute episodes of illness, starting in childhood, with an attempt to distinguish subtypes of the disorder depending on the parent's response to prophylactic lithium treatment.

In the initial section of the present paper, clinical, neurobiological, and neurocognitive components of staging in BD will be discussed. Special attention will be paid to mechanism of allostasis and resilience in the context of staging models. Since the staging of BD is closely related to the treatment of this disorder, the effect of staging on the efficacy of various methods of treatment will be discussed. In the final section, it will be demonstrated that successful treatment and prophylaxis with lithium may favourably influence illness progression, hampering the progress of the disorder into late stages.

Clinical components of staging

Clinical symptoms make the main feature of staging classification. In their review of staging in BD, Cosci and Fava (2013) point to a relative lack of evidence supporting the definition of a stage 0 (at risk) for BD. According to them, stage 1 includes mild or non-specific symptoms of mood disorder, characteristic of the prodromal phase (e.g. increased self-confidence, energy and elated mood, mood swings), or cyclothymia. In stage 2, acute manifestations of major depressive disorder and mania/hypomania are present. In stage 3, residual phase symptoms occur with marked impairment in cognition and functioning despite mood-stabilizing treatment, and during stage 4, acute episodes appear despite mood-stabilizing treatment.

Other clinical concepts of BD staging put more emphasis on the early or prodromal period of the development of this disorder. Kapczinski et al. (2009a) have put forward, before stage 1, a latent phase, including patients with family load of bipolar disorder (ultra-high-risk) and hyperthymic or cyclothymic temperament, as well as with anxiety or subsyndromal depressive or hypomanic symptoms. In a similar vein, Duffy et al. (2010) point to an excess of anxiety and sleep disorders in the offspring of patients with BD as well as psychoactive substance use in the period before overt clinical presentation of mood symptoms. In the Kapczinski et al. (2009a) model, the staging is based on the clinical and functional assessment during interepisodic periods. Therefore in stage 1, patients would present a well-established euthymia and absence of interepisodic overt psychiatric symptomatology; in stage 2, psychiatric symptomatology is present between episodes; in stage 3, patients present a clinically relevant pattern of cognitive and functional deterioration; and in stage 4, patients are incapable of living autonomously.

An important element of staging in recurrent mood disorder is duration of illness and number of episodes. It has been postulated that each subsequent affective episode may exert deleterious effect on brain function in terms of neuroanatomic and cognitive changes. This issue was first raised 20 years ago (Altshuler 1993) and the review of the correlates of illness progression in the recurrent affective disorders has been recently performed by Post et al. (2012). Magalhaes et al. (2012) analysed 3,345 bipolar patients participating in the Systematic Treatment Enhancement Program for Bipolar Disorder (STEP-BD) and showed that patients with multiple previous episodes had consistently poorer cross-sectional and prospective outcomes: functioning and quality of life were worse, disability was more common, and symptoms were more chronic and severe. Guitierrez-Rojas et al. (2011) reported that the number of previous manic episodes was associated with work disability and family disability, while the number of previous depressive episodes was associated with disability in the social domain. Recently, Reinares et al. (2013), identifying two subtypes of bipolar patients presenting 'good' and 'poor' outcomes, have shown that episode density and level of residual depressive symptoms emerged as the most significant clinical predictors of the given subtype.

Since about 50% of BD patients present with their first episode as major depressive disorder (MDD), a special case related to staging is the phenomenon of unipolar–bipolar conversion. The dynamics of such conversion may be about 1.5% per year of patients diagnosed either as first episode of depression or recurrent depression (Angst et al. 2005b). In a recent study carried out in our group, the rate of the conversion from MDD to BD in 122 patients followed for 30 years was 1.8% per year and the conversion occurred in 1/3 patients first hospitalized due to a depressive episode, with mean time to conversion being 9 years (Dudek et al. 2013). The last figure may be similar to the period of a delay of BD diagnosis found in some epidemiological studies (Baethge et al. 2003). Most probably, depressive episodes preceding the first (hypo)manic one during the course of BD should be included in stage 1.

Another issue is the effect of subthreshold bipolarity occurring in patients diagnosed as MDD, which may be detected by new tools for hypomania, such as the Mood Disorder Questionnaire (MDQ) (Hirshfeld at al. 2000) and the Hypomania Checklist-32 (HCL-32) (Angst et al. 2005a). In the Polish TRES-DEP study including 1,051 patients with MDD, we showed that patients with bipolarity features (37.5% by HCL-32 and 20% by MDQ) had more family history of depression, bipolar disorder, alcoholism, and suicide, a more severe course of disease (earlier onset of illness, more depressive episodes, more psychiatric hospitalizations, and more resistance to treatment with antidepressants), as well as worse social functioning (e.g. less frequently married) (Rybakowski et al. 2012). Therefore, the course of illness in MDD patients with subthreshold bipolarity is more akin to those with BD, which may also have therapeutic implications (e.g. necessity of more frequent use of mood-stabilizing drugs).

Neurobiological components of staging: allostasis and resilience

Neurobiological elements of staging are closely related to the concept of 'allostasis', used for the first time by Sterling and Eyer (1988), and then expanded by McEwen and Stellar (1993), forming a new perspective for research on stress and its consequences. According to this concept, allostatic (adaptive) systems are set into motion in response to destabilizing environmental changes and pathogenic factors. The cumulative cost of these processes is called 'allostatic load' (AL). As allostasis is the process used to achieve stability in the face of environmental perturbations, resilience is the ability of an organism to withstand threats to stability in the environment (Karatoreos and McEwen 2013).

The concept of AL may explain vulnerability to stress and cognitive impairment in bipolar patients (Vieta et al. 2013). Biochemical mediators of AL include glucocorticoids, neurotrophic factors, the immune-inflammatory system, and oxidative stress. AL increases progressively as mood episodes occur over time, and its biochemical mediators may behave differently in subsequent stages of the illness. As consequences of AL, anatomical and functional changes in the brain may also occur, reflected in neuroimaging studies. It is, however, possible that some factors connected with resilience may influence these biochemical mediators, and, consequently, exert an effect on the processes of staging. These factors may include both inherited or acquired vulnerability as well as therapeutic interventions, both psycho- and pharmacological ones.

The hypothalamic-pituitary-adrenal (HPA), axis connected with the stress response and glucocorticoid regulation, plays an important role in the processes of AL and staging. It has been found that increased cortisol response, escape from dexamethasone suppression, or response to the dexamethasone/corticotrophin releasing hormone (dex/CRH) combination may have a relationship with increased number of prior episodes (Rybakowski and Twardowska 1999; Kunzel et al. 2003; Hennings et al. 2009).

Kapczinski et al. (2009b) have put forward the notion that other biochemical markers could be relevant in the characterization of staging. They suggest that the brain-derived neurotrophic factor (BDNF), cytokines, and elements of the antioxidant system could serve as such markers. In the early stage of bipolar illness, state-dependent changes of BDNF are observed (decrease during acute episode, increase after treatment), increase of cytokines such as interleukin (IL-6), IL-10, and tumour necrosis factor alpha (TNF-α), and increase of 3-nitrotyrosine levels. In the late stage, a decrease of BDNF is observed, an increase of inflammatory cytokines (IL-6 and TNF-α), and an increase of 3-nitrotyrosine, as well as glutathione reductase (GR) and glutathione-S-transferase (GST) activity (Andreazza et al. 2009; Kauer-Sant'Anna et al. 2009). In this same vein, our group has suggested that another potential marker of staging could be matrix metalloproteinase-9 (MMP-9), an enzyme implicated in a number of pathological conditions such as cardiovascular disease, cancer, and neuropsychiatric disorders. In our first study of serum MMP-9 in psychiatric illness we have found that younger patients with depression (below or equal to 45 years of age), both during an acute episode and in remission after depression, had significantly higher MMP-9 levels, compared to those with an acute episode and remission after mania, and control subjects (Rybakowski et al. 2013a).

Neuroanatomical correlates of BD staging include the indices of decreased volume of several brain structures, such as prefrontal cortex, anterior cingulate, and hippocampus with greater number of mood episodes and/or greater duration of the illness (Harrison and Eastwood 2001; Farrow et al. 2005; Blumberg et al. 2006). Decreases in white matter volume in bipolar patients were also reported as a function of the number of prior hospitalizations (Moore et al. 2001). In contrast to these findings, a number of studies have shown increases in amygdala volume in bipolar patients, which correlated with age and greater number of hospitalizations for mania (Altshuler et al. 2000; Usher et al. 2010).

Cognitive components of staging

In their meta-analysis, Robinson et al. (2006) found that euthymic bipolar patients show an important impairment in aspects of executive function and verbal memory. However, they did not conclude whether greater cognitive dysfunction was related to a greater number of episodes or to increased duration of illness. In addition, a number of studies performed on bipolar patients while in the euthymic state have shown correlation between existing neuropsychological deficits and a greater number of affective episodes and more severe course of illness. The first suggestions in this respect were made by Altshuler (1993) 20 years ago, stating that recurrent affective episodes may cause insults to the central nervous system, resulting in cognitive decline. Several years later, it was demonstrated that scores of executive functioning in bipolar patients were negatively correlated with the number of episodes of mania and depression (Zubieta et al. 2001). McQueen et al. (2001) showed that visual backward masking task impairment in bipolar patients was connected with past burden of illness, particularly past number of depressions; in another study, impairments of verbal learning and memory correlated with the number of manic episodes (Cavanagh et al. 2002). Clark et al. (2002) observed that sustained attention deficit was related to progression of bipolar illness. Martinez-Aran et al. (2004) have also provided evidence of neuropsychological impairment in euthymic bipolar patients in the domain of verbal memory and executive dysfunctions. Verbal memory impairment was related to a longer duration of illness, a higher number of manic episodes, and prior psychotic symptoms. More recently, verbal intelligence was shown to be the most significant predictor of the subtype of bipolar patients presenting 'good' or 'poor' outcomes (Reinares et al. 2013).

Besides causing neuropsychological deficits, recurrent affective episodes in bipolar illness constitute a risk factor for subsequent dementia. Using the Danish case registry, Kessing and Andersen (2004) found that the rate of dementia tended to increase 6% with every episode leading to admission, for patients with BD. If there was a history of four prior unipolar or bipolar depressions over one's lifetime, this was associated with a doubling of the risk for a dementia diagnosis. In American studies, including mostly patients with MDD, it was found that even the occurrence of two prior episodes of depression increased the risk of dementia (Dotson et al. 2010; Saczynski et al. 2010).

Effect of staging on the efficacy of treatment

A significant consequence of staging models is the possibility of tailoring treatment according to the stage of illness. The staging model underlines the need of early psychotherapeutic or pharmacologic intervention and defines the first episode of illness as the critical target for intervention. That would potentially be a means of prevention against clinical, neurobiological, and cognitive consequences of the illness.

As to psychotherapeutic interventions, Scott et al. (2006) reported that bipolar patients with fewer than 12 previous episodes had better response to cognitive behavioural therapy compared to those with 12 or more episodes. In a recent assessment of family psychoeducation in bipolar illness, Reinares et al. (2010) showed that patients in early stages benefitted from caregiver psychoeducation and achieved longer times to recurrence. At the same time, no significant benefits from family psychoeducation were found in patients on advanced stages.

In a review of olanzapine studies, Berk et al. (2011) showed that the response rates for the mania were significantly higher for patients having lower number of episodes (52–69% and 10–50%), for 1–5 and >5 previous episodes, respectively. For the depression studies, response rates were also higher for the 1–5 episode group. Response rates for the maintenance studies were 29–59% and 11–40% for 1–5 and >5 previous episodes, respectively, and the chance of relapse to either mania or depression was reduced by 40–60% for those who had experienced 1–5 episodes or 6–10 episodes, compared to the >10 episode group, respectively.

A number of studies have shown that lithium efficacy may be connected with the number of previous episodes. Swann et al. (1999) found a negligible effect of lithium in acute mania in patients having more than 10 previous episodes. Franchini et al. (1999) demonstrated that beginning lithium therapy within the first 10 years of bipolar illness predicts better preventive outcomes than beginning prophylaxis later. On the other hand, Ketter et al. (2006) demonstrated that early-stage (but not intermediate or later-stage) bipolar patients had a significantly lower rate of relapse/recurrence of manic/mixed episodes with olanzapine compared to lithium.

A rapid cycling course of BD has been regarded as the more severe type of trajectory, and usually occurs at later stages of the illness. A number of studies pointed to significantly worse results of monotherapy with mood stabilizers such as lithium (Dunner and Fieve 1974; Abu-Saleh and Coppen 1986), carbamazepine (McKeon et al. 1992), and valproate (Calabrese et al. 2005) in rapid cycling bipolar patients.

Lithium treatment and excellent lithium responders

In 2013, we celebrated the 50th anniversary of the first publication on lithium's prophylactic effect in affective disorder (Hartigan 1963). In 1970–1973, the results of eight controlled studies researching the prophylactic effectiveness of lithium were published. Most of these studies employed a method of comparing the course of illness in subjects in whom lithium was discontinued and replaced with a placebo, with a group of subjects who continued to receive lithium (discontinuation design). The analyses showed that the percentage of patients in whom recurrences of depression or mania occurred was significantly lower while receiving lithium (on average 30%) than while receiving placebo (on average 70%) (Schou and Thompsen 1976). However, in the late 1990s, the results of these studies were criticized on methodological grounds (Moncrieff 1997).

The prophylactic effectiveness of lithium has been confirmed in two meta-analyses performed in the first decade of the twenty-first century. Geddes et al. (2004) studied five randomized controlled trials involving 770 patients, and showed that lithium was more effective than placebo in preventing all relapses, with a relative risk (RR) of 0.65, being slightly better against manic recurrences (RR = 0.62) than against depressive recurrences (RR = 0.72). Nivoli et al. (2010) performed a systematic research of long-term treatment enrolling 1,561 bipolar patients with at least 6 months of follow-up, of whom 534 were randomized to lithium. They concluded that, while earlier studies suggested effectiveness of lithium against both mania and depression, more recent ones show greater evidence of the effectiveness of lithium prophylaxis against manic relapses. Nowadays, lithium is still regarded as the cornerstone of the long-term therapy of BD (Rybakowski 2011).

In 1999, the Canadian psychiatrist, Paul Grof (1999) introduced the term 'excellent lithium responders' for patients in whom lithium monotherapy can dramatically change their life, by a total prevention of further episodes. Two years later we attempted to compare bipolar patients entering lithium prophylaxis in two subsequent decades (the 1970s and 1980s). Sixty bipolar patients who entered lithium prophylaxis in the 1970s, and 49 entering prophylaxis in the 1980s, received the drug over a 10-year period. Patients not experiencing affective episodes for 10 or more years (excellent lithium responders) constituted 35% of the '1970' group of patients and 27% of those in the '1980' group. That represents overall, roughly one-third of lithium-treated bipolar patients (Rybakowski et al. 2001). In a recent paper, Grof (2010) concluded that the best response to lithium is associated with a clinical profile of an episodic clinical course, complete remission, bipolar family history, and low psychiatric comorbidity. This would reflect a 'classic' form of the bipolar disorders, whose features are similar to those described by Emil Kraepelin (1899) as *manisch-depressives Irresein*. That would also be consistent with the description of stage I patients according to Kapczinski et al. (2009a).

A meta-analysis of clinical factors associated with lithium efficacy was performed by Kleindienst et al. (2005). They investigated 42 potential clinical predictors of lithium prophylactic efficacy, based on the results of

43 studies. Two factors connected with better effect of lithium were found, namely later illness onset and an episodic pattern of mania–depression sequences. On the other hand, three factors were identified that may weaken the prophylactic effect of lithium: a high number of previous hospitalizations, continuous cycling, and an episodic pattern of depression–mania sequence. This may correspond to other studies showing that lithium is more efficacious at earlier stages of the disorder and in lower severity of the disorder. In these terms, patients at earlier stages of the illness would have a higher probability of being excellent responders to lithium.

Recently, we have performed an experimental study to delineate a specific personality profile for the best lithium response. In 71 patients treated with lithium carbonate for 5–37 years (mean 18 years), an assessment of temperamental affective profiles was carried out using the Temperament Scale of the Memphis, Pisa, Paris, and San Diego-Autoquestionnaire (TEMPS-A) (Akiskal et al. 2005), while schizotypic traits were assessed using the Oxford-Liverpool Inventory of Feelings and Experiences (O-LIFE) (Mason and Claridge 2006). The scores obtained on these scales were correlated with the assessment of prophylactic lithium efficacy using the Alda scale (Grof et al. 2002). The response to lithium correlated significantly positively with the hyperthymic temperament score, and negatively with the anxiety, cyclothymic, and depressive temperament scores (Rybakowski et al. 2013b). A significant negative correlation of lithium efficacy with cognitive disorganization was also demonstrated (Dembinska-Krajewska et al. 2012). A dimension of cognitive disorganization is highly associated with 'psychoticism' and increases the risk for schizophrenia and BD with psychotic symptoms (Schurhoff et al. 2005).

Effect of successful lithium treatment on the staging process

Successful lithium therapy may favourably influence clinical, neurobiological, and neurocognitive components of staging. Such an effect is particularly evident in the group of 'excellent lithium responders'. Due to a complete prevention of affective recurrences in excellent lithium responders, the progress of illness is halted. Significant decrease of recurrences in partial lithium responders may also result in slowing down the process of staging. However, it is also possible that excellent lithium responders, even before the treatment, may constitute a subgroup of BD with most favourable clinical course and outcome. Anyway, the clinical characteristics of excellent lithium responders, including less comorbidity and an interepisodic period free of symptoms, would place the excellent lithium responders as early-stage patients.

The effect of lithium on neurobiological components of staging may be mostly due to its neurotrophic and neuroprotective effect and to resilience promotion. Recently, Gray and McEwen (2013) suggested that lithium improves clinical symptoms by blocking stress-induced changes and facilitating neural plasticity. The most important neurobiological processes in this respect are stimulation of the BDNF system, and inhibition of glucogen synthase kinase-3beta (GSK-3β) (Quiroz et al. 2010). In molecular-genetic studies, an association of lithium efficacy with polymorphism of *BDNF* and *GSK-3β* genes was found (Benedetti et al. 2005; Rybakowski et al. 2005). In our own study we also observed an association between lithium efficacy and polymorphism of glucocorticoid receptor *(NR3C1)* gene, involved in stress regulation (Szczepankiewicz et al. 2011).

In a proposal of biochemical markers of staging, a decrease in serum BDNF has been postulated as a marker of later stage of BD (Kauer-Sant'Anna et al. 2009). In our study we have found that excellent lithium responders with long-term BD, with a mean of 21 years of lithium treatment, have normal serum BDNF levels (Rybakowski and Suwalska 2010). We have also demonstrated that sustained remission in bipolar patients, achieved mostly by lithium maintenance, brings the inflammatory cytokine status to a level similar to healthy control subjects (Remlinger-Molenda et al. 2012). A recent study showed that lithium may exert a favourable effect on oxidative stress parameters (Khairova et al. 2012).

A neuroprotective effect of lithium was also shown in neuroimaging studies, by means of an increase in cerebral grey matter volume in lithium-treated BD patients. Such an effect has not been demonstrated for any other mood-stabilizing drug. A greater cortical grey matter density in lithium-treated patients with BD was observed, especially in the dorsolateral prefrontal cortex and the anterior cingulate region (Monkul et al. 2007). In addition, a recent study (Moore et al. 2009) has shown an increase in total grey matter volume in the prefrontal cortex after 4 weeks of treatment among lithium responders. Moreover, a bilateral increase in hippocampal volume after both short term (up to 8 weeks) and long term (2–4 years) lithium administration was also shown in patients with BD (Yucel et al. 2007, 2008). In this same vein, total hippocampal volume in lithium-treated bipolar patients was significantly larger as compared to that of both unmedicated bipolar patients and healthy control subjects (Bearden et al. 2008). However, there is still controversy in the topic, as a recent study of Hajek et al. (2013) showed that the increase of hippocampal volume in bipolar patients was independent of long-term lithium response.

Comparison of the effect of lithium and valproate in 22 bipolar patients showed that lithium caused an increase in grey matter volume, associated with a positive clinical response, while valproate-treated patients did not show such an effect (Lyoo et al. 2010). A cross-sectional structural brain magnetic resonance imaging study of 74 remitted bipolar patients receiving long-term prophylactic treatment with lithium, valproate, carbamazepine, or antipsychotics showed that volume of grey matter in the subgenual anterior cingulate gyrus on the right and in the postcentral gyrus, the hippocampus/amygdala complex and the insula on the left was greater in patients on lithium treatment compared to all other treatments (Germana et al. 2010).

The enhancement of learning and memory by lithium in experimental animals has been shown in many studies (Yazlowitskaya et al. 2006; Nocjar et al. 2007; Zhang et al. 2012). On the other hand, some degree of cognitive impairment has been demonstrated in lithium-treated patients (Senturk et al. 2007; Mora et al. 2013). The studies performed by our research group showed that the preservation, or even improvement, of cognitive functions may be connected with the quality of the lithium prophylaxis. This is, to a great extent, observed in excellent lithium responders, who, even after long-term lithium treatment, have normal cognitive functions when compared to healthy matched controls (Rybakowski et al. 2009; Rybakowski and Suwalska 2010).

Several mechanisms may be responsible for a favourable effect of lithium on cognitive functions in excellent lithium responders. A possible mechanism may be connected with some antiviral properties of lithium. Dickerson et al. (2004) demonstrated that infection with herpex simplex virus may be associated with cognitive deficits in BD, whereas in our study, long-term lithium administration was connected with attenuation, or remission, of herpes infection (Rybakowski and Amsterdam 1991).

Related to the lithium effect on cognitive functions, there is a possibility that lithium could present a preventive effect against dementia in patients with BD. Nunes et al. (2007) found in their group of 114 bipolar patients that those receiving long-term lithium therapy had a decreased prevalence of Alzheimer's disease compared with patients not receiving recent lithium therapy. In the Danish epidemiological study of Kessing et al. (2010), a total of 4,856 patients with a diagnosis of a manic or mixed episode or BD at their first psychiatric contact were investigated over the study period (1995–2005). Among these patients, 50.4% were exposed to lithium, 36.7% to anticonvulsants, 88.1% to antidepressants, and 80.3% to antipsychotics. A total of 216 patients received a diagnosis of dementia during follow-up (103.6/10,000 person-years). Analysis revealed that continued treatment with lithium was associated with a reduced rate of dementia in patients with BD, in contrast to continued treatment with anticonvulsants, antidepressants, or antipsychotics.

In conclusion, a host of data obtained from clinical and neurobiological studies, and especially from the experience with so-called excellent lithium responders, suggests that successful treatment and prophylaxis with lithium may favourably influence the staging process in BD, hampering the progress of the disease. This may be reflected in the domains of clinical status, neurobiological markers, and cognitive functioning.

References

Abou-Saleh MT and Coppen A (1986) Who responds to prophylactic lithium? J Affect Disorders 10:115–125.

Akiskal HS, Akiskal KK, Haykal RF, et al. (2005) TEMPS-A: progress towards validation of a self-rated clinical version of the Temperament Evaluation of the Memphis, Pisa, Paris, and San Diego Autoquestionnaire. J Affect Disorders 85:3–16.

Altshuler LL (1993) Bipolar disorder: are repeated episodes associated with neuroanatomic and cognitive changes? Biol Psychiat 33:563–565.

Altshuler LL, Bartzokis G, Grieder T, et al. (2000) An MRI study of temporal lobe structures in men with bipolar disorder or schizophrenia. Biol Psychiat **48**:147–162.

Andreazza AC, Kapczinski F, Kauer-Sant'Anna M, et al. (2009) 3-Nitrotyrosine and glutathione and glutathione antioxidant system in patients in the early and late stages of bipolar disorder. Neuroscience **34**:263–271.

Angst J, Adolfsson R, Benazzi F, et al. (2005a) The HCL-32: towards a self-assessment tool for hypomanic symptoms in outpatients. J Affect Disorders **88**:217–233.

Angst J, Sellaro R, Stassen HH, et al. (2005b) Diagnostic conversion from depression to bipolar disorders: results of a long-term prospective study of hospital admissions. J Affect Disorders **84**:149–157.

Baethge C, Tondo L, Bratti IM, et al. (2003) Prophylaxis latency and outcome in bipolar disorders. Can J Psychiat **48**:449–457.

Bearden CE, Thompson PM, Dutton RA, et al. (2008) Three-dimensional mapping of hippocampal anatomy in unmedicated and lithium-treated patients with bipolar disorder. Neuropsychopharmacology **33**:1229–1238.

Benedetti F, Serretti A, Pontigia A, et al. (2005) Long-term response to lithium salts in bipolar illness is influenced by the glycogen synthase kinase 3-beta- 50T/C SNP. Neurosci Lett **376**:51–55.

Berk M (2009) Neuroprogression: pathways to progressive brain changes in bipolar disorder. Int J Neuropsychoph **12**:441–445.

Berk M, Brnabic A, Dodd S, et al. (2011) Does stage of illness impact treatment response in bipolar disorder? Empirical treatment data and their implication for the staging model and early intervention. Bipolar Disord **13**:87–98.

Blumberg HP, Krystal JH, Bansal R, et al. (2006) Age, rapid cycling, and pharmacotherapy effects on ventral prefrontal cortex in bipolar disorder: a cross-sectional study. Biol Psychiat **59**:611–618.

Calabrese JR, Shelton MD, Rapport DJ, et al. (2005) A 20-month, double-blind, maintenance trial of lithium versus divalproex in rapid-cycling bipolar disorder. Am J Psychiat **162**:2152–2161.

Cavanagh JT, Van Beck M, Muir W, et al. (2002) Case-control study of neurocognitive function in euthymic patients with bipolar disorder: an association with mania. Brit J Psychiat **180**:320–326.

Clark L, Iversen SD, and Goodwin GM (2002) Sustained attention deficit in bipolar disorder. Brit J Psychiat **180**:313–319.

Cosci F and Fava GA (2013) Staging of mental disorders: systematic review. Psychother Psychosom **82**:20–34.

Dembinska-Krajewska D, Kliwicki S, Chlopocka-Wozniak M, et al. (2012) Efficacy of prophylactic lithium administration in bipolar affective illness and schizotypic traits (in Polish). Farmakoterapia w Psychiatrii i Neurologii **28**:153–158.

Dickerson FB, Boronow JJ, Stallings C, et al. (2004) Infection with herpes simplex virus type 1 is associated with cognitive deficits in bipolar disorder. Biol Psychiat **55**:588–593.

Dotson VM, Beydoun MA, and Zonderman AB (2010) Recurrent depressive symptoms and the incidence of dementia and mild cognitive impairment. Neurology 75:27–34.

Dudek D, Siwek M, Zielinska D, et al. (2013) Diagnostic conversions from major depressive disorder into bipolar disorder in an outpatient setting: results of a retrospective chart review. J Affect Disorders 144:112–115.

Duffy A, Alda M, Hajek T, et al. (2010) Early stages in the development of bipolar disorder. J Affect Disorders 121:127–135.

Dunner DL and Fieve RR (1974) Clinical factors in lithium carbonate prophylaxis failure. Arch Gen Psychiat 30:229–233.

Farrow TF, Whitford TJ, Williams LM, et al. (2005) Diagnosis-related regional gray matter loss over two years in first episode schizophrenia and bipolar disorder. Biol Psychiat 58:713–723.

Franchini L, Zanardi R, Smeraldi E, et al. (1999) Early onset of lithium prophylaxis as a predictor of good long-term outcome. Eur Arch Psychiat Clin Neurosci 249:227–230.

Geddes JR, Burgess S, Kawton K, et al. (2004) Long-term lithium therapy for bipolar disorder: systematic review and meta-analysis of randomized controlled trials. Am J Psychiat 161:217–222.

Germana C, Kempton MJ, Sarnicola A, et al. (2010) The effects of lithium and anticonvulsants on brain structure in bipolar disorder. Acta Psychiat Scand 122:481–487.

Gray JD and McEwen BS (2013) Lithium's role in neural plasticity and its implications for mood disorders. Acta Psychiat Scand 128:347–361.

Grof P (1999) Excellent lithium responders: people whose lives have been changed by lithium prophylaxis. In: Birch NJ, Gallicchio VS, and Becker RW, eds. Lithium: 50 Years of Psychopharmacology, New Perspectives in Biomedical and Clinical Research. Cheshire, Connecticut: Weidner Publishing Group, pp. 36–51.

Grof P (2010) Sixty years of lithium responders. Neuropsychobiology 62:27–35.

Grof P, Duffy A, Cavazzoni P, et al. (2002) Is response to prophylactic lithium a familial trait? J Clin Psychiat 63:942–947.

Gutierrez-Rojas L, Jurado D, and Gurpegui M (2011) Factors associated with work, social life and family life disability in bipolar disorder patients. Psychiat Res 186:254–260.

Hajek T, Bauer M, Simhandl C, et al. (2013) Neuroprotective effect of lithium on hippocampal volumes in bipolar disorder independent of long-term lithium response. Psychol Med 44:507–517.

Harrison PJ and Eastwood SL (2001) Neuropathological studies of synaptic connectivity in the hippocampal formation in schizophrenia. Hippocampus 11:508–519.

Hartigan G (1963) The use of lithium salts in affective disorders. Brit J Psychiat 109:810–814.

Hennings JM, Owashi T, Binder EB, et al. (2009) Clinical characteristics and treatment outcome in a representative sample of depressed inpatients—findings from the Munich antidepressant response signature (MARS) project. J Psychiat Res **43**:215–229.

Hirschfeld RMA, Williams JBW, Spitzer RL, et al. (2000) Development and validation of a screening instrument for bipolar spectrum disorder: the Mood Disorder Questionnaire. Am J Psychiat **157**:1873–1875.

Kapczinski F, Dias VV, Kauer-Sant'Anna M, et al. (2009a) Clinical implications of a staging model for bipolar disorders. Expert Rev Neurother **9**:957–966.

Kapczinski F, Dias VV, Kauer-Sant'Anna M, et al. (2009b) The potential use of biomarkers as an adjunctive tool for staging bipolar disorder. Prog Neuro-Psychoph **33**:1366–1371.

Karatoreos IN and McEwen BS (2013) Annual Research Review: the neurobiology and physiology of resilience and adaptation across the life course. J Child Psychol Psychiat **54**:337–347.

Kauer-Sant'Anna M, Kapczinski F, Andreazza AC, et al. (2009) Brain derived neurotrophic factor and inflammatory markers in patients with early vs. late stage bipolar disorder. Int J Neuropsychoph **12**:447–458.

Kessing LV and Andersen PK (2004) Does the risk of developing dementia increase with the number of episodes in patients with depressive disorder and in patients with bipolar disorder? J Neurol Neurosurg Psychiat **75**:1662–1666.

Kessing LV, Forman JL, and Andersen PK (2010) Does lithium protect against dementia? Bipolar Disord **12**:97–94.

Ketter TA, Houston JP, Adams DH, et al. (2006) Differential efficacy of olanzapine and lithium in preventing manic or mixed recurrence in patients with bipolar I disorder based on number of previous manic or mixed episodes. J Clin Psychiat **67**:95–101.

Khairova R, Pawar R, Salvadore G, et al. (2012) Effect of lithium on oxidative stress parameters in healthy subjects. Mol Med Rep **5**:680–682.

Kleindienst N, Engel RR, and Greil W (2005) Which clinical factors predict response to prophylactic lithium? A systematic review for bipolar disorders. Bipolar Disord **7**:404–417.

Kraepelin E (1899) Psychiatrie. Ein Lehrbuch für Studierende und Ärzte. 6 Auflage. Leipzig: Barth.

Kunzel HE, Binder EB, Nickel T, et al. (2003) Pharmacological and nonpharmacological factors influencing hypothalamic-pituitary-adrenocortical axis reactivity in acutely depressed psychiatric in-patients, measured by the Dex-CRH test. Neuropsychopharmacology **28**:2169–2178.

Lyoo K, Dager SR, Kim JE, et al. (2010) Lithium-induced grey matter volume increase as a neural correlate of treatment response in bipolar disorder: a longitudinal brain imaging study. Neuropsychopharmacology **35**:1743–1750.

MacQueen GM, Young LT, Galway TM, et al. (2001) Backward masking task performance in stable, euthymic outpatients with bipolar disorder. Psychol Med **31**:1269–1277.

Magalhães PV, Dodd S, Nierenberg AA, et al. (2012) Cumulative morbidity and prognostic staging of illness in the Systematic Treatment Enhancement Program for Bipolar Disorder (STEP-BD). Aust N Z J Psychiat 46:1058–1067.

Martinez-Aran A, Vieta E, Colom F, et al. (2004) Cognitive impairment in euthymic bipolar patients: implications for clinical and functional outcome. Bipolar Disord 6:224–232.

Mason O and Claridge G (2006) The Oxford-Liverpool Inventory of Feelings and Experiences (O-LIFE): further description and extended norms. Schizophr Res 82:203–211.

McEwen BS and Stellar E (1993) Stress and the individual. Mechanisms leading to disease. Arch Intern Med 153:2093–2101.

McKeon P, Manley P, and Swanwick G (1992) Manic-depressive illness. Treatment outcome in bipolar disorder subtypes. Irish J Psychol Med 9:9–12.

Moncrieff J (1997) Lithium: evidence reconsidered. Brit J Psychiat 171:113–119.

Monkul ES, Matsuo K, Nicoletti MA, et al. (2007) Prefrontal gray matter increases in healthy individuals after lithium treatment: a voxel-based morphometry study. Neurosci Lett 429:7–11.

Moore GJ, Cortese BM, Glitz DA, et al. (2009) A longitudinal study of the effects of lithium treatment on prefrontal and subgenual prefrontal gray matter volume in treatment-responsive bipolar disorder patients. J Clin Psychiat 70:699–705.

Moore PB, Shepherd DJ, Eccleston D, et al. (2001) Cerebral white matter lesions in bipolar affective disorder: relationship to outcome. Brit J Psychiat 178:172–176.

Mora E, Portella MJ, Forcada I, et al. (2013) Persistence of cognitive impairment and its negative impact on psychosocial functioning in lithium-treated, euthymic bipolar patients: a 6-year follow-up study. Psychol Med 43:1187–1196.

Nivoli AMA, Murru A, and Vieta E (2010) Lithium: still a cornerstone in the long-term treatment in bipolar disorder? Neuropsychobiology 62:27–35.

Nocjar C, Hammonds MD, and Shim SS (2007) Chronic lithium treatment magnifies learning in rats. Neuroscience 150:774–788.

Nunes PV, Forlenza OV, and Gattaz WF (2007) Lithium and risk for Alzheimer's disease in elderly patients with bipolar disorder. Brit J Psychiat 190:359–360.

Post RM (1992) Transduction of psychosocial stress into the neurobiology of recurrent affective disorder. Am J Psychiat 149:999–1010.

Post RM, Fleming J, and Kapczinski F (2012) Neurobiological correlates of illness progression in the recurrent affective disorders. J Psychiat Res 46:561–573.

Quiroz JA, Machado-Vieira R, Zarate CA, et al. (2010) Novel insights in lithium's mechanism of action: neurotrophic and neuroprotective effects. Neuropsychobiology 62:50–60.

Reinares M, Colom F, Rosa AR, et al. (2010) The impact of staging bipolar disorder on treatment outcome of family psychoeducation. J Affect Disorders 123:81–86.

Reinares M, Papachristou E, Harvey P, et al. (2013) Towards a clinical staging for bipolar disorder: defining patient subtypes based on clinical outcome. J Affect Disorders 144:65–71.

Remlinger-Molenda A, Wojciak P, Michalak M, et al. (2012) Selected cytokine profiles during remission in bipolar patients. Neuropsychobiology 66:193–198.

Robinson LJ, Thompson JM, Gallagher P, et al. (2006) A meta-analysis of cognitive deficits in euthymic patients with bipolar disorder. J Affect Disorders 93:105–115.

Rybakowski JK (2011) Lithium in neuropsychiatry: a 2010 update. World J Biol Psychiat 12:340–348.

Rybakowski JK and Amsterdam JD (1991) Lithium prophylaxis and recurrent labial herpes infections. Lithium 2:43–47.

Rybakowski JK, Chłopocka-Woźniak M, and Suwalska A (2001) The prophylactic effect of long-term lithium administration in bipolar patients entering lithium treatment in the 1970s and 1980s. Bipolar Disord 3:63–67.

Rybakowski JK, Dembinska D, Kliwicki S, et al. (2013b) TEMPS-A and long-term lithium response: positive correlation with hyperthymic temperament. J Affect Disorders 145:187–189.

Rybakowski JK, Dudek D, Pawlowski T, et al. (2012) Use of the Hypomania Checklist-32 and the Mood Disorder Questionnaire for detecting bipolarity in 1,051 patients with major depressive disorder. Eur Psychiat 27:577–581.

Rybakowski JK, Permoda-Osip A, and Borkowska A (2009) Response to prophylactic lithium in bipolar disorder may be associated with a preservation of executive cognitive functions. Eur Neuropsychopharm 19:791–795.

Rybakowski JK, Remlinger-Molenda A, Czech-Kucharska A, et al. (2013a) Increased serum matrix metalloproteinase-9 (MMP-9) levels in young patients during bipolar depression. J Affect Disorders 146:286–289.

Rybakowski JK and Suwalska A (2010) Excellent lithium responders have normal cognitive functions and plasma BDNF levels. Int J Neuropsychoph 13:617–622.

Rybakowski JK, Suwalska A, Skibinska M, et al. (2005) Prophylactic lithium response and polymorphism of the brain-derived neurotrophic factor gene. Pharmacopsychiatry 38:166–170.

Rybakowski JK and Twardowska K (1999) The dexamethasone/corticotropin-releasing hormone test in depression in bipolar and unipolar affective illness. J Psychiat Res 33:363–370.

Saczynski JS, Beiser A, Seshadri S, et al. (2010) Depressive symptoms and risk of dementia: the Framingham heart study. Neurology 75:35–41.

Schou M and Thompsen K (1976) Lithium prophylaxis of recurrent endogenous affective disorders. In: Johnson FN, ed. Lithium Research and Therapy. London: Academic Press, pp. 63–84.

Schurhoff F, Laguerre A, Szoke A, et al. (2005) Schizotypal dimensions: continuity between schizophrenia and bipolar disorders. Schizophr Res 80:235–242.

Scott J, Paykel E, Morriss R, et al. (2006) Cognitive behavioural therapy for severe and recurrent bipolar disorders: randomised controlled trial. Brit J Psychiat **188**:313–320.

Senturk V, Goker C, Bilgic A, et al. (2007) Impaired verbal memory and otherwise spared cognition in remitted bipolar patients on monotherapy with lithium or valproate. Bipolar Disord **9**(Suppl. 1):136–144.

Sterling P and Eyer J (1988) Allostasis: a new paradigm to explain arousal pathology. In: Fisher S and Reason J, eds. Handbook of Life Stress, Cognition and Health. New York: Wiley, pp. 629–649.

Swann AC, Bowden CL, Calabrese JR, et al. (1999) Differential effect of number of previous episodes of affective disorder on response to lithium or divalproex in acute mania. Am J Psychiat **156**:1264–1266.

Szczepankiewicz A, Rybakowski JK, Suwalska A, et al. (2011) Glucocorticoid receptor polymorphism is associated with lithium response in bipolar patients. Neuro Endocrinol Lett **32**:545–551.

Usher J, Leucht S, Falkai P, et al. (2010) Correlation between amygdala volume and age in bipolar disorder e a systematic review and meta-analysis of structural MRI studies. Psychiat Res **182**:1–8.

Vieta E, Popovic D, Rosa AR, et al. (2013) The clinical implications of cognitive impairment and allostatic load in bipolar disorder. Eur Psychiat **28**:21–29.

Yazlovitskaya EM, Edwards E, Thotala D, et al. (2006) Lithium treatment prevents neurocognitive deficit resulting from cranial irradiation. Cancer Res **66**:11179–11186.

Yucel K, McKinnon MC, Taylor VH, et al. (2007) Bilateral hippocampal volume increases after long-term lithium treatment in patients with bipolar disorder: a longitudinal MRI study. Psychopharmacology 2007; **195**: 357–367.

Yucel K, Taylor VH, McKinnon MC, et al. (2008) Bilateral hippocampal volume increase in patients with bipolar disorder and short-term lithium treatment. Neuropsychopharmacology **13**:361–367.

Zhang L, Chen X, Feng W, et al. (2012) Enhancing effects of chronic lithium treatment on detour learning in chicks. Biol Trace Elem Res **148**:38–43.

Zubieta JK, Huguelet P, O'Neil RL, et al. (2001) Cognitive function in euthymic bipolar I disorder. Psychiat Res **102**:9–20.

Chapter 15

Staging and early intervention in bipolar disorder

Vicent Balanzá-Martínez, María Lacruz, and Rafael Tabarés-Seisdedos

Introduction

In psychiatry, the major focus of early intervention has been in schizophrenia, and this approach has not received comparable attention in bipolar disorder (BD) (Berk et al. 2014). At the turn of the millennium, first-episode mania was seen as 'a neglected priority for early intervention' (Conus and McGorry 2002). However, BD is associated with progressive worsening over time, as well as high rates of morbidity and mortality, and this clearly represents a persuasive rationale for early detection and intervention strategies (Berk et al. 2009).

To that end, the essential first step is early and accurate diagnosis of BD. This has proven to be a particularly complex task in clinical practice, due to the low specificity of prodromal features. In addition, patients with BD are often initially misdiagnosed with schizophrenia, personality disorders, or major depressive disorder (MDD). Reasons for misdiagnosis include the index episode being typically depressive and frequent comorbidities. Moreover, manic episodes are frequently atypical in adolescence and early adulthood, with high rates of mixed episodes and psychotic symptoms. As a result, average gaps between symptom onset and initiation of suitable treatments may be as long as a decade (Post et al. 2003). Both delayed diagnosis and introduction of mood stabilizers have a wide range of negative consequences, including increased rates of suicide, comorbidities, and hospitalizations, as well as worse psychosocial functioning and therapeutic response. Moreover, the use of non-effective medications, particularly antidepressant monotherapy, may be associated with rapid cycling and manic switching (Berk et al. 2007).

Towards earlier diagnosis of bipolar disorder

The identification of the bipolar prodromes and subjects at high risk to develop BD may clearly move the focus towards prevention in BD. On the one hand, the depiction of the clinical and neurocognitive prodromal features is an active area of research in BD. The 'prodrome' is a period of disturbance, representing a deviation from a person's previous behaviour, prior to the development of the florid manifestations of a disorder (Conus et al. 2006). There is growing evidence that symptoms can pre-date the onset of BD by months or even years. The bipolar prodrome consists of: (i) subthreshold or attenuated forms of full-blown mania and depression symptoms; (ii) personality traits, such as cyclothymia; and (iii) a wide range of symptoms common to several mental disorders, such as sleep disturbances, anxiety, irritability, or hyperactivity (Skjelstad et al. 2010; Howes et al. 2011). The initial prodrome of BD is character-ized by dysregulation of mood and energy, whereas symptoms of mania and depression seem to increase closer to the full onset of BD (Skjelstad et al. 2010). Obviously, the specificity of these prodromal symptoms is low and, compared to schizophrenia, the prodrome in BD is more pleomor-phic and non-specific. Recent data suggest that neurocognitive deficits may also precede first-episode mania (Ratheesh et al. 2013). High-risk subjects for BD may show widespread deficits in the broad domains of verbal memory and executive function, although to a lesser degree than patients (Balanzá-Martínez et al. 2008; Olvet et al. 2013).

In addition, the development of at-risk criteria for first-episode mania/BD has attracted a similar research interest. The Melbourne group has recently proposed a set of 'bipolar at-risk' (BAR) criteria, including the peak age range of the first onset of BD (aged 15–25 years), genetic risk (having a first-degree relative with BD type I (BD-I)), and presenting with subthreshold mania, cyclothymic features, or depressive symptoms (Bechdolf et al. 2012). Similarly, clusters of risk factors have been sug-gested by other groups (Leopold et al. 2012). Large-scale prospective studies are warranted to establish the validity, specificity, and sensitivity of these criteria. Although challenging, refinement of the clinical and neurocognitive prodromes/high-risk state of BD may guide the devel-opment of early intervention strategies.

The specific strategies of early intervention in bipolar disorder

Early intervention may provide a 'window of opportunity' to develop early pharmacological and psychosocial interventions that may prevent, or at least minimize, some of the morbidity associated with repeated episodes and chronicity (Macneil et al. 2012). One of the aims of staging models is to assist in treatment selection and individualized care. Specific treatments should be tailored to the clinical and therapeutic needs of subjects in each stage of the disorder. The earlier stages tend to have a better prognosis and tend to require simpler treatments. Moreover, response to treatment is generally better early in the illness course. Hence, monotherapy with mood stabilizers might be the first choice early in the course, whereas combination strategies may be necessary later on, especially for more refractory cases (Berk et al. 2014).

In the following sections, the specific strategies of early intervention are presented according to (i) their pharmacological or psychosocial nature, and (ii) their application to high-risk subjects or early stage/first episode of BD.

Pharmacological interventions in subjects at high risk for bipolar disorder

The most common age of onset of BD is adolescence. Therefore, effective and safe interventions for youth at high risk for BD could potentially delay progression to full-blown illness and improve long-term functional outcomes (DelBello and Kowatch 2006). Moreover, without early intervention, the social and emotional development of high-risk youth may be seriously compromised (Miklowitz et al. 2011). Despite the rationale for early intervention, few pharmacological trials have targeted at-risk bipolar youth. The potential iatrogenic effects of antidepressant and stimulant medications in at-risk bipolar youth prompted clinical trials of mood stabilizers and antipsychotics for the treatment of prodromal mood symptoms in this population (McNamara et al. 2012). In these studies, risk factors for developing BD have typically included having a family history and/or an early-onset mood disorder other than BD-I.

Geller et al. (1998) conducted a 6-week, double-blind, placebo-controlled trial of lithium and recruited 30 prepubescent children with MDD and family history predictors of future bipolarity, including BD-I in first- or second-degree relatives or a multigenerational/loaded MDD family history without BD. For the 24 study completers, lithium was not more effective than placebo in alleviating prepubertal MDD, as assessed with the Children's Global Assessment Scale. Four subjects receiving lithium withdrew due to adverse events, mostly cognitive impairment. Of note, only 40% of patients had a parent with BD, whereas 40% had a second-degree relative with BD and 20% a family history of MDD only. Thus, the heterogeneous pattern of family risk may have resulted in reduced response rate to lithium in this study. Moreover, the treatment period was as short as 6 weeks, and drug titration reached the targeted lithium levels only at week 3.

In a 6-week, double-blind, placebo-controlled randomized trial (Dickstein et al. 2009), lithium treatment was not associated with significant clinical improvement in 25 youth (7–17 years) suffering from severe, functionally impairing, non-episodic irritability and hyperarousal, a syndrome defined as severe mood dysregulation (SMD). Results of this study should be considered with caution because SMD may represent a developmental variant of mania, but does not map well onto any *Diagnostic and Statistical Manual of Mental Disorders* (DSM)/*International Classification of Diseases* (ICD) diagnostic category, including BD.

Chang et al. (2003) conducted a 12-week, open trial of divalproex treatment for 24 BD offspring aged 6–18 years with mood or behavioural disorders (MDD, dysthymia, cyclothymia, or attention deficit hyperactivity disorder (ADHD)) and subthreshold, mild mood symptoms. They found that 18 subjects (78% of study completers) were considered good responders to divalproex based on primary outcome criteria of 'very much improved' or 'much improved' on the Clinical Global Impressions-Improvement (CGI-I) scale. In addition, significant reductions in mood symptoms were found. No patient discontinued the study due to adverse effects, but weight gain was observed.

Moreover, open-label divalproex reduced aggression in 24 BD offspring with MDD, cyclothymia, ADHD, and oppositional defiant disorder (Saxena et al. 2006). Most patients (71%) were responders to divalproex, as defined by an improvement on the Overt Aggression Scale over the 12-week study.

In a subsequent double-blind trial, 56 children and adolescents (5–17 years) with bipolar spectrum disorders (BD not otherwise specified or cyclothymia) who had at least one biological parent with BD were randomly assigned to receive either divalproex sodium or placebo for up to 5 years (Findling et al. 2007). In contrast to previous open trials, this study failed to show any benefit for valproate monotherapy. Survival time to discontinuation for any reason or discontinuation due to a mood event (primary outcome measures) did not significantly differ between treatment groups. Moreover, decreases in mood symptoms and improvements in psychosocial functioning were also similar in both groups, suggesting that divalproex did not produce clinically meaningful improvements in this high-risk population. Divalproex was well tolerated with no patient discontinuing the trial due to adverse effects.

So far, only one study has examined the efficacy of a second-generation antipsychotic (SGA) for the treatment of mood symptoms in BD offspring. In a 12-week, single-blind trial of quetiapine, DelBello et al. (2007) recruited 20 symptomatic adolescents (12–18 years) with an early-onset mood disorder other than BD-I (BD type II, BD not otherwise specified, cyclothymia, dysthymia, and MDD) and at least one first-degree relative with BD-I. They found that 87% of subjects were responders to quetiapine (300–600 mg/day) as defined by a CGI-I score of 'very much improved' or 'much improved' at endpoint. Moreover, manic and depressive symptoms decreased and overall functioning improved over time. Overall, quetiapine was well tolerated. Significant increase in body weight and somnolence were common, but did not result in study discontinuation. These findings require replication with placebo-controlled studies of quetiapine and other SGAs. A further limitation of the latter two studies is that most of participants might no longer be considered 'high risk', since they already suffered from a bipolar spectrum disorder.

To date, six early intervention trials have examined the efficacy, safety, and tolerability of pharmacological agents in at-risk bipolar youth. Most trials have involved mood stabilizers, such as lithium and valproate. The methodological differences between these studies, including sample characteristics and primary outcome measures, limit establishing recommendations for specific pharmacotherapies in early stages of BD. In addition, study duration was longer than 12 weeks in only one case (Findling et al. 2007). Overall, modal duration of studies is insufficient to examine the long-term safety and efficacy of medications. This is a critical issue, given that early interventions targeting the prodrome/high-risk state need to be safe and well tolerated with long-term administration. Moreover, the long-term effects of medications on brain development are largely ignored (McNamara et al. 2012). Randomized trials with larger samples are warranted to examine the effectiveness of medications in these populations.

Pharmacological interventions in first-episode and early-stage bipolar disorder

Stage-related differences in the efficacy of treatments at various phases in the course of BD have been shown in several studies (Berk et al. 2013). The efficacy of lithium is consistently reduced with successive episodes (Gelenberg et al. 1989; Swann et al. 1999; for a discordant result, see Baldessarini et al. 2003). Similarly, patients at the earliest stages of BD showed a more favourable response to treatment with the SGA olanzapine on measures of mania, depression, overall global impression, and relapse (Berk et al. 2011a). Thus, response to certain medications would be greater in early-stage BD. Moreover, pharmacological interventions in early-stage BD may slow the progression of BD, reverse some biological abnormalities, and improve the overall prognosis (Salvadore et al. 2008). The first episode is thus seen as a critical window for early intervention. Despite this evidence and the distinguishing features of first-episode BD, there is relatively lack of detailed information about the most suitable pharmacological treatments at this stage (Berk et al. 2007; Scott 2012). Overall, clinical guidelines for BD have not addressed this topic. Nevertheless, prophylactic medication should be considered following a single severe manic episode (Goodwin 2009).

Early psychosocial interventions

Cognitive behavioural therapy (CBT), psychoeducation, family-focused therapy (FFT), and interpersonal therapy have consistently shown to improve clinical course and outcomes in BD. To date, controlled trials of these psychotherapies have focused almost entirely on patients with a chronic BD. Interestingly, these evidence-based psychological interventions may be particularly effective on early-stage BD (Berk et al. 2014). A review by Lam et al. (2009) suggested that CBT is effective in preventing or delaying relapse regardless the number of previous episodes. However, a large trial ($n = 252$) found that CBT was more effective in patients in the early stages of BD (between episodes 1 and 6), whereas those with more than 12 episodes deteriorated with CBT compared to treatment as usual (Scott et al. 2006). Moreover, Reinares et al. (2010) reported that patients with the smallest number of previous episodes obtained the greatest benefit from psychoeducation. Accordingly, response to both medications and adjunctive psychotherapies seems to decrease as the illness becomes more chronic, which reinforces the key role of early intervention. However, such interventions should be adapted to the specific needs and features of high-risk and early-stage subjects.

Psychosocial interventions in high-risk subjects

Psychotherapies, particularly those involving psychoeducation and skill training, may provide a treatment alternative for high-risk youth, especially if children and adolescents decline medications or experience significant side effects (Miklowitz et al. 2011). So far, very few early intervention trials have examined psychosocial effects in subjects at risk for BD.

In a 1-year open trial, family-focused treatment adapted for youth at high risk for BD (FFT-HR) was tested among 13 subjects with: (i) at least one biological parent with BD; (ii) DSM 4th edition (DSM-IV) criteria for MDD, cyclothymia, or BD not otherwise specified; and (iii) active mood symptoms in the past month (Miklowitz et al. 2011). The 4-month FFT-HR consisted of 12 sessions of psychoeducation, and training in communication and problem-solving skills. The intervention proved to be feasible and acceptable. FFT-HR resulted in significant reductions in depression and hypomania symptoms and improvements in global functioning over 1 year.

These results have been recently confirmed by the same group in a randomized trial (Miklowitz et al. 2013). Using the same inclusion criteria, 40 youth at high risk for BD were randomly allocated to a 4-month FFT-HR programme or a control group consisting of brief psychoeducation (1–2 family sessions). FFT-HR was associated with more rapid recovery from depression, less time ill, and less severe manic symptoms over 1 year. Thus, family intervention may help sustain recovery from mood symptoms among youth at high risk for BD. Moreover, greater benefits of FFT-HR were found in families with high expressed emotion (EE) versus families with low EE. Nevertheless, randomized trials with longer follow-up periods (e.g. following participants into young adulthood) are needed to establish whether the addition of early psychosocial interventions to usual care can reduce the risk of syndromal conversion to BD among genetically vulnerable youth.

In addition, Nadkarni and Fristad (2010) found that psychoeducational interventions may protect depressed children from conversion to bipolar spectrum disorders. In an 18-month study, 165 prepubertal children (8–11 years at baseline) with a mood disorder diagnosis participating in the Multi-Family Psychoeducational Psychotherapy (MF-PEP) treatment study were assigned to immediate treatment with MF-PEP or a 1-year wait-list control condition. Participation in the MF-PEP group was associated with a four-fold reduction in risk for conversion.

Psychosocial interventions in the first episode and early stages of bipolar disorder

Despite the use of evidence-based pharmacotherapies, studies of first-episode mania have shown a gap between syndromal and functional recovery (e.g. Tohen et al. 2003). Adjunctive psychotherapies may help bridge this gap. The core elements of psychosocial interventions in early-stage BD should encompass psychoeducation, CBT, vocational and educational functioning, relapse prevention, and FFT (McMurrich et al. 2012). Multicomponent, comprehensive programmes need to specifically target subthreshold mood symptoms and comorbid conditions, especially substance misuse, as well as educational and vocational counselling, medication adherence, and issues of functional recovery (Berk et al. 2007; McMurrich et al. 2012).

Very few studies have addressed psychological interventions at subjects in the early stages of BD. In a small, open trial of CBT for seven individuals recently diagnosed with BD-I (Jones and Burrell-Hodgson 2008), patients were able to identify significantly more early 'warning signs' of both mania and depression, and used significantly more adaptive coping strategies for the management of mania. Moreover, substantial reductions in subsyndromal symptoms were observed along with stability of sleep/wake cycles. The intervention proved to be acceptable and feasible. However, results of this pilot study are limited by its small sample size, and the lack of both objective measures of mood and a comparison group. The same group is currently conducting a single-blind, randomized trial for individuals within the first 5 years since onset of BD (Jones et al. 2012). Moreover, a manualized psychological intervention has recently shown to be feasible in clinical practice for young patients with a first episode of psychotic mania (Macneil et al. 2012).

Future prospects and conclusions

There is growing evidence that early identification and treatment may improve long-term outcomes of BD. Given the significant developments during the last decade, early intervention in BD has already a robust dataset suggesting its clinical validity. However, a handful clinical trials have specifically targeted subjects at risk or in the early stage of BD and, notably, there has been no prospective prevention study in this area. The following suggestions may help move the field forward.

First, early intervention strategies should have neuroprotective properties aimed to potentially minimize the neurostructural and neurocognitive changes associated with neuroprogression and ultimately their impact on functional outcomes. Several medications, such as lithium, valproate, and some atypical antipsychotics, share many effects on pathways regulating neurogenesis, inflammation, and oxidative stress (Berk et al. 2011b).

Second, nutritional and lifestyle interventions may also hold the promise to arrest the progression of the disorder. For instance, supplementation with omega-3 polyunsaturated fatty acids (n-3 PUFAs) has shown protective effects in youth at ultra-high-risk for psychosis (Amminger et al. 2010). Thus, monotherapy with n-3 PUFAs may offer similar benefits in early-stage BD, and clinical trials are warranted (McNamara and Strawn 2013). These nutrients have demonstrated efficacy to improve bipolar depression and may also improve the physical health of BD patients (Balanzá-Martínez et al. 2011).

Third, early psychological intervention should also target neurocognitive impairment, which represents a core feature of BD and, notably, leads to functional impairment also in early-stage BD (Torres et al. 2011). Neurocognitive deficits have been correlated with several indicators of illness severity, particularly the number of past episodes. Therefore, the early use of cognitive and functional remediation (Martínez-Arán et al. 2011; Fuentes-Durá et al. 2012) may also improve long-term functional outcomes.

Fourth, a more comprehensive model of staging has recently posited that early, non-specific intervention, such as non-pharmacological and self-managing strategies, may be efficacious to prevent the transition to psychiatric disorders in general, not only psychosis (McGorry and van Os 2013). In general, non-pharmacological strategies, such as family intervention, cognitive remediation, supplementation with omega-3 PUFAs, and education in healthy lifestyle habits, are recommended for the earliest stages, while antipsychotic medication and supported employment are suggested for the late prodromal stage (Scott et al. 2013).

Fifth, evidence from programmes of first-episode schizophrenia could be transferred to first-episode BD. In schizophrenia, the early use of evidence-based interventions has shown a reduction in transition rates to the first episode of psychosis. Moreover, programmes including long-term family interventions and psychosocial interventions obtained better results in terms of treatment adherence, social functioning, and durability of therapeutic effects (McFarlane 2011).

Finally, all these interventions are to be implemented in mental health services. Early detection and intervention services for psychosis have been successfully developed in several countries. Whether similar specialized services are useful in BD is currently under investigation. According to a recent trial, treatment in a specialized mood disorder clinic early in the course of BD proved superior to treatment as usual, reduced readmission to a psychiatric hospital and increased patients satisfaction with care (Kessing et al. 2013). Early access to services providing structured, comprehensive, and age-appropriate interventions, including evidence-based medications psychosocial approaches, is enthusiastically recommended (Scott 2012).

In summary, it is hoped that further development of early intervention strategies and services will transform the prognosis and care of BD in the next decades.

References

Amminger GP, Schäfer MR, Papageorgiou K, et al. (2010) Long-chain omega-3 fatty acids for indicated prevention of psychotic disorders: a randomized, placebo-controlled trial. Arch Gen Psychiat **67**:146–154.

Balanzá-Martínez V, Fries GR, Colpo GD, et al. (2011) The therapeutic use of omega-3 fatty acids in bipolar disorder. Exp Rev Neurother **11**:1029–1047.

Balanzá–Martínez V, Rubio C, Selva–Vera G, et al. (2008) Neurocognitive endophenotypes (endophenocognitypes) from studies of relatives of bipolar disorder subjects: a systematic review. Neurosci Biobehav R **32**:1426–1438.

Baldessarini RJ, Tondo L, and Hennen J (2003) Treatment latency and previous episodes: relationship to pretreatment morbidity and response to maintenance treatment in bipolar I and II disorders. Bipolar Disord **5**:169–179.

Bechdolf A, Ratheesh A, Wood SJ, et al. (2012) Rationale and first results of developing at-risk (prodromal) criteria for bipolar disorder. Curr Pharm Des **18**:358–375.

Berk M, Berk L, Dodd S, et al. (2014) Stage managing bipolar disorder. Bipolar Disord **16**(5):471–457.

Berk M, Brnabic A, Dodd S, et al. (2011a) Does stage of illness impact treatment response in bipolar disorder? Empirical treatment data and their implication for the staging model and early intervention. Bipolar Disord **13**:87–98.

Berk M, Hallam K, Lucas N, et al. (2007) Early intervention in bipolar disorders: opportunities and pitfalls. Med J Aust **187**(7 Suppl):S11–S14.

Berk M, Kapczinski F, Andreazza AC, et al. (2011b) Pathways underlying neuroprogression in bipolar disorder: focus on inflammation, oxidative stress and neurotrophic factos. Neurosci Biobehav R **35**:804–817.

Berk M, Malhi GS, Hallam K, et al. (2009) Early intervention in bipolar disorders: clinical, biochemical and neuroimaging imperatives. J Affect Disorders **114**:1–13.

Chang KD, Dienes K, Blasey C, et al. (2003) Divalproex monotherapy in the treatment of bipolar offspring with mood and behavioral disorders and at least mild affective symptoms. J Clin Psychiat 64:936–942.

Conus P, Berk M, and McGorry PD (2006) Pharmacological treatment in the early phase of bipolar disorders: what stage are we at? Aust N Z J Psychiat 40:199–207.

Conus P and McGorry PD (2002) First-episode mania: a neglected priority for early intervention. Aust N Z J Psychiat 36:158–172.

DelBello MP, Adler CM, Whitsel RM, et al. (2007) A 12-week single-blind trial of quetiapine for the treatment of mood symptoms in adolescents at high risk for developing bipolar I disorder. J Clin Psychiat 68:789–795.

DelBello MP and Kowatch RA (2006) Pharmacological interventions for bipolar youth: developmental considerations. Dev Psychopathol 18:1231–1246.

Dickstein DP, Towbin KE, Van Der Veen JW, et al. (2009) Randomized double-blind placebo-controlled trial of lithium in youths with severe mood dysregulation. J Child Adol Psychop 19:61–73.

Findling RL, Frazier TW, Youngstrom EA, et al. (2007) Double-blind, placebo-controlled trial of divalproex monotherapy in the treatment of symptomatic youth at high risk for developing bipolar disorder. J Clin Psychiat 68:781–788.

Fuentes-Durá I, Balanzá-Martínez V, Ruiz-Ruiz JC, et al. (2012) Neurocognitive training in patients with bipolar disorders—current status and perspectives. Psychother Psychosom 81:250–252.

Gelenberg AJ, Kane JM, Keller MB, et al. (1989) Comparison of standard and low serum levels of lithium for maintenance treatment of bipolar disorder. N Engl J Med 321:1489–1493.

Geller B, Cooper TB, Zimerman B, et al. (1998) Lithium for prepubertal depressed children with family history predictors of future bipolarity: a double-blind, placebo-controlled study. J Affect Disorders 51:165–175.

Goodwin GM (2009) Evidence-based guidelines for treating bipolar disorder: revised second edition—recommendations from the British Association for Psychopharmacology. J Psychopharmacol 23:346–388.

Howes OD, Lim S, Theologos G, et al. (2011) A comprehensive review and model of putative prodromal features of bipolar affective disorder. Psychol Med 41:1567–1577.

Jones SH and Burrell-Hodgson G (2008) Cognitive-behavioural treatment of first diagnosis bipolar disorder. Clin Psychol Psychother 15:367–377.

Jones S, Mulligan LD, Law H, et al. (2012) A randomised controlled trial of recovery focused CBT for individuals with early bipolar disorder. BMC Psychiat 12:204.

Kessing LV, Hansen HV, Hvenegaard A, et al. (2013) Treatment in a specialised out-patient mood disorder clinic v. standard out-patient treatment in the early course of bipolar disorder: randomised clinical trial. Brit J Psychiat 202:212–219.

Lam DH, Burbeck R, Wright K, et al. (2009) Psychological therapies in bipolar disorder: the effect of illness history on relapse prevention–a systematic review. Bipolar Disord 11:474–482.

Leopold K, Ritter P, Correll CU, et al. (2012) Risk constellations prior to the development of bipolar disorders: rationale of a new risk assessment tool. J Affect Disorders **136**:1000–1010.

Macneil CA, Hasty M, Cotton S, et al. (2012) Can a targeted psychological intervention be effective for young people following a first manic episode? Results from an 18-month pilot study. Early Interv Psychiat **6**:380–388.

Martínez-Arán A, Torrent C, Solé B, et al. (2011) Functional remediation for bipolar disorder. Clin Pract Epidemiol Ment Health **7**:112–116.

McFarlane WR (2011) Prevention of the first episode of psychosis. Psychiatr Clin N Am **34**:95–107.

McGorry P and van Os J (2013) Redeeming diagnosis in psychiatry: timing versus specificity. Lancet **381**:343–345.

McMurrich S, Sylvia LG, Dupuy JM, et al. (2012) Course, outcomes, and psychosocial interventions for first-episode mania. Bipolar Disord **14**:797–808.

McNamara RK and Strawn JR (2013) Role of long-chain omega-3 fatty acids in psychiatric practice. Pharma Nutrition **1**:41–49.

McNamara RK, Strawn JR, Chang KD, et al. (2012) Interventions for youth at high risk for bipolar disorder and schizophrenia. Child Adol Psych Cl **21**:739–751.

Miklowitz DJ, Chang KD, Taylor DO, et al. (2011) Early psychosocial intervention for youth at risk for bipolar I or II disorder: a one-year treatment development trial. Bipolar Disord **13**:67–75.

Miklowitz DJ, Schneck CD, Singh MK, et al. (2013) Early intervention for symptomatic youth at risk for bipolar disorder: a randomized trial of family-focused therapy. J Am Acad Child Adolesc Psy **52**:121–131.

Nadkarni RB and Fristad MA (2010) Clinical course of children with a depressive spectrum disorder and transient manic symptoms. Bipolar Disord **12**:494–503.

Olvet DM, Burdick KE, and Cornblatt BA (2013) Assessing the potential to use neurocognition to predict who is at risk for developing bipolar disorder: a review of the literature. Cogn Neuropsychiat **18**:129–145.

Post RM, Leverich GS, Altshuler L, et al. (2003) An overview of recent findings of the Stanley Foundation Bipolar Network (Part I). Bipolar Disord **5**:310–319.

Ratheesh A, Lin A, Nelson B, et al. (2013) Neurocognitive functioning in the prodrome of mania—an exploratory study. J Affect Disorders **147**:441–445.

Reinares M, Colom F, Rosa AR, et al. (2010) The impact of staging bipolar disorder on treatment outcome of family psychoeducation. J Affect Disorders **123**:81–86.

Salvadore G, Drevets WC, Henter ID, et al. (2008) Early intervention in bipolar disorder, part I: clinical and imaging findings. Early Interv Psychiat **2**:122–135.

Saxena K, Howe M, Simeonova D, et al. (2006) Divalproex sodium reduces overall aggression in youth at high risk for bipolar disorder. J Child Adol Psychop **16**:252–259.

Scott J (2012) Beyond psychosis: the challenge of early intervention in bipolar disorders. Rev Psiquiatr Salud Ment (Barc.) **5**:1–4.

Scott J, Leboyer M, Hickie I, et al. (2013) Clinical staging in psychiatry: a cross-cutting model of diagnosis with heuristic and practical value. Brit J Psychiat 202:243–245.

Scott J, Paykel E, Morriss R, et al. (2006) Cognitive-behavioural therapy for severe and recurrent bipolar disorders: randomised controlled trial. Brit J Psychiat 188:310–320.

Skjelstad DV, Malt UF, and Holte A (2010) Symptoms and signs of the initial pro-drome of bipolar disorder: a systematic review. J Affect Disorders 126:1–13.

Swann AC, Bowden CL, Calabrese JR, et al. (1999) Differential effect of number of previous episodes of affective disorder on response to lithium or divalproex in acute mania. Am J Psychiat 156:1264–1266.

Tohen M, Zarate CA Jr, Hennen J, et al. (2003) The McLean-Harvard First-Episode Mania Study: prediction of recovery and first recurrence. Am J Psychiat 160:2099–2107.

Torres IJ, DeFreitas CM, DeFreitas VG, et al. (2011) Relationship between cognitive functioning and 6-month clinical and functional outcome in patients with first manic episode bipolar I disorder. Psychol Med 41:971–982.

Chapter 16

Pharmacological treatment of late-stage bipolar disorder

Aline André Rodrigues and Mauricio Kunz

Introduction

The concept of illness progression and clinical staging in bipolar disorder (BD) is a relatively new idea. Therefore, clinical evidence on the pharmacological treatment of late-stage bipolar disorder is still scarce.

The course of bipolar disorder is considerably heterogeneous—while some patients recover well even after several episodes, others show increased illness severity from the onset of symptoms (Berk et al. 2007b; Kapczinski et al. 2009). These contrasting findings may be due, at least in part, to different patterns of vulnerability and resilience found in this population (McEwen and Wingfield 2003; Caspi and Moffit 2006; Vieta et al. 2012).

For many patients, especially if associated with inadequate treatment, BD presents a progressively deteriorating course. Based on this assumption, a clinical staging model for BD has been proposed (Berk et al. 2007a; Kapczinski ct al. 2009; Reinares et al. 2013). Different models have been suggested for BD, always relying on the premise that the illness progresses from latent, asymptomatic stages to more advanced, chronic stages, in which symptoms do not completely remit (Berk et al. 2007b; Kapczinski et al. 2009). Early stages of illness are characterized by a history of few previous mood episodes and full functional recovery in the euthymic interval between them. Late stages are characterized by chronic cognitive and functional impairment, often with subsyndromal mood symptoms. In this vein, progression of BD has been associated with higher rates of comorbidity (Matza et al. 2005), higher risk of hospitalization (Goldberg and Ernst 2002), and suicide (Hawton et al. 2005), as well as with lower responsiveness to treatment (Ketter et al. 2006; Scott et al. 2006).

The objective of this chapter is to review the cognitive and functional impairment in the late stage, as well as the few studies examining the impact of illness progression on treatment response.

Late stage: cognition and function

Cognitive deficits are related to a worse clinical course and poorer psychosocial functioning (Mur et al. 2009; Bonnín et al. 2012). These deficits are primarily observed during acute episodes, but some of them persist, in a milder form, during clinical remission (Torres et al. 2007; Bora et al. 2010). Findings such as impaired working memory and visual memory are more likely to remit during euthymia, whereas problems in executive function, verbal memory, and selective attention can be present even during remission of mood states (Goldberg and Chengappa 2009). These cognitive impairments seem to become especially significant with cumulative episodes, and have been demonstrated mainly for executive functions (Torres et al. 2007). Moderate cognitive deficits were observed in other domains such as verbal memory, response inhibition, sustained attention, psychomotor speed, abstraction, and set-shifting (Robinson and Ferrier 2006; Mur et al. 2007).

BD has been initially thought to show functional recovery in interepisode periods but most of the current studies point to marked cognitive impairments, even during euthymia. Impairment may affect various areas of functioning—for example, autonomy, work, cognition, interpersonal relationships, and financial status (Rosa et al. 2008)—and seems to take place already at the initial phases of illness, during the first mood episode (Nehra et al. 2006), becoming more pronounced as the illness progresses (Rosa et al. 2012). Impairment in remembering long-term information has been associated with lower occupational functioning in BD (Martinez-Aran et al. 2007).

Torrent et al. (2013) recently published the first randomized controlled trial of the efficacy of a new therapy called 'functional remediation'. This therapy includes neurocognitive techniques, training, psychoeducation on cognition-related issues, and problem solving and had a large effect on functioning—notably on occupational and interpersonal domains. Furthermore, the identification of these cumulative impairments of functioning (Rosa et al. 2012) and cognition (Kessing and Andersen 2004), associated with multiple episodes has led to a new understanding of the natural course of BD.

Future research is necessary to identify new therapeutic strategies focused on preventing the progression of bipolar disorder, as well as on restoring the cognitive and functional ability of these patients.

Treatment in the late stage

Only a few studies have investigated the impact of stage of illness on treatment response rates. The first investigated the relationship between number of lifetime episodes of affective disorder and the antimanic response to lithium, divalproex, or placebo. An apparent transition in the relationship between number of previous episodes and response to antimanic medication occurred at about 10 previous episodes. Patients with a history of many previous episodes presented a poor response to lithium, but not divalproex (Swann et al. 1999).

A more recent study performed a pooled data analysis of several trials of olanzapine for mania, depression, and maintenance. Individuals were categorized as having had 0, 1–5, 6–10, or >10 prior illness, and data were analysed across these groups. Participants in the 1–5 episode group presented significantly higher response rates when compared with participants who had >10 previous episodes for either mania or depression trials. In maintenance trials of olanzapine, there was a 60% reduction in the chance of relapse into mania, and a 40% reduction in the chance of relapse into depression for participants with 1–5 previous episodes, compared with participants who had recorded >10 previous episodes. However, only relapse into mania was statistically significant. In general terms, the study found a clear association between a larger number of episodes and a poorer response to therapy in patients with BD during treatment with olanzapine (Berk et al. 2011). Not a single clinical trial has examined the impact of this particular definition of staging on response to treatment with medication. Nevertheless, one study has investigated the impact of staging on treatment outcome of family psychoeducation. In a post hoc analysis from a 15-month randomized controlled trial showing the efficacy of group psychoeducation for caregivers in the prophylaxis of recurrences of mood episodes, patients in the early stage clearly benefitted from the intervention by having a longer time to recurrence. On the other hand, no significant benefits from caregiver psychoeducation were found in patients in the late stage (Reinares et al. 2010). In addition, Colom et al. (2010) highlighted the importance of early intervention, showing the lack of efficacy of group psychoeducation in patients with more than 15 previous episodes, who were euthymic at the study onset.

These few studies allow for one general conclusion: individuals with BD at the earliest stages of illness consistently have a more favourable response to treatment. In light of current evidences of neuroprogression (Berk et al. 2007b; Kapczinski et al. 2009), this conclusion highlights the importance of early diagnosis and early intervention. However, it does not add to the important task of adequately managing and treating late-stage patients. In fact, the paucity of data only evidences the need for clinical trials assessing the efficacy of treatments in different stages of BD. In addition, the assessment of the literature makes clear the need for the development of specific interventions for late-stage patients, focusing not only on acute treatment or prevention of mood recurrences but also on cognitive and functional remediation (see Fig. 16.1).

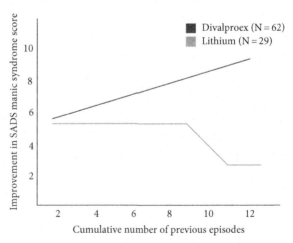

Fig. 16.1 Previous episodes of affective disorder and response to treatment in patients with acute mania.

Source data from Swann et al., 1999.

Treatment-resistant patients

Defining refractoriness in BD is complex and should concern and include either every phase and pole, or the disorder as a whole (Foun-toulakis 2012). Even though there are no specific trials with late-stage patients, the notion of treatment-resistant patients might add to the clinical management. Frequent episodic recurrences can lead to progressive treatment failures and development of treatment refractoriness. Therefore, there are data on treatment-resistant patients that deserve consideration. A recent literature review found that therapeutic trials for treatment-resistant mania are uncommon, and provide few promising leads other than the use of clozapine—which will be discussed later (Poon et al. 2012).

Bipolar disorders (types I and II) show an excess of depressive morbidity (Tondo et al. 2014). Therapeutic trials for treatment-resistant bipolar depression have assessed a wide range of treatment options, including anticonvulsants, modern antipsychotics, NMDA antagonists, dopamine agonists, calcium-channel blockers, and thyroid hormones, as well as behavioural therapy, sleep deprivation, light therapy, electroconvulsive therapy (ECT), and transcranial magnetic stimulation. We found just five controlled trials of treatment-resistant depression. The studies examined the effects of ketamine, modafinil, pramipexole, lamotrigine, inositol, and risperidone (Tondo et al. 2014). Although treatment resistance is highly prevalent in bipolar depression, there is a paucity in level I evidence, highlighting the urgent need for further studies.

Sienaert et al. (2009) compared unilateral and bifrontal ECT in patients with unipolar ($n = 51$) and bipolar depression ($n = 13$). Response rates did not differ between the groups, but the group with bipolar depression received fewer ECT treatments than unipolar patients. Another study compared unilateral, bifrontal, and bitemporal ECT in unipolar and bipolar disorder patients and all the techniques observed were equally effective in both groups (Bailine et al. 2010). ECT has proven antimanic properties, and can be used in the maintenance treatment of BD (Sienaert and Peuskens 2006). The review concludes that all of these seem promising but limited in effectiveness. Also, several of these

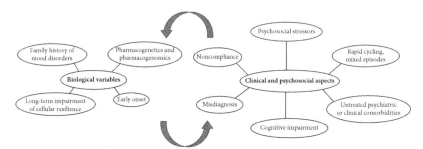

Fig. 16.2 Biological, clinical, and environmental factors involved in the pathophysiology of treatment-resistant mood disorders.

Source data from Machado-Vieira et al., 2007.

pharmacological treatments have some support for the long-term treatment of resistant BD, but most of these trials have been methodologically limited. Another important issue raised in this review is that the definition of treatment resistance may vary among investigators, making comparisons of interventions difficult (see Fig. 16.2).

Clozapine in late-stage bipolar disorder

The nature of the relationship between BD and schizophrenia is controversial. Schizoaffective disorder falls on a spectrum between BD and schizophrenia, and some common characteristics like therapeutic response, brain imaging findings, and phenomenology are consistent with a dimensional view (Ketter et al. 2004). In patients with treatment-resistant schizophrenia, clozapine is considered the 'gold standard' therapy, efficient in both positive and negative symptomatology (Meltzer 2012).

Initially restricted due to safety concerns, the turning point in the history of clozapine came in 1988 with publication of two landmark comparative trials demonstrating its efficacy and with its approval by the Food and Drug Administration (FDA) in 1990, which lead to the subsequent reintroduction into clinical practice (Hippius 1999). Since then, further advantages of clozapine have been identified, including improvement in cognitive function and symptoms of disorganization, improved quality of life, improved compliance, reduction in suicidality, reduction in aggression, absence of depressive effects, and continued efficacy in long-term treatment (Kang and Simpson 2010).

In fact, clozapine was the first atypical antipsychotic to be reported to improve some domains of cognition (Hagger et al. 1993) and it seems to have the ability to restore function in even the most refractory of patients (Meltzer 2012). The reason for the superior efficacy of clozapine and its positive effects on cognition are unknown, but it seems to involve modulation of neuroplasticity and connectivity, through induction of interconnected mitogenic signalling pathways, which seems to be a distinct feature from other antipsychotic drugs (Pereira et al. 2012). In animal models, clozapine significantly facilitated the potentiation of synaptic transmission and plasticity in the prefrontal cortex (Gemperle et al. 2003). Synaptic plasticity, expressed as long-term potentiation in the hippocampal–medial prefrontal cortex pathway, is considered to be involved in cognitive function and learning and memory processes (Matsumoto et al. 2008).

Müller and Heipertz (1977) treated 52 manic patients with clozapine—one half of them in monotherapy—and observed that clozapine appears to be superior in the treatment of mania. The use of atypical antipsychotics in the management of BD has increased considerably over the last decade. There is consistent evidence for atypical antipsychotics use as adjunctive therapy and monotherapy in all phases of illness (Yatham et al. 2009). Most evidence for the use of olanzapine and quetiapine comes from large randomized controlled efficacy trials sponsored by the pharmaceutical industry. Evidence for the use of clozapine in BD, however, is largely based on uncontrolled naturalistic trials and retrospective studies. Several of them have supported its efficacy in treatment-resistant BD, including mixed episodes, and rapid cycling (Frye et al. 1998) and even in reducing rehospitalization rates in patients with long-term treatment (Chang et al. 2006).

While results from retrospective chart reviews and naturalistic trials provide suggestive evidence on clozapine's utility in BD, they must be considered with caution. Probably in part because of clozapine's profile of adverse effects and lack of interest from pharmaceutical companies, no blinded clozapine trials have been conducted in patients with BD. However, two randomized trials have examined its effectiveness using open-label designs. In the first study, Barbini et al. (1997) prospectively compared adjunctive chlorpromazine to adjunctive clozapine in acutely manic patients. While the study duration was only three weeks, significant decreases in Young Mania Rating Scale (YMRS) scores were observed in both conditions, with clozapine patients showing faster responses. This study demonstrated that adjunctive clozapine was as effective as, and quicker than, an adjunctive first-generation antipsychotic in the treatment of acute mania.

In the second study, Suppes et al. (1999) compared adjunctive clozapine with treatment as usual (that is, no clozapine) in a sample of patients diagnosed with bipolar I disorder or schizoaffective disorder, bipolar type in a prospective, naturalistic, randomized 1-year study. Clinical response was defined as 30% reduction in Brief Psychiatric Rating Scale (BPRS) scores. By 6 months, response rates were 82% and 57%, in the clozapine groups and treatment as usual groups, respectively. The authors suggest that these findings demonstrate the mood-stabilizing properties for clozapine. Results from these randomized trials provide some information about clozapine's comparative utility in BD, suggesting antimanic and mood-stabilizing properties. However, though randomized, several limitations must be considered when interpreting their conclusions.

More interesting findings come from retrospective studies. For instance, in a pharmacoepidemiological study conducted in Denmark with 21,473 BD patients treated with clozapine (mean dose 307.4 mg), patients treated with the medication had a clinically significant reduction in the number of bed-days, psychiatric admissions, psychotropic co-medications, and hospital contact for self-harm/overdose, without the need for increased medical treatments (Nielsen et al. 2012). Therefore, these unique properties of clozapine on cognitive and functional outcomes of patients with schizophrenia might be particularly beneficial for patients with late-stage BD. However, evidence for this assumption is urgently needed.

Conclusion

Late-stage BD is associated with refractoriness to standard treatment options. There is a paucity of clinical trials examining the differential impact of treatments on different stages of illness, or even assessing the effectiveness of treatment strategies specifically targeted for late-stage patients.

Current evidence only highlights the need for early diagnosis and early treatment to avoid illness progression and refractoriness to treatment. Of the different agents evaluated in patients with treatment-resistant bipolar disorder, clozapine might be an interesting option given its unique effects on cognition and functionality and patients with refractory schizophrenia—further studies to demonstrate its benefits in bipolar disorder are needed though.

Future studies for late-stage BD might benefit from adding psychosocial approaches, in combination with pharmacotherapy. This may provide a means to prevent episodes but also to reduce interepisode symptoms and improve cognition and functioning.

References

Bailine S, Fink M, Knapp R, et al. (2010) Electroconvulsive therapy is equally effective in unipolar and bipolar depression. Acta Psychiat Scand 121(6):431–436.

Barbini B, Scherillo P, Benedetti F, et al. (1997) Response to clozapine in acute mania is more rapid than that of chlorpromazine. Int Clin Psychopharmacol 12(2):109–112.

Berk M, Brnabic A, Dodd S, et al. (2011) Does stage of illness impact treatment response in bipolar disorder? Empirical treatment data and their implication for the staging model and early intervention. Bipolar Disord 13(1):87–98.

Berk M, Conus P, Lucas N, et al. (2007b) Setting the stage: from prodrome to treatment resistance in bipolar disorder. Bipolar Disord 9(7):671–678.

Berk M, Hallam KT, and McGorry PD (2017a) The potential utility of a staging model as a course specifier: a bipolar disorder perspective. J Affect Disorders 100(1–3):279–281.

Bonnín CM, Sánchez-Moreno J, Martínez-Arán A, et al. (2012) Subthreshold symptoms in bipolar disorder: impact on neurocognition, quality of life and disability. J Affect Disorders 136(3):650–659.

Bora E, Fornito A, Yücel M, et al. (2010) Voxelwise meta-analysis of gray matter abnormalities in bipolar disorder. Biol Psychiat 67(11):1097–1105.

Caspi A and Moffit TE (2006) Gene–environment interactions in psychiatry: joining forces with neuroscience. Nat Rev Neurosci 7(7):583–590.

Chang JS, Ha KS, Young Lee K, et al. (2006) The effects of long-term clozapine add-on therapy on the rehospitalization rate and the mood polarity patterns in bipolar disorders. J Clin Psychiat 67(3):461–467.

Colom F, Reinares M, Pacchiarotti I, et al. (2010) Has number of previous episodes any effect on response to group psychoeducation in bipolar patients? A 5-year follow-up post-hoc analysis. Acta Neuropsychiatr 22:50–53.

Fountoulakis KN (2012) Refractoriness in bipolar disorder: definitions and evidence-based treatment. CNS Neurosci Ther 18(3):227–237.

Frye MA, Ketter TA, Altshuler LL, et al. (1998) Clozapine in bipolar disorder: treatment implications for other atypical antipsychotics. J Affect Disorders 48(2–3):91–104.

Gemperle AY, Enz A, Pozza MF, et al. (2003) Effects of clozapine, haloperidol and iloperidone on neurotransmission and synaptic plasticity in prefrontal cortex and their accumulation in brain tissue: an in vitro study. Neuroscience 117(3):681–695.

Goldberg JF and Chengappa KN (2009) Identifying and treating cognitive impairment in bipolar disorder. Bipolar Disord 11(Suppl 2):123–137.

Goldberg JF and Ernst CL (2002) Features associated with the delayed initiation of mood stabilizers at illness onset in bipolar disorder. J Clin Psychiat 63(11):985–991.

Hagger C, Buckley P, Kenny JT, et al. (1993) Improvement in cognitive functions and psychiatric symptoms in treatment-refractory schizophrenic patients receiving clozapine. Biol Psychiat 34(10):702–712.

Hawton K, Sutton L, Haw C, et al. (2005) Suicide and attempted suicide in bipolar disorder: a systematic review of risk factors. J Clin Psychiat 66(6):693–704.

Hippius H (1999) A historical perspective of clozapine. J Clin Psychiat 60(Suppl 12):22–23.

Kang X and Simpson GM (2010) Clozapine: more side effects but still the best antipsychotic. J Clin Psychiat 71(8):982–983.

Kapczinski F, Dias VV, Kauer-Sant'Anna M, et al. (2009) Clinical implications of a staging model for bipolar disorders. Expert Rev Neurother 9(7):957–966.

Kessing LV and Andersen PK (2004) Does the risk of developing dementia increase with the number of episodes in patients with depressive disorder and in patients with bipolar disorder? J Neurol Neurosurg Psychiat 75(12):1662–1666.

Ketter TA, Houston JP, Adams DH, et al. (2006) Differential efficacy of olanzapine and lithium in preventing manic or mixed recurrence in patients with bipolar I disorder based on number of previous manic or mixed episodes. J Clin Psychiat 67(1):95–101.

Ketter TA, Wang PW, Becker OV, et al. (2004) Psychotic bipolar disorders: dimensionally similar to or categorically different from schizophrenia? J Psychiat Res (1):47–61.

Martinez-Aran A, Vieta E, Torrent C, et al. (2007) Functional outcome in bipolar disorder: the role of clinical and cognitive factors. Bipolar Disord 9(1–2):103–113.

Matsumoto M, Shikanai H, Togashi H, et al. (2008) Characterization of clozapine-induced changes in synaptic plasticity in the hippocampal-mPFC pathway of anesthetized rats. Brain Res 21;1195:50–55.

Matza LS, Rajagopalan KS, Thompson CL, et al. (2005) Misdiagnosed patients with bipolar disorder: comorbidities, treatment patterns, and direct treatment costs. J Clin Psychiat 66(11):1432–1440.

McEwen BS and Wingfield JC (2003) The concept of allostasis in biology and biomedicine. Horm Behav 43(1):2–15.

Meltzer HY (2012) Clozapine. Clin Schizophr Relat Psychoses 6(3):134–144.

Muller P and Heipertz R (1977) [Treatment of manic psychosis with clozapine (author's transl)]. Fortschr Neurol Psychiatr Grenzgeb 45:420–424.

Mur M, Portella MJ, Martínez-Arán A, et al. (2007) Persistent neuropsychological deficit in euthymic bipolar patients: executive function as a core deficit. J Clin Psychiat 68(7):1078–1086.

Mur M, Portella MJ, Martinez-Aran A, et al. (2009) Influence of clinical and neuropsychological variables on the psychosocial and occupational outcome of remitted bipolar patients. Psychopathology 42(3):148–156.

Nehra R, Chakrabarti S, Pradhan BK, et al. (2006) Comparison of cognitive functions between first- and multi-episode bipolar affective disorders. J Affect Disorders 93(1–3):185–192.

Nielsen J, Kane JM, and Correll CU (2012) Real-world effectiveness of clozapine in patients with bipolar disorder: results from a 2-year mirror-image study. Bipolar Disord 14(8):863–869.

Pereira A, Sugiharto-Winarno A, Zhang B, et al. (2012) Clozapine induction of ERK1/2 cell signalling via the EGF receptor in mouse prefrontal cortex and striatum is distinct from other antipsychotic drugs. Int J Neuropsychoph 15(8):1149–1160.

Poon SH, Sim K, Sum MY, et al. (2012) Evidence-based options for treatment-resistant adult bipolar disorder patients. Bipolar Disord 14(6):573–584.

Reinares M, Colom F, Rosa AR, et al. (2010) The impact of staging bipolar disorder on treatment outcome of family psychoeducation. J Affect Disorders 123(1–3):81–86.

Reinares M, Papachristou E, Harvey P, et al. (2013) Towards a clinical staging for bipolar disorder: defining patient subtypes based on functional outcome. J Affect Disorders 144(1–2):65–71.

Robinson LJ and Ferrier IN (2006) Evolution of cognitive impairment in bipolar disorder: a systematic review of cross-sectional evidence. Bipolar Disord 8(2):103–116.

Rosa AR, Franco C, Martínez-Aran A, et al. (2008) Functional impairment in patients with remitted bipolar disorder. Psychother Psychosom 77(6):390–392.

Rosa AR, González-Ortega I, González-Pinto A, et al. (2012) One-year psychosocial functioning in patients in the early vs. late stage of bipolar disorder. Acta Psychiat Scand 125(4):335–341.

Scott J, Paykel E, Morriss R, et al. (2006) Cognitive-behavioural therapy for severe and recurrent bipolar disorders: randomised controlled trial. Brit J Psychiat 188:313–320.

Sienaert P and Peuskens J (2006) Electroconvulsive therapy: an effective therapy of medication-resistant bipolar disorder. Bipolar Disord 8(3):304–306.

Sienaert P, Vansteelandt K, Demyttenaere K, et al. (2009) Ultra-brief pulse ECT in bipolar and unipolar depressive disorder: differences in speed of response. Bipolar Disord 11(4):418–424.

Suppes T, Webb A, Paul B, et al. (1999) Clinical outcome in a randomized 1-year trial of clozapine versus treatment as usual for patients with treatment-resistant illness and a history of mania. Am J Psychiat **156**(8):1164–1169.

Swann AC, Bowden CL, Calabrese JR, et al. (1999) Differential effect of number of previous episodes of affective disorder on response to lithium or divalproex in acute mania. Am J Psychiat **156**(8):1264–1266.

Tondo L, Vázquez GH, and Baldessarini RJ (2014) Options for pharmacological treatment of refractory bipolar depression. Curr Psychiat Rep **16**(2):431.

Torrent C, Bonnin Cdel M, Martınez-Aran A, et al. (2013) Efficacy of functional remediation in bipolar disorder: a multicenter randomized controlled study. Am J Psychiat **170**:852–859.

Torres IJ, Boudreau VG, and Yatham LN (2007) Neuropsychological functioning in euthymic bipolar disorder: a meta-analysis. Acta Psychiat Scand Suppl **434**:17–26.

Vieta E, Popovic D, Rosa AR, et al. (2012) The clinical implications of cognitive impairment and allostatic load in bipolar disorder. Eur Psychiat **28**:21–29.

Yatham LN, Kennedy SH, Schaffer A, et al. (2009) Canadian Network for Mood and Anxiety Treatments (CANMAT) and International Society for Bipolar Disorders (ISBD) collaborative update of CANMAT guidelines for the management of patients with bipolar disorder: update 2009. Bipolar Disord **11**(3):225–255.

Chapter 17

Illness progression and psychosocial interventions in bipolar disorder

María Reinares and Francesc Colom

Introduction

In contrast to the original thought that bipolar patients achieved overall recovery between episodes, it is now clear that persistent clinical and subthreshold symptomatology (Judd et al. 2002, 2003), cognitive deficits (Martínez-Arán et al. 2004), and functional impairment (Rosa et al. 2010) are common characteristics of the course of the illness in a high percentage of patients, even when they receive adequate treatment. It is clear, on the basis of the years lost due to premature mortality and the years lived with disability, that bipolar disorder is one of the conditions causing a higher global burden (Murray et al. 2012). Though it is evident that long-term pharmacological treatment is essential to manage the illness, and that adjunctive psychosocial interventions can also play a positive part, as highlighted by evidence-based studies (for a review see Geddes and Miklowitz 2013), many patients do not receive an early diagnosis and/ or adequate treatment. However, even in those who do so, adherence is a frequent issue in bipolar disorder (Berk et al. 2010). As a consequence of treatment delay, there can be a higher risk of poorer social adjustment, hospitalizations, suicide, comorbidities, forensic complications, and global impairment of the capacity to face developmental tasks in bipolar patients (Conus et al. 2006).

Although the course of the disorder is not uniform and there is a high heterogeneity amongst patients, some data suggest that bipolar disorder may be a potentially progressively deteriorating illness, if not properly treated. This view is based on the findings of stress-, episode- and stimulant-induced sensitization processes, cognitive dysfunction, poor response to medications, medical comorbidities, and neurological correlates to the number of episodes or duration of illness (Post et al. 2012). The risk of recurrence seems to increase with each new affective episode (Kessing et al. 2004). In addition, recent studies show that the higher the number of relapses, particularly manic episodes, the greater the deficits in cognition (López-Jaramillo et al. 2010; Elshahawi et al. 2011). Despite longitudinal studies that have shown a stable progression or slight worsening of cognitive impairment over time (Mora et al. 2012; Torrent et al. 2012), what seems unquestionable is that cognitive deficits are higher in bipolar disorder and have a significant prognostic value on functional outcomes (Depp et al. 2012). Mood episodes prevention would stop— or at least slow down—the cycle of allostatic load and neuroprogression, which complicates the illness course by contributing to cognitive impairment and comorbid pathologies (Vieta et al. 2012). As suggested by McGorry et al. (2007), a disorder that is potentially severe and which may progress if untreated is likely to be most appropriate for staging models, early treatment should demonstrably increase the chance of a cure or at least of reducing mortality and disability. Therefore, early diagnosis and treatment are crucial in limiting these processes and improving the prognosis of the illness.

The introduction of appropriate pharmacological treatment—taking into consideration the use of medications with less neurocognitive side-effects and directing attention to the potential neuroprotective properties of existing agents (Dias et al. 2012)—and adjunctive psychological treatments are crucial to reduce the risk of recurrences. The advantages of adjunctive psychosocial approaches are that they work on aspects that medication cannot reach and that are equally essential for relapse prevention, such as detection of early signs of relapse, avoidance of substance use, enhancement of medication adherence, promotion of a healthy lifestyle (including habits and regularity), improvement of cognition and social skills, work on family attitudes and communication, and improvement of stress management. They can also contribute to reducing functional impairment, which tends to persist even after syndromal recovery (Tohen et al. 2000; Rosa et al. 2011). However, the response to any treatment could be more or less successful depending on the stage of the illness.

Staging models in bipolar disorder

The staging model in bipolar disorder suggests a progression from pro-dromal to more severe and refractory presentations (Kapczinski et al. 2009a). Staging models may help to clarify the mechanisms underlying the progression of the disorder and assist in treatment planning and prognosis. Staging differs from the conventional diagnostic practice in that it not only defines the extent of progression of a disorder at a particular point in time but also where a person is currently located along the continuum of the course of the illness (Cosci and Fava 2013). The provision of stage-appropriate treatment would modify the individual's risk of disease progression; there is, however, a need to clarify the optimum timing and use of stage-specific interventions, compared with disorder-specific treatments (Scott et al. 2013). The timing of neuro-biological changes suggests that the optimal period for neuroprotective interventions is either the prodromal phase or during the early stages of the illness (Salvadore et al. 2008). In the later stages the emphasis would be more focused on rehabilitative treatments.

The knowledge of the determinants of outcome and prognosis is critical for staging classification and optimization of individualized treatment. In an attempt to identify empirical groups of bipolar patients with common functional outcomes, Reinares et al. (2013) used latent class analysis. Two classes were identified representing a 'good' and 'poor' functional outcome class. The advantage of this classification is that classes were derived directly from data, rather than defined a priori, based on theoretical assumptions, and that they account for multiple disease dimensions. Consistent with previous literature, multiple clinical and cognitive variables were individually related to functional outcome. However, only episode density (number of episodes divided by years of illness), level of residual depressive symptoms, estimated verbal intelligence, and inhibitory control significantly differentiated between prognostic classes. The results suggest that variability in functional outcome derives from true heterogeneity within the patient population, which can be captured by at least two dimensions representing clinical severity and cognitive dysfunction. In a 1-year follow-up study, patients with multiple episodes showed worse psychosocial functioning than first-episode patients; baseline subsyndromal depressive symptoms were also associated with poor functional recovery (Rosa et al. 2012).

Theoretical proposals of staging models, including different disease dimensions such as biological correlates, have been suggested (Fries et al. 2012), incorporating a longitudinal appraisal of cognition, psychosocial functioning, and clinical variables, together with biomarkers and neuroimaging data, to guide both prognosis and effective therapeutic strategies (Berk et al. 2007; Kapczinski et al. 2009a). Berk et al. (2007) have suggested that the disorder begins with an at-risk, asymptomatic period, where a range of risk factors may be operating (stage 0). Individuals begin to exhibit mild or non-specific symptoms of mood disorder (stage 1a), and may progress to manifest the range of prodomal patterns (stage 1b). These may culminate in a first threshold episode of illness (stage 2), which can be of either polarity, but is more commonly depressive. This may be followed by a first relapse, either subthreshold (stage 3a), or threshold illness (stage 3b), followed by a subsequent pattern of remission and recurrences (stage 3c). While some individuals may recover syndromally or symptomatically, others may have an unremitting or treatment-refractory course (stage 4). Pharmacological and psychotherapeutic treatments relevant to each illness stage differ substantially. In contrast to the early phases, in which the focus would be on early intervention and neuroprotective strategies, in the later stages the emphasis would be more on rehabilitative treatments, dealing with the disabilities associated to the illness. The model proposed by Kapczinski et al. (2009a) suggests a progression from an at-risk period to more severe and refractory presentations engendered by cumulative exposure to acute episodes, substance abuse, life stress, and inherited vulnerability. The model includes a latent phase followed by four stages: mood and anxiety symptoms and increased risk for developing threshold bipolar disorder (latent phase), well-established periods of euthymia and absence of overt psychiatric morbidity between episodes, without cognitive impairment (stage I), patients with rapid cycling or current axis I or II comorbidities, transient impairment (stage II), patients with a clinically relevant pattern of cognitive and functioning deterioration (stage III), and patients with cognitive and functional impairment, unable to live autonomously (stage IV). Some phases are related to specific altered brain-scans and biomarkers. The authors have also made some therapeutic and prognostic suggestions linked to the illness stage. Whereas in early stages mood stabilizer monotherapy or a combined treatment would be enough, complex regimens or palliative measures would be required in advanced stages. Table 17.1 shows the potential interventions suggested for each stage by Berk et al. (2007) and Kapczinski et al. (2009a). These models identify the first illness episode as a

Table 17.1 Potential interventions based on clinical staging models

Berk et al. (2007)	
Clinical stage	**Potential intervention**
1a	Formal mental health literacy
	Family psychoeducation
	Substance abuse reduction
	Cognitive behavioural therapy
1b	1a plus therapy for episode: phase specific or mood stabilizer
2	1b plus case management, vocational rehabilitation
3a	2 plus emphasis on maintenance medication and psychosocial strategies for full remission
3b	2a plus relapse prevention strategies
3c	3b plus combination mood stabilizers
4	3c plus clozapine and other tertiary therapies, social participation despite disability
Kapczinski et al. (2009a)	
Latent	Reduce exposure to pathogens
I	Mood stabilizer monotherapy; psychoeducation
II	Combined treatment (pharmacotherapy + psychotherapy; focus on the treatment of comorbidities)
III	Complex regimens usually required; consider innovative strategies
IV	Palliative; daycare centre

Source: Data from Berk et al. (2007) and Kapczinski et al. (2009a).

critical target for early intervention, creating the opportunity to prevent some of the neuroanatomical, neuropsychological, clinical, and functional consequences of the illness (Kapczinski et al. 2009b). These proposals represent an important contribution within the framework of an individualized needs-based approach, although they need to be better operationalized and validated by empirical research (Vieta et al. 2010).

Illness progression and response to psychosocial treatment

Some studies have shown that the earlier the intervention is implemented, the better the response to treatment. In pharmacological trials, the early introduction of lithium prophylaxis was found to be a predicting factor of good long-term outcome in a sample of patients with mood disorders (Franchini et al. 1999). Similarly, a differential effect regarding the number of previous affective episodes on response to lithium (Swann et al. 1999) and olanzapine (Ketter et al. 2006) has been reported. Recently, after categorizing the sample on the basis of the number of previous recurrences, a better response to olanzapine was observed in acute mania and prevention of mania maintenance studies in individuals with the fewest number of episodes (Berk et al. 2011). Another study showed that, although no differences were found in the antidepressant response on the basis of previous episodes, functioning and quality of life were worse, disability more common, and symptoms more chronic and severe in those with a higher number of previous episodes (Magalhães et al. 2012).

The efficacy of adjunctive psychological treatments such as cognitive-behavioural therapy, psychoeducation, interpersonal and social rhythm therapy, systematic-care management, and family intervention has been demonstrated in bipolar disorder (for a recent review see Reinares et al. 2014). However, not all the trials have shown positive results (Miller et al. 2004; Scott et al. 2006; Meyer and Hautzinger 2012; de Barros Pellegrinelli et al. 2013), with some data indicating that the benefits of the treatment may vary in different subgroups of patients (Reinares et al. 2014). Similar to pharmacological studies, some psychological trials have shown that a higher number of previous episodes could be related to a reduction of the treatment response (Scott et al. 2006; Colom et al. 2010). In an 18-month follow-up randomized controlled trial, Scott et al. (2006) did not find significant differences in terms of recurrences between two groups: one that received 22 sessions of cognitive-behavioural therapy and another that received treatment as usual. A post-hoc analysis demonstrated a significant interaction, with adjunctive cognitive-behavioural therapy being more effective compared with treatment as usual only in those patients with fewer than 12 previous episodes. The targeted individuals of this study were characterized by a highly recurrent course and complex presentations, with 30% of the sample being in acute episode and 47% showing lifetime or current comorbidity with substance misuse or dependence. The importance of introducing psychological interventions as soon as possible has also been highlighted in a subanalysis by Colom et al. (2010) who showed the lack of efficacy of group psychoeducation in more veteran patients who were euthymic at the study onset. Those patients with more than 15 episodes at study entry showed no benefit at all from psychoeducation (Fig. 17.1). As the authors suggest, both the likelihood of suffering from cognitive impairment and the difficulties of changing habits may be more common in more veteran patients, which could contribute to the lack of efficacy of psychoeducation in this subgroup. Coping abilities may modulate the relationship between stress and recurrence of episodes; it is possible that there is a progressive impairment of coping mechanisms in those patients in advanced stages, increasing vulnerability and decreasing resilience as the illness progresses (Kapczinski et al. 2008). In contrast to previous findings, Lam et al. (2009), applying meta-regression of six studies, using the number of episodes as a predictor variable, did not find that the number of previous episodes moderated the effect of psychological treatments in bipolar disorder. However, there is a high variability in the methodology among studies. There is a need for designing methodologically rigorous studies to assess this issue, as most data come from post-hoc analyses. Aside from the number of previous episodes, other aspects related to the illness may be associated with treatment response. In an attempt to divide the sample into stages considering the number of episodes, comorbidities, and the level of interepisode functional

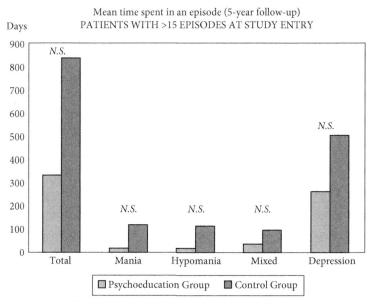

Fig. 17.1 Lack of efficacy of group psychoeducation on individuals with more than 15 episodes at study entry.

N.S.: Non-significant

Reprinted from Acta Neuropsychiatrica, 22:, Colom F, Reinares M, Pacchiarotti I, Popovic D, Mazzarini L, Martínez-Arán A, Torrent C, Rosa A, Palomino-Otianiano R, Franco C, Bonnín CM, Vieta E, Has number of previous episodes any effect on response to group psychoeducation in bipolar patients?, 50–53, Copyright (2010), with permission from Cambridge University Press.

impairment, Reinares et al. (2010) performed a post-hoc analysis of a trial on family psychoeducation. Following clinical and functional criteria suggested by Kapczinski et al. (2009a), the sample was divided into stage I (patients with well-established periods of euthymia who returned to their baseline level of functioning in the absence of overt psychiatric morbidity between episodes) and the other stages (II, III, and IV) that in this study were included under the category of advanced stages. Findings showed that psychoeducation delivered to caregivers resulted in an increase of the time to recurrences, particularly in those cases of bipolar patients at early stages. In the same way that long-standing maladaptive coping strategies and habits may become more difficult to change in more severe patients, caregivers' attitudes, behaviours, and family functioning as a whole may be more difficult to modify in relatives of those patients with higher chronicity and severity. In addition, it is possible that more severe patients would need to be directly involved in the treatment, which was not the case in this intervention.

However, all the findings mentioned above do not mean that veteran patients would not benefit from psychosocial interventions, only that these treatments should be reformulated for this population. They could take advantage of further developments, paying special attention to functional problems derived from the illness. All these results have therefore important implications in the management of bipolar disorders and highlight that resources offered to different subgroups of patients should differ.

As long as the evidence of sustained cognitive and functional impairment in bipolar patients increases, the interest in strategies that lead to reducing or mitigating its impact will grow. Promising data of cognitive (Deckersbach et al. 2010) and functional remediation in bipolar disorder (Torrent et al. 2013) have been recently reported, although the former was not a randomized-controlled trial. Functional remediation involves the use of neurocognitive techniques and training as well as psychoeducation on cognition issues and problem-solving within an ecological framework (Martínez-Arán et al. 2011). Torrent et al. (2013) carried out a multicentre trial with euthymic bipolar patients who were randomized into three groups to receive 21 sessions of group functional remediation ($n = 77$), 21 sessions of group psychoeducation ($n = 82$), or treatment as usual ($n = 80$). All participants were required to have a moderate to severe degree of functional impairment at baseline (Functional Assessment Short Test: FAST≥18). The primary outcome measure of the study was improvement in psychosocial functioning from baseline to the end of the intervention, assessed by the FAST. Compared with those who received treatment as usual, only the functional remediation programme showed efficacy in improving the functional outcome of the patients, particularly in the interpersonal and occupational domains. There was no significant effect of treatment group on the clinical or neurocognitive variables, but the main effect of time was significant. An improvement was found, probably as a result of learning, in all the measures of the California Verbal Learning Test, and in perseverative errors on the Wisconsin Card Sorting Test and Trail Making Test, part A. The authors suggest that, even though some cognitive deficits may persist, patients who received the remediation training might exhibit greater ability and more strategies to cope with those deficits in daily life. The promising findings with these modalities of cognitive and functional remediation that have started to be developed and tested for bipolar disorders may represent a potential resource for some patients with poorer outcomes.

From a preventive point of view, earlier and more sustained long-term prophylaxis could contribute to the reduction of the potentially severe consequences of episode recurrence and progression for morbidity and treatment non-responsiveness (Post et al. 2012). In fact, there is gradually more research focused on high-risk populations and patients with first episodes. Uncertainties regarding whether an individual with prominent risk factors will develop mania, the lag between the onset of prodromal mood symptoms and manic onset, and the lack of specificity of risk factors and prodromal clinical features for mania require that potential interventions introduced during the prodromal phase be safe and well tolerated with long-term administration (McNamara et al. 2010). As McGorry et al. (2009) have reported, the advantages of the use of psychological therapies over medication as a first-line treatment in ultra-high-risk population include: (a) being more acceptable, tolerable and less stigmatizing; (b) having no risk of exposing false-positive subjects to pharmacological side effects; (c) providing effective treatment for false-positives, who, although they do not go on to develop psychosis, generally suffer from other disorders, such as mood and anxiety disorders. Although the evidence is still not conclusive, a recent meta-analysis indicates that interventions that delay or prevent transition to psychosis from the prodromal syndrome could be clinically and economically important to avoid the development of more severe disorders (Stafford et al. 2013). Preliminary studies have been carried out in bipolar disorder with promising results for young people at risk of bipolar disorder (Miklowitz et al. 2011), bipolar children and adolescents (Miklowitz et al. 2008; Fristad et al. 2009), and patients with a first manic episode (Macneil et al. 2012).

Determining at what stage of the disorder the intervention is more effective and consequently adjusting therapeutic strategies on the basis of the user's stage are aims for future research. However, there are different outcomes for patients and it is also possible that given the same conditions there may be subgroups that show a poorer outcome. If this is the case, these subgroups should be identified and therapeutic interventions introduced as soon as possible in order to improve prognosis. There is a need for long-term prospective studies about illness progression in order to complement the findings obtained in cross-sectional studies.

Conclusions: a stage-oriented treatment guideline

The clinical relevance of the previous studies underlies the importance of introducing adjunctive therapeutic interventions as soon as possible in bipolar disorder and the need for designing tailored specific intervention in patients with different levels of impairment in order to improve illness prognosis, functional recovery, and quality of life. The staging model for bipolar disorder needs, no doubt, more empirical support and the rapid advances in the field of biomarkers might provide it in the next few years. Thus, this is the time to start organizing our therapeutic resources on the basis of the already existing staging proposals and evidence. Psychological and psychosocial interventions will play an outstanding role, probably on both extremes of the staging span: early stages and very advanced stages. In the former, psychosocial strategies are crucial to: (1) detect high risk individuals; (2) increase social sensitivity for detection and against stigma, particularly amongst key/significant individuals such as teachers, general practitioners, sport coaches, and religious counsellors; (3) develop healthy lifestyle programmes amongst young people. In the most advanced stages of the illness, there is a role for cognitive and functional remediation, support for the family, and palliative care oriented towards specific areas such as social skills, weight gain, etc. In early and intermediate stages, clinical care should be based on well-known and effective treatments, starting with patient and family psychoeducation and cognitive approaches validated in the area of bipolar disorder.

References

Berk L, Hallam KT, Colom F, et al. (2010) Enhancing medication adherence in patients with bipolar disorder. Hum Psychopharmacol 25:1–16.

Berk M, Conus P, Lucas N, et al. (2007) Setting the stage: from prodrome to treatment resistance in bipolar disorder. Bipolar Disord 9:671–678.

Berk M, Brnabic A, Dodd S, et al. (2011) Does stage of illness impact treatment response in bipolar disorder? Empirical treatment data and their implication for the staging model and early intervention. Bipolar Disord 13:87–98.

Colom F, Reinares M, Pacchiarotti I, et al. (2010) Has number of previous episodes any effect on response to group psychoeducation in bipolar patients? Acta Neuropsychiatr 22:50–53.

Conus P, Berk M, and McGorry PD (2006) Pharmacological treatment in the early phase of bipolar disorders: what stage are we at? Aust N Z J Psychiatry 40:199–207.

Cosci F and Fava GA (2013) Staging of mental disorders: systematic review. Psychother Psychosom 82:20–34.

de Barros Pellegrinelli K, de O Costa LF, Silval KI, et al. (2013) Efficacy of psychoeducation on symptomatic and functional recovery in bipolar disorder. Acta Psychiatr Scand 127:153–158.

Deckersbach T, Nierenberg AA, Kessler R, et al. (2010) RESEARCH: Cognitive rehabilitation for bipolar disorder: An open trial for employed patients with residual depressive symptoms. CNS Neurosci Ther 16:298–307.

Depp CA, Mausbach BT, Harmell AL, et al. (2012) Meta-analysis of the association between cognitive abilities and everyday functioning in bipolar disorder. Bipolar Disord 14:217–226.

Dias V, Balanzá-Martinez V, Soeiro-de-Souza MG, et al. (2012) Pharmacological approaches in bipolar disorders and the impact on cognition: a critical overview. Acta Psychiatr Scand 126:315–331.

Elshahawi HH, Essawi H, Rabie MA, et al. (2011) Cognitive functions among euthymic bipolar I patients after a single manic episode versus recurrent episodes. J Affect Disord 130:180–191.

Franchini L, Zanardi R, Smeraldi E, et al. (1999) Early onset of lithium propylaxis as a predictor of good long-term outcome. Eur Arch Psychiatry Clin Neurosci 249:227–230.

Fries GR, Pfaffenseller B, Stertz L, et al. (2012) Staging and neuroprogression in bipolar disorder. Curr Psychiatry Rep 14:667–675.

Fristad MA, Verducci JS, Walters K, et al. (2009) Impact of multifamily psychoeducational psychotherapy in treating children aged 8 to 12 years with mood disorders. Arch Gen Psychiatry 66: 1013–1021.

Geddes JR and Miklowitz DJ (2013) Treatment of bipolar disorder. Lancet 381:1672–1682.

Judd LL, Akiskal HS, Schettler PJ, et al. (2002) The long-term natural history of the weekly symptomatic status of bipolar I disorder. Arch Gen Psychiatry 59:530–537.

Judd LL, Akiskal HS, Schettler PJ, et al. (2003) A prospective investigation of the natural history of the long-term weekly symptomatic status of bipolar II disorder. Arch Gen Psychiatry **60**:261–269.

Kapczinski F, Dias VV, Kauer-Sant'Anna M, et al. (2009a) Clinical implications of a staging model for bipolar disorders. Expert Rev Neurother **9**:957–966.

Kapczinski F, Dias VV, Kauer-Sant'anna M, et al. (2009b) The potential use of biomarkers as an adjunctive tool for staging bipolar disorder. Prog Neuropsychopharmacol Biol Psychiatry **33**:1366–1371.

Kapczinski F., Vieta E, Andreazza AC, et al. (2008) Allostatic load in bipolar disorder: implications for pathophysiology and treatment. Neurosci Biobehav Rev **32**:675–692.

Kessing LV, Hansen MG, Andersen PK, et al. (2004) The predictive effect of episodes on the risk of recurrence in depressive and bipolar disorders—a life-long perspective. Acta Psychiatr Scand **109**:339–344.

Ketter TA, Houston JP, Adams DH, et al. (2006) Differential efficacy of olanzapine and lithium in preventing manic or mixed recurrence in patients with bipolar I disorder based on number of previous manic or mixed episodes. J Clin Psychiatry **67**:95–101.

Lam DH, Burbeck R, Wright K, et al. (2009) Psychological therapies in bipolar disorder: the effect of illness history on relapse prevention—a systematic review. Bipolar Disord **11**:474–482.

López-Jaramillo C, Lopera-Vásquez J, Gallo A, et al. (2010) Effects of recurrence on the cognitive performance of patients with bipolar I disorder: implications for relapse prevention and treatment adherence. Bipolar Disord **12**:557–567.

Macneil CA, Hasty M, Cotton S, et al. (2012) Can a targeted psychological intervention be effective for young people following a first manic episode? Results from an 18-month pilot study. Early Interv Psychiatry **6**:380–388.

Magalhães PV, Dodd S, Nierenberg AA, et al. (2012) Cumulative morbidity and prognostic staging of illness in the Systematic Treatment Enhancement Program for Bipolar Disorder (STEP-BD). Aust N Z J Psychiatry **46**:1058–1067.

Martínez-Arán A, Torrent C, Solé B, et al. (2011) Functional remediation for bipolar disorder. Clin Pract Epidemiol Ment Health **7**:112–116.

Martínez-Arán A, Vieta E, Reinares M, et al. (2004) Cognitive function across manic or hypomanic, depressed, and euthymic status in bipolar disorder. Am J Psychiatry **161**:262–270.

McGorry PD, Nelson B, Amminger GP, et al. (2009) Intervention in individuals at ultra-high risk for psychosis: a review and future directions. J Clin Psychiatry **70**:1206–1212.

McGorry PD, Purcell R, Hickie IB, et al. (2007) Clinical staging: a heuristic model for psychiatry and youth mental health. Med J Aust **187**(7 Suppl):S40–42.

McNamara RK, Nandagopal JJ, Strakowski SM, et al. (2010) Preventative strategies for early-onset bipolar disorder: towards a clinical staging model. CNS Drugs **24**:983–996.

Meyer TD and Hautzinger M (2012) Cognitive behaviour therapy and supportive therapy for bipolar disorders: relapse rates for treatment period and 2-year follow-up. Psychol Med **42**:1429–1439.

Miklowitz DJ, Axelson DA, Birmaher B, et al. (2008) Family-focused treatment for adolescents with bipolar disorder: results of a 2-year randomized trial. Arch Gen Psychiatry **65**:1053–1061.

Miklowitz DJ, Chang KD, Taylor DO, et al. (2011) Early psychosocial intervention for youth at risk for bipolar I or II disorder: a one-year treatment development trial. Bipolar Disord **13**:67–75.

Miller IW, Solomon DA, Ryan CE, et al. (2004) Does adjunctive family therapy enhance recovery from bipolar I mood episodes? J Affect Disord **82**:431–436.

Mora E, Portella MJ, Forcada I, et al. (2012) Persistence of cognitive impairment and its negative impact on psychosocial functioning in lithium-treated, euthymic bipolar patients: a 6-year follow-up study. Psychol Med **31**:1–10.

Murray CJ, Vos T, Lozano R, et al. (2012) Disability-adjusted life years (DALYs) for 291 diseases and injuries in 21 regions, 1990–2010: a systematic analysis for the Global Burden of Disease Study 2010. Lancet **380**:2197–2223.

Post RM, Fleming J, and Kapczinski F (2012) Neurobiological correlates of illness progression in the recurrent affective disorders. J Psychiatr Res **46**:561–573.

Reinares M, Colom F, Rosa AR, et al. (2010) The impact of staging bipolar disorder on treatment outcome of family psychoeducation. J Affect Disord **123**:81–86.

Reinares M, Papachristou E, Harvey P, et al. (2013) Towards a clinical staging for bipolar disorder: Defining patient subtypes based on functional outcome. J Affect Disord **144**:65–71.

Reinares M, Sánchez-Moreno J, and Fountoulakis KN (2014) Psychosocial interventions in bipolar disorder: what, for whom, and when. J Affect Disord **156**:46–55.

Rosa AR, González-Ortega I, González-Pinto A, et al. (2012) One-year psychosocial functioning in patients in the early vs. late stage of bipolar disorder. Acta Psychiatr Scand **125**:335–341.

Rosa AR, Reinares M, Amann B, et al. (2011) Six-month functional outcome of a bipolar disorder cohort in the context of a specialized-care program. Bipolar Disord **13**:679–686.

Rosa AR, Reinares M, Michalak EE, et al. (2010) Functional impairment and disability across mood states in bipolar disorder. Value Health **13**:984–988.

Salvadore G, Drevets WC, Henter ID, et al. (2008) Early intervention in bipolar disorder, Part II: Therapeutics. Early Interv Psychiatry **2**:136–146.

Scott J, Leboyer M, Hickie I, et al. (2013) Clinical staging in psychiatry: a cross-cutting model of diagnosis with heuristic and practical value. Br J Psychiatry **202**:243–245.

Scott J, Paykel E, Morriss R, et al. (2006) Cognitive-behavioural therapy for severe and recurrent bipolar disorders: randomised controlled trial. Br J Psychiatry **188**:310–320.

Stafford MR, Jackson H, Mayo-Wilson E, et al. (2013) Early interventions to prevent psychosis: systematic review and meta-analysis. Br Med J **18**; 346:f185(1–13).

Swann AC, Bowden CL, Calabrese JR, et al. (1999) Differential effect of number of previous episodes of affective disorder on response to lithium or divalproex in acute mania. Am J Psychiatry **156**:1264–1266.

Tohen M, Hennen J, Zarate CM Jr, et al. (2000) Two-year syndromal and functional recovery in 219 cases of first-episode major affective disorder with psychotic features. Am J Psychiatry **157**:220–228.

Torrent C, Bonnin CM, Martínez-Arán A, et al. (2013) Efficacy of functional remediation in bipolar disorder: a multicenter randomized controlled study. Am J Psychiatry **170**:852–859.

Torrent C, Martínez-Arán A, Bonnín CM, et al. (2012) Long-term outcome of cognitive impairment in bipolar disorder. J Clin Psychiatry **73**:e899–905.

Vieta E, Popovic D, Rosa AR, et al. (2012) The clinical implications of cognitive impairment and allostatic load in bipolar disorder. Eur Psychiatry **28**:21–29.

Vieta E, Reinares M, and Rosa AR (2010) Staging bipolar disorder. Neurotox Res **19**:279–285.

Chapter 18

Staging systems in bipolar disorder: current findings, future directions, and implications for clinical practice

Flavio Kapczinski, Eduard Vieta,
Pedro V. S. Magalhães, and Michael Berk

Staging within psychiatry and in bipolar disorder

Albert Broders's initiative to grade tumours numerically with the purpose of indicating prognosis was a fundamental step towards the widespread adoption of staging in medicine since the 1920s (Wright 2012). The numerous systems available in fields as diverse as oncology and rheumatology, neurology, and nephrology attest to the utility of the principle. A staging system is a heuristic tool intended to add prognostic significance to clinical diagnoses. In doing so, the clinician is armed with information capable of aiding selection of stage-specific strategies for treatment.

We can refer to Kraepelin the initial descriptions of illness progression in bipolar disorder. He noticed that episodes tended to recur at shorter intervals in the long-term follow up of patients. In that, probably Kraepelin was influenced by the German authors that anteceded him. In 1861, Griesinger stated that: 'it generally happens, that with patients who fall into insanity, (. . .) the attacks, as time advances, become longer and more serious . . . the lucid interval shorter, and with each new attack the prognosis become more unfavorable.' Neumann (1859) even used the word staging (*Stadien*), describing the hyperaesthesia psychica as a prodromal stage (*Vorlauferstadium*) of severe mental illness. Kahlbaum also used the term 'stage' as he mentioned that no form of disease exists, but stages (*Stadien*) of one and the same disease process.

However, prognostic staging has been gaining traction in psychiatry in the past 10 years, mainly due to its potential utility (McGorry et al. 2006). After the original proposals of staging for psychotic disorders by Fava and Kellner (1993), this has been adapted and refined by McGorry and colleagues. A few systems have been put forward specifically for people with other disorders, such as bipolar disorder. There is now consistent evidence that, at least for a significant portion of people with this disease, clinical course and outcome are not as benign as initially described (Goodwin and Jamison 2007). The evidence thus far points to relevant differences between early and late stages of bipolar disorders in clinical course of illness, neurobiology, systemic pathology, and treatment responsiveness. These all suggest staging is a viable addition to clinical care in bipolar disorder.

McGorry and his colleagues were the first to comprehensively discuss its implications and benefits (McGorry et al. 2006, 2007; McGorry 2007). In a series of articles they argue that staging has the potential of enhancing diagnostic practice by strengthening the clinician's capacity to select stage appropriate treatments. Clinical staging, as they discuss in their initial formulation, is useful in any disease that tends to progress or may progress, making it potentially valuable for many psychiatric disorders. They put forward two assumptions as fundamental for clinical staging. The first is that early stages have a better prognosis and response to treatment than later stages. The second is that early treatment is more effective, and that simpler and less toxic treatments may suffice early, whereas riskier treatments are often needed later; clozapine being an exemplar. Thus, the main argument for staging is its potential to bridge research and clinical practice, allowing for better illness models that have the potential to intervene early, potentially reducing the risk of illness progression.

In the framework suggested by McGorry, bipolar disorder should tend to progress, or at least some patients should progress to be amenable to staging. There is a long-standing debate on whether bipolar disorder is a generally progressive illness (Goodwin and Jamison 2007). Even if the evidence on cycle length is inconclusive at the moment (Baldessarini et al. 2012), the possibility that a substantial proportion of patients present a progressive course makes staging relevant. Furthermore, cycle length is only one aspect of progression, and not necessarily germane to treatment selection. Treatment response may differ across stage, and the phenomenology may subtly evolve. Differences in illness biology and consequent treatment resistance, for instance, may suggest different stage-specific strategies. As one particularly salient illustration, the pharmacotherapy of outpatients with bipolar disorders tends to be complex, and non-responders tend to be exposed to a greater number of medications (Post et al. 2010). It should also be made explicit that the first goal of staging is enhancing the clinical utility of interventions, not describing the natural history of illness. Thus, the fact that not all patients have a neat progression between stages should not be an insurmountable difficulty for a particular model.

In bipolar disorder, the two most relevant systems of staging were put forward by Berk (Berk et al. 2007a, b) and then Kapczinski (Kapczinski et al. 2009). Berk's system is directly derived from McGorry's formulation for psychosis (McGorry et al. 2006). It proposes a model that begins with risk states and progresses to subthreshold, then threshold, multiple relapses, to persistent and unremitting illness. It is fundamentally built on episode recurrence. The starting point in Kapczinski's model is also an at-risk state, but it progresses to no impairment during euthymia, to marked impairment to the inability to live autonomously. It is thus a model based on functioning during euthymia (Table 18.1). The models converge on the relevance of having an 'at risk' stage, and there should be substantial overlap between the two systems. Some of their assumptions differ, however, and, to our knowledge, their relative merits in terms of utility and validity have not been formally tested. The available data, as discussed next, are based on one of the two systems.

Both models have strengths and limitations; a limitation of the former model is that not all people show deterioration in a linear manner predicated on number of episodes, whereas a limitation of the latter is a degree of circularity in argument predicating stage on functional outcome. The former model has strengths in capturing the early stages, whereas the latter has strengths in defining functional capacity and prognosis.

Table 18.1 Disease stages according to the Berk and Kapczinski models

Stage	Berk	Kapczinski
0	Increased risk of mood disorder	At risk, positive family history, mood or anxiety symptoms
1a	Mild or non-specific symptom	Well-defined periods of euthymia without symptoms
1b	Prodromal features (ultra-high risk)	
2	First threshold episode	Interepisodic symptoms related to comorbidities
3a	Recurrence of subthreshold mood symptoms	Marked impairment in cognition or functioning
3b	First threshold relapse	
3c	Multiple relapses	
4	Persistant unremitting illness	Unable to live autonomously due to impairment

Source: Data from Berk et al. (2007a) and Kapczinski et al. (2009).

A brief review of the supporting clinical evidence in bipolar disorder

Ideally, a staging system would be supported by randomized data coming from studies specifically designed to test the utility of the model. Such data should be able to demonstrate differential prognosis and effects of interventions according to stage. Definitive studies are not available in bipolar disorder, due to the secondary nature of data analysis and the fact that studies usually use proxies of staging and not fully fledged systems.

Recently, Magalhaes and colleagues (Magalhaes et al. 2012b) published an analysis of the STEP-BD (Sachs et al. 2003) database, using number of episodes as a proxy of staging. In that large dataset ($n = 3,345$), patients naturalistically treated in specialized facilities followed for up to 2 years were stratified according the number of previous episodes (fewer than 5, between 5 and 9, 10 or more). Controlling for a host of possible clinical and demographic confounders, they were able to demonstrate that those with multiple episodes indeed had a worse prognosis on symptom scores and functioning and quality of life. They were generally more impaired at baseline and tended not to improve as much in clinical and functional measures. This analysis was able to demonstrate that a proxy of staging—number of episodes—is able to prospectively stratify clinical and functional outcomes. It has the advantage of having a very large sample felt to be representative of those treated for bipolar disorder in the United States, and outcomes that are relevant to bipolar disorder. Also of relevance, Rosa and colleagues (Rosa et al. 2012) published an analysis of a 1-year follow-up of inpatients with bipolar disorder. Similarly to the STEP-BD patients, those with multiple episodes had many significant differences at baseline and also displayed a worse recovery rate at the end of the 1-year follow-up. These data converge with those from the Stanley Foundation Bipolar Collaborative network (Post et al. 2003, 2010).

Secondary data from two randomized psychotherapy trials also support the second assumption behind staging (Scott et al. 2006; Reinares et al. 2013). Both show that patients in earlier stages have a better response to psychotherapy. In the first, Scott and colleagues (Scott et al. 2006) reported that patients with fewer than 12 previous episodes had a positive response to cognitive behavioural therapy (CBT) compared to those with 12 or more episodes. In this trial, patients ($n = 253$) were randomized to CBT or treatment as usual, and only those with fewer than 12 episodes had a smaller rate of recurrence on CBT. This analysis, however, was conducted post hoc. In another post-hoc analysis, Reinares and colleagues (Reinares et al. 2010) clinically stratified patients ($n = 113$) in early or late stages, and compared the outcomes in a randomized trial of family psychoeducation. Again, they only found a positive response, in terms of time to recurrence, for those in early stage bipolar disorder. Berk and colleagues used pooled data from olanzapine trials to evaluate stage-related differences in treatment response (Berk et al. 2011a). Within this large dataset (12 studies, 4,346 participants in total), they were able to demonstrate that treatment response was higher with fewer episodes in the acute mania studies, and a similar effect in relapse prevention. There were no differences in responses in depression studies. Finally, in the same report mentioned earlier, Magalhaes and colleagues (Magalhaes et al. 2012b) tested a differential response to adjunctive antidepressant in the randomized arm of STEP-BD (Sachs et al. 2007). They were also not able to demonstrate significant inter-actions with depressive symptoms, which is not surprising in the context of the negative overall findings of that study. However, there is negative data in depression, suggesting that treatment response is not associated with number of depressive episodes (Dodd et al. 2013). Pacchiarotti et al. though, did find a significant association between the number of previous hypomanic episodes and poor response to antidepressants (Pacchiarotti et al. 2011). Greater exploration of this phenomenon is clearly necessary.

There is increasing evidence showing that people with bipolar disorder experience persistent cognitive deficits and poor psychosocial functioning, even when they are euthymic (Goldberg et al. 1995; Martinez-Aran et al. 2004; Judd et al. 2005). It is now recognized that functional and symptom-atic outcome in bipolar disorder are not synonymous (Tohen et al. 2000; Nolen et al. 2004). Psychosocial functioning describes a person's ability to function socially and occupationally, and to live independently (Zarate et al. 2000; Ustun and Kennedy 2009). In this regard, several studies have shown a marked functional impairment associated with bipolar disorder (Altshuler et al. 2006; Cacilhas et al. 2009; Rosa et al. 2009). Patients show difficulties in multiple areas of functioning (independent living, interpersonal relation-ships, occupational and educational achievement, recreational enjoyment, and sexual activity), and such impairment appears to occur in early stages of the illness (Nehra et al. 2006; Kauer-Sant'Anna et al. 2009a; Jansen et al. 2012). For instance, the European Mania in Bipolar Longitudinal Evaluation of Medication (EMBLEM) study ($n = 3,115$) reported that a greater propor-tion of first-episode patients achieve symptomatic and functional recovery compared to those with multiple episodes (Tohen et al. 2010). Likewise, a recent 1-year functioning study reported that patients at late stages were significantly more impaired than those at early stage of bipolar disorder in distinct domains of functioning (Rosa et al. 2012). Significant clinical dif-ferences, mainly in terms of severity of depression, suicide attempts and the number of years before receiving a correct diagnosis have been observed between patients with first and multiple episodes (Azorin et al. 2011). Taken together, these findings suggest that the episode frequency has an impact on the patient's outcome, and particularly on psychosocial functioning.

Furthermore, cognitive impairment has been related to a worse clinical course and poor psychosocial functioning (Tabares-Seisdedos et al. 2008; Martino et al. 2011). Greater cognitive deficits are not only associated with illness severity (Robinson et al. 2006; Martinez-Aran et al. 2007), but also with cumulative mood episodes (Torres et al. 2010). In this regard, worse overall neurocognitive performance in euthymic patients who had at least three manic episodes compared to those with only one mania have been found (Lopez-Jaramillo et al. 2010). Other clinical features such as hospitalizations, duration of the illness, and psychiatric comorbidities appear to contribute to the cognitive impairment (Martinez-Aran et al. 2007; Sanchez-Moreno et al. 2009).

Research on biologically relevant peripheral markers has increased in the past decade (Magalhaes et al. 2012d; Frey et al. 2013). This line of work is useful in that these markers are either correlated with central nervous system changes, but also because it suggests that bipolar disorder is associated with systemic pathophysiology (Grande et al. 2012). Peripheral biomarkers are pertinent to the theme of staging, inasmuch as they are conceptualized as mediators of allostasis (Kapczinski et al. 2008; Juster et al. 2010; Magalhaes et al. 2012d), and their demonstration in different stages is one of the fundamental hypotheses of neuroprogression (Berk 2009; Berk et al. 2011b). Ultimately, they might be useful in selecting staged interventions. For instance, the presence of relevant medical comorbidity is often associated with indications of late-stage bipolar disorder (Magalhaes et al. 2012c). Recently, patients with such comorbidities were shown to have a better response to N-acetylcysteine (NAC) than those without medical conditions (Magalhaes et al. 2012a). There is also unpublished recent data of potential greater efficacy of NAC in the later stages of schizophrenia. If confirmed, these findings would suggest the use of adjunctive antioxidants in those with comorbidities and in more chronic disorders, which could be proxies of greater allostatic load and higher levels of circulating free radicals.

Perhaps the pivotal study on the association of biomarkers with staging was conducted by Kauer-Sant'Anna and colleagues (Kauer-Sant'Anna et al. 2009b). In that case–control study, the authors were able to demonstrate that patients in a late stage (i.e. after multiple episodes) had a multitude of differences in peripheral inflammation biomarkers as compared to controls, which was not the case in early-stage patients. Furthermore, even in the case of tumour necrosis factor-α (TNF-α), where both groups of patients had elevated circulating levels, patients in late stages had a several-fold increase. Further exploration of this sample also revealed that gluthatione-S-transferase and reductase are increased in late-stage patients, as well as 3-nitrotyrosine; only the latter was found increased in early-stage patients (Andreazza et al. 2009). These alterations in oxidative biology imply a pro-oxidant pathology in bipolar disorder. Further increases in protein and lipid damage have been reported in patients with bipolar disorder seen at tertiary facilities, which are generally late-stage patients (Kapczinski et al. 2011). A recent report of a community-based sample also demonstrated early-stage increases in protein damage (Magalhaes et al. 2012e). Other biological foundations of progression have been explored in depression, including autoimmunity secondary to oxidatively damaged neo-epitopes, and altered gut permeability leading also to amplification of immune cascades (Maes et al. 2012a, b). These are as yet unexplored pathways in bipolar disorder.

Neurotrophins are also relevant to staging, as they are pertinent to the kindling hypothesis (Post 2007a, b). In the aforementioned study, Kauer-Sant'Anna and colleagues (Kauer-Sant'Anna et al. 2009b) demonstrated a relevant decrease in brain-derived neurotrophic factor (BDNF) in late-stage patients, but not in those in an early stage. A later meta-analysis was able to demonstrate a correlation between the age and length of illness and serum BDNF across seven studies (Fernandes et al. 2010). A similar significance can be attributed when data of a 'systemic toxicity index' was examined in late-stage patients and people in early-stage bipolar disorder from the general population (Kapczinski et al. 2010; Magalhaes et al. 2011). Those studies used principal component analysis to derive an index, with inflammation markers, BDNF, and oxidative stress markers. Again, in late stages changes were much more pronounced, albeit they were present in early stages. Table 18.2 contains a summary of available findings regarding peripheral markers.

Lin and colleagues recently reviewed neuroimaging evidence for staging in severe mental disorders, including bipolar disorder (Lin et al. 2013).

Table 18.2 Biomarkers in early and late-stage bipolar disorder

Marker	Early stage	Late-stage
BDNF (Kauer-Sant'Anna et al. 2009b; Fernandes et al. 2010)	≈	↓↓
TNF (Kauer-Sant'Anna et al. 2009b)	↑	↑↑
IL-6 (Kauer-Sant'Anna et al. 2009b)	↑	↑
IL-10 (Kauer-Sant'Anna et al. 2009b)	↑	≈
PCC (Andreazza et al. 2009; Kapczinski et al. 2011; Magalhaes et al. 2012e)	↑≈	≈
TBA (Kapczinski et al. 2011)	≈	↑↑
Systemic toxicity (Kapczinski et al. 2010; Magalhaes et al. 2011)	↑	↑↑

Source: Data from Kauer-Sant'Anna et al. (2009b), Fernandes et al. (2010), Andreazza et al. (2009), Kapczinski et al. (2011), and Magalhaes et al. (2012e).

They highlight the possibility that structural and functional networks could be differently affected in each illness stage. White matter pathology could be responsible for early stage dysconnectivity. In first-episode patients, for instance, recent meta-analysis show significant white matter reductions, but not grey matter (Vita et al. 2009). Another meta-analysis of voxelwise studies also demonstrated fewer alterations in grey matter in first-episode patients (Bora et al. 2010). Stage changes were specifically investigated in only a few cross-sectional studies. In one mafnetic resonance imaging study, the total number of episodes were correlated with the size of the left hippocampus, and only patients with fewer than 10 episodes had a larger hippocampus compared to controls (Javadapour et al. 2007). Lagopoulus compared a mixed cohort of people with 'attenuated syndromes' (stage 1) with patients with 'discrete disorders' (psychosis, bipolar disorder, or depression, stages 2 or 3) (Lagopoulos et al. 2012). Patients on stages 2 or 3 had a more widespread pattern of grey matter loss. In a region of interest (ROI) study, Nery et al. (2009) showed similar orbitofrontal cortex grey matter volumes in individuals with bipolar disorder and controls. The total number of episodes did not significantly influence the result.

A recent systematic review of longitudinal neuroimaging studies notes several caveats and a general dearth of prospective data (Lim et al. 2013). Among structural neuroimaging studies, neuroprogressive changes were more robustly noted in prefrontal, cingulate and subgenual cortices, and fusiform gyrus, although total brain volume seems to be stable.

Current applications, areas of uncertainty, and future directions

Most of extant evidence relevant to staging models is cross-sectional. This is surely the source of much of the heterogeneity in the biomarker and neuroimaging data. It is also a source of disagreement among investigators and a major cause of open questions on issues such as whether neurocognitive is actually progressive or stable. Having been included in cross-sectional studies, those patients with more episodes, especially manic and psychotic episodes, are more likely to be impaired, and therefore an assumption of some neuroprogression can be made. However, the first longitudinal studies do not support cognitive neuroprogression (Samamé 2014). As these changes probably evolve over many years, and with repeated episodes, it may well be that longitudinal studies are too short and may actually enrol precisely those patients who are more likely to stay in a long-term study and, therefore, be more adherent and less impaired, but we do not have a final answer as yet. Another source of weakness in the current published literature is the small sample size of the studies, most of which are pilot studies in nature. These generate further difficulties in generalization of results. With the caveat that most data at present is either cross-sectional in nature, based on post-hoc analysis (or both), most studies converge to confirm staging assumptions in bipolar disorder. Whether the illness is generally progressive or not, stage-based interventions have the potential benefit of providing the most effective and less toxic intervention in a time-sensitive manner.

The most evident direction of staging research in bipolar disorder should then be the design of adequately powered longitudinal studies that incorporate biomarker data. Transitions between stages should be studied and validated. Staging proposals can also be formally compared. For instance, a new method for staging non-small cell lung cancer was recently compared with the one traditionally used (Fukui et al. 2008). The new system was considered superior because of its ability to separate between stage IB and IIA regarding survival. This also demonstrates how relevant it is collecting meaningful endpoints and avoiding tauto-logical demonstrations. A staging system should be able to predict and stratify relevant outcomes—hospitalization, recurrence, etc.—in a con-sistent way. In this fashion, merely predicting future functioning based on functioning, or future relapses based on previous relapses, may con-tain an element of circularity that should be avoided.

One attractive alternative would be the formal investigation of staging in a randomized controlled trial. One possibility would be to confirm the results of secondary analyses that suggest psychotherapy is more effect-ive in early stages than in late stages. It is equally plausible that people at the divergent ends of the spectrum may need quite different types of psychotherapy. Specific models of therapy for first-episode individuals have been developed, and therapies such as acceptance and commit-ment therapy have been argued as a good therapeutic fit for late-stage disorders (Macneil et al. 2011; Berk et al. 2012). Additionally, functional remediation clearly makes more sense in patients who are significantly disabled (Torrent et al. 2013). However, there is some potential for inter-ventions targeting cognitive reserve to work in the prevention of cog-nitive decline, and those would then fit much better in patients at early stages, Alternatively, patients could be randomized to either receive treatment as usual or staged interventions. This latter option would be more pragmatic, albeit requiring a much larger sample size.

Clinically, the early versus late distinction may appear obvious, in the sense that such patients have overtly different needs. Clinicians prob-ably have their own, probably idiosyncratic ways in dealing with this issue (Cosci and Fava 2013). Nevertheless, confirming these effects and estimating their size matters. Also of consequence, such different cohorts of patients are usually lumped in clinical trials, which could obscure relevant treatment differences. There is a growing consensus that early intervention is valuable in individuals with severe mental dis-orders (Berk et al. 2010). Interventions for individuals in late stages have been more problematic and less often studied (Berk et al. 2012). We know that functional remediation may work in late stages, but we do not have similar information for drug therapy such as clozapine, for example. Having a schema that includes various levels of treatment resistance could also have the benefit of directing new research efforts. This would be especially important, as it is becoming widely recognized that there is a very high degree of inadequate response to most monotherapies, more studies of what might be more effective for this majority of individuals would be desirable. The same argument could be made of also examining the role of comorbidities is a staging model, as both anxiety and substance abuse comorbidities appear to convey a relative poor prognosis in a great many of naturalistic follow-up studies, but there are virtually no prospective data about what treatment strategies might be more effective.

Most available data to date confirm that generally defined late-stage patients have a worse overall prognosis and poorer response to standard treatment. Although refinement of staging systems is certainly in need of further study, we would affirm it is proper at this juncture to speak broadly of 'early' and 'late' stages. Early stages are at the first, or the first few, episodes and are in aggregate associated with better functioning after recovery. Late stages are associated with multiple episodes and tend to have impairment in multiple areas of functioning. In other words, the models proposed by Kapczinski and Berk concur on the importance of 'early' or 'late' stage disease. The next steps require consideration of the details of intermediary stages and how many additional stages are optimal. The ultimate goal should be linking staging models with optimally tailored therapy. This should be the subject of further local and global collaborative efforts.

Staging and neuroprogression: conclusion

Since German authors noted that some psychiatric disorders may have a progressive course, this is the first time that the concept of staging has received a thoughtful discussion and an organized attempt to assess its clinical validity in psychiatry. As mentioned earlier in this chapter, the efforts of McGorry and his group to include staging as a meaningful dimension in psychiatric diagnose have caught momentum in the context of the current debate about psychiatric classification. The McGorry group has put the emphasis of the concept of staging in populations at risk and those in prodromal phases.

This approach derives from the notion that available treatments may not be effective to rescue many patients to a state of full remission. Thus, interventions that could be placed earlier in the course of illness could carry a higher potential for preventing ultra-high-risk patients from converting into full-blown clinical presentations. However, this is a new field and the potential of such interventions to benefit patients is yet to be tested. Meanwhile, new research evidence shows that many bipolar disorder patients, particularly those who experience multiple episodes, stress, and exposure to drugs of abuse, may have a more unfavourable course (see Chapter 1). Also, such late-stage patients may benefit from more intensive care to recover functionality. In this manner, staging can inform clinicians about prognosis and help tailoring treatments according to the patients' needs.

In the case of bipolar disorder, cumulative wear and tear of the whole body and brain tissue seems to take place as disorder progresses. That has been previously acknowledged with the notion that increased allostatic load among these patients could lead into more unfavourable clinical outcomes (see Chapter 3). More recently, Berk et al. have described the concept of neuroprogression that captures the notion that a more unfavourable course of illness would have a biological underpinnings (see Chapter 4 for a more detailed account of neuroprogression). These biological underpinnings would hold the potential to inform translational researchers for the development of new targets for interventions aiming at preventing or reversing neuroprogression. The putative pathways of neuroprogression overlap with the ones described for allostatic load. Thus, neuroprogression, as conceptualized so far, may be a more general mechanism underlying the progression of several psychiatric disorders. In fact, since the original description of the term, 52 papers have been published covering different fields of psychiatry (for instance, see Davis et al. (2014)).

Hopefully, new research focused on the biological mechanisms of neuroprogression will enlighten us as to how prevent the consequences of progression of severe mental disorders. The clinical validation of staging in the bipolar disorder field may help clinicians to tailor individualized treatment and better inform patients and families about prognosis and means for rehabilitation.

References

Altshuler LL, Post RM, Black DO, et al. (2006) Subsyndromal depressive symptoms are associated with functional impairment in patients with bipolar disorder: results of a large, multisite study. J Clin Psychiatry **67**:1551–1560.

Andreazza AC, Kapczinski F, Kauer-Sant'anna M, et al. (2009) 3-Nitrotyrosine and glutathione antioxidant system in patients in the early and late stages of bipolar disorder. J Psychiatry Neurosci **34**(4):263–271.

Azorin JM, Kaladjian A, Adida M, et al. (2011) Correlates of first-episode polarity in a French cohort of 1089 bipolar I disorder patients: role of temperaments and triggering events. J Affect Disord **129**(1–3):39–46.

Baldessarini RJ, Salvatore P, Khalsa HM, et al. (2012) Episode cycles with increasing recurrences in first-episode bipolar-I disorder patients. J Affect Disord **136**(1–2):149–154.

Berk M (2009) Neuroprogression: pathways to progressive brain changes in bipolar disorder. Int J Neuropsychopharmacol **12**:441–445.

Berk M, Berk L, Udina M, et al. (2012) Palliative models of care for later stages of mental disorder: maximizing recovery, maintaining hope, and building morale. Aust N Z J Psychiatry **46**:92–99.

Berk M, Brnabic A, Dodd S, et al. (2011a) Does stage of illness impact treatment response in bipolar disorder? Empirical treatment data and their implication for the staging model and early intervention. Bipolar Disord **13**:87–98.

Berk M, Conus P, Lucas N, et al. (2007a) Setting the stage: from prodrome to treatment resistance in bipolar disorder. Bipolar Disord **9**:671–678.

Berk M, Hallam KT, and McGorry PD (2007b) The potential utility of a staging model as a course specifier: a bipolar disorder perspective. J Affect Disord **100**:279–281.

Berk M, Hallam K, Malhi GS, et al. (2010) Evidence and implications for early intervention in bipolar disorder. J Ment Health **19**:113–126.

Berk M, Kapczinski F, Andreazza AC, et al. (2011b) Pathways underlying neuroprogression in bipolar disorder: focus on inflammation, oxidative stress and neurotrophic factors. Neurosci Biobehav Rev **35**:804–817.

Bora E, Fornito A, Yucel M, et al. (2010) Voxelwise meta-analysis of gray matter abnormalities in bipolar disorder. Biol Psychiatry **67**(11):1097–1105.

Cacilhas AA, Magalhaes PVD, Cereser KM, et al. (2009) Validity of a Short Functioning Test (FAST) in Brazilian outpatients with bipolar disorder. Value Health **12**:624–627.

Cosci F and Fava GA (2013) Staging of mental disorders: systematic review. Psychother Psychosom **82**(1):20–34.

Davis J, Moylan S, Harvey BH, et al. (2014) Neuroprogression in schizophrenia: pathways underpinning clinical staging and therapeutic corollaries. Aust N Z J Psychiatry **48**(6):512–529.

Dodd S, Berk M, Kelin K, et al. (2013) Treatment response for acute depression is not associated with number of previous episodes: lack of evidence for a clinical staging model for major depressive disorder. J Affect Disord 150(2):344–349.

Fava GA and Kellner R (1993) Staging—a neglected dimension in psychiatric classification. Acta Psychiatr Scand 87:225–230.

Fernandes BS, Gama CS, Cereser KM, et al. (2010) Brain-derived neutrotrophic in mania, depression, and euthymia in bipolar disorders: a systematic review and meta-analysis. Bipolar Disord 12:19–19.

Frey BN, Andreazza AC, Houenou J, et al. (2013) Biomarkers in bipolar disorder: a positional paper from the International Society for Bipolar Disorders Biomarkers Task Force. Aust N Z J Psychiatry 47(4):321–332.

Fukui T, Mori S, Hatooka S, et al. (2008) Prognostic evaluation based on a new TNM staging system proposed by the International Association for the Study of Lung Cancer for resected non-small cell lung cancers. J Thorac Cardiovasc Surg 136(5):1343–1348.

Goldberg JF, Harrow M, and Grossman LS (1995) Course and outcome in bipolar affective disorder: a longitudinal follow-up study. Am J Psychiatry 152:379–384.

Goodwin FK and Jamison KR (2007) Manic-Depressive Illness: Bipolar Disorders and Recurrent Depression. New York: Oxford University Press.

Grande I, Magalhaes PV, Kunz M, et al. (2012) Mediators of allostasis and systemic toxicity in bipolar disorder. Physiol Behav 106:46–50.

Jansen K, Magalhaes PV, Tavares Pinheiro R, et al. (2012) Early functional impairment in bipolar youth: a nested population-based case-control study. J Affect Disord 142:208–212.

Javadapour A, Malhi GS, Ivanovski B, et al. (2007) Increased anterior cingulate cortex volume in bipolar I disorder. Aust N Z J Psychiatry 41:910–916.

Judd LL, Akiskal HS, Schettler PJ, et al. (2005) Psychosocial disability in the course of bipolar I and II disorders—a prospective, comparative, longitudinal study. Arch Gen Psychiatry 62:1322–1330.

Juster RP, Mcewen BS, and Lupien SJ (2010) Allostatic load biomarkers of chronic stress and impact on health and cognition. Neurosci Biobehav Rev 35:2–16.

Kapczinski F, Dal-Pizzol F, Teixeira AL, et al. (2010) A systemic toxicity index developed to assess peripheral changes in mood episodes. Mol Psychiatry 15:784–786.

Kapczinski F, Dal-Pizzol F, Teixeira AL, et al. (2011) Peripheral biomarkers and illness activity in bipolar disorder. J Psychiatr Res 45:156–161.

Kapczinski F, Dias VV, Kauer-Sant'anna M, et al. (2009) Clinical implications of a staging model for bipolar disorders. Expert Rev Neurother 9:957–966.

Kapczinski F, Vieta E, Andreazza AC, et al. (2008) Allostatic load in bipolar disorder: Implications for pathophysiology and treatment. Neurosci Biobehav Rev 32:675–692.

Kauer-Sant'anna M, Bond DJ, Lam RW, et al. (2009a) Functional outcomes in first-episode patients with bipolar disorder: a prospective study from the Systematic Treatment Optimization Program for Early Mania project. Comprehens Psychiatry 50:1–8.

Kauer-Sant'anna M, Kapczinski F, Andreazza AC, et al. (2009b) Brain-derived neurotrophic factor and inflammatory markers in patients with early- vs. late-stage bipolar disorder. Int J Neuropsychopharmacol 12:447–458.

Lagopoulos J, Hermens DF, Naismith SL, et al. (2012) Frontal lobe changes occur early in the course of affective disorders in young people. BMC Psychiatry 12:4.

Lim CS, Baldessarini RJ, Vieta E, et al. (2013) Longitudinal neuroimaging and neuropsychological changes in bipolar disorder patients: review of the evidence. Neurosci Biobehav Rev 37:418–435.

Lin A, Reniers RL, and Wood SJ (2013) Clinical staging in severe mental disorder: evidence from neurocognition and neuroimaging. Br J Psychiatry Suppl 54:s11–17.

Lopez-Jaramillo C, Lopera-Vasquez J, Gallo A, et al. (2010) Effects of recurrence on the cognitive performance of patients with bipolar I disorder: implications for relapse prevention and treatment adherence. Bipolar Disord 12:557–567.

Macneil CA, Hasty MK, Berk M, et al. (2011) Psychological needs of adolescents in the early phase of bipolar disorder: implications for early intervention. Early Interv Psychiatry 5:100–107.

Maes M, Kubera M, Leunis JC, et al. (2012a) Increased IgA and IgM responses against gut commensals in chronic depression: further evidence for increased bacterial translocation or leaky gut. J Affect Disord 141:55–62.

Maes M, Ringel K, Kubera M, et al. (2012b) Increased autoimmune activity against 5-HT: a key component of depression that is associated with inflammation and activation of cell-mediated immunity, and with severity and staging of depression. J Affect Disord 136:386–392.

Magalhaes PV, Dean OM, Bush AI, et al. (2012a) Systemic illness moderates the impact of N-acetyl cysteine in bipolar disorder. Prog Neuropsychopharmacol Biol Psychiatry 37:132–135.

Magalhaes PV, Dodd S, Nierenberg AA, et al. (2012b) Cumulative morbidity and prognostic staging of illness in the Systematic Treatment Enhancement Program for Bipolar Disorder (STEP-BD). Aust N Z J Psychiatry 46:1058–1067.

Magalhaes PVS, Jansen K, Pinheiro RT, et al. (2011) Systemic toxicity in early-stage mood disorders. J Psychiatr Res 45:1407–1409.

Magalhaes PV, Kapczinski F, Nierenberg AA, et al. (2012c) Illness burden and medical comorbidity in the Systematic Treatment Enhancement Program for Bipolar Disorder. Acta Psychiatr Scand 125:303–308.

Magalhaes PVS, Fries GR, and Kapczinski F (2012d) Peripheral markers and the pathophysiology of bipolar disorder. Rev Psiquiatr Clin 39:60–67.

Magalhaes PV S, Jansen K, Pinheiro RT, et al. (2012e) Peripheral oxidative damage in early-stage mood disorders: a nested population-based case-control study. Int J Neuropsychopharmacol 15:1043–1050.

Martinez-Aran A, Vieta E, Reinares M, et al. (2004) Cognitive function across manic or hypomanic, depressed, and euthymic states in bipolar disorder. Am J Psychiatry **161**:262–270.

Martinez-Aran A, Vieta E, Torrent C, et al. (2007) Functional outcome in bipolar disorder: the role of clinical and cognitive factors. Bipolar Disord **9**(1–2):103–113.

Martino DJ, Igoa A, Marengo E, et al. (2011) Neurocognitive impairments and their relationship with psychosocial functioning in euthymic bipolar II disorder. J Nerv Ment Dis **199**(7):459–464.

McGorry PD (2007) Issues for DSM-V: Clinical staging: a heuristic pathway to valid nosology and safer, more effective treatment in psychiatry. Am J Psychiatry **164**:859–860.

McGorry PD, Hickie IB, Yung AR, et al. (2006) Clinical staging of psychiatric disorders: a heuristic framework for choosing earlier, safer and more effective interventions. Aust N Z J Psychiatry **40**:616–622.

McGorry PD, Purcell R, Hickie IB, et al. (2007) Clinical staging: a heuristic model for psychiatry and youth mental health. Med J Aust **187**:S40–S42.

Nehra R, Chakrabarti S, Pradhan BK, et al. (2006) Comparison of cognitive functions between first- and multi-episode bipolar affective disorders. J Affect Disord **93**:185–192.

Nery FG, Chen HH, Hatch JP, et al. (2009) Orbitofrontal cortex gray matter volumes in bipolar disorder patients: a region-of-interest MRI study. Bipolar Disord **11**:145–153.

Nolen WA, Luckenbaugh DA, Altshuler LL, et al. (2004) Correlates of 1-year prospective outcome in bipolar disorder: results from the Stanley Foundation Bipolar Network. Am J Psychiatry **161**(8):1447–1454.

Pacchiarotti I, Valenti M, Bonnin CM, et al. (2011) Factors associated with initial treatment response with antidepressants in bipolar disorder. Eur Neuropsychopharmacol **21**:362–369.

Post RM (2007a) Kindling and sensitization as models for affective episode recurrence, cyclicity, and tolerance phenomena. Neurosci Biobehav Rev **31**:858–873.

Post RM (2007b) Role of BDNF in bipolar and unipolar disorder: Clinical and theoretical implications. J Psychiatr Res **41**:979–990.

Post RM, Altshuler LL, Frye MA, et al. (2010) Complexity of pharmacologic treatment required for sustained improvement in outpatients with bipolar disorder. J Clin Psychiatry **71**:1176–1186.

Post RM, Denicoff KD, Leverich GS, et al. (2003) Morbidity in 258 bipolar outpatients followed for 1 year with daily prospective ratings on the NIMH life chart method. J Clin Psychiatry **64**:680–690; quiz 738–739.

Reinares M, Colom F, Rosa AR, et al. (2010) The impact of staging bipolar disorder on treatment outcome of family psychoeducation. J Affect Disord **123**:81–86.

Reinares M, Papachristou E, Harvey P, et al. (2013) Towards a clinical staging for bipolar disorder: defining patient subtypes based on functional outcome. J Affect Disord **144**:65–71.

Robinson LJ, Thompson JM, Gallagher P, et al. (2006) A meta-analysis of cognitive deficits in euthymic patients with bipolar disorder. J Affect Disord 93(1–3):105–115.

Rosa AR, Gonzalez-Ortega I, Gonzalez-Pinto A, et al. (2012) One-year psychosocial functioning in patients in the early vs. late stage of bipolar disorder. Acta Psychiatr Scand 125(4):335–341.

Rosa AR, Reinares M, Franco C, et al. (2009) Clinical predictors of functional outcome of bipolar patients in remission. Bipolar Disord 11:401–409.

Sachs GS, Nierenberg AA, Calabrese JR, et al. (2007) Effectiveness of adjunctive antidepressant treatment for bipolar depression. N Engl J Med 356:1711–1722.

Sachs GS, Thase ME, Otto MW, et al. (2003) Rationale, design, and methods of the systematic treatment enhancement program for bipolar disorder (STEP-BD). Biol Psychiatry 53:1028–1042.

Samamé C, Martino DJ, and Strejilevich SA (2014) Longitudinal course of cognitive deficits in bipolar disorder: a meta-analytic study. J Affect Disord 164:130–108.

Sanchez-Moreno J, Martinez-Aran A, Tabares-Seisdedos R, et al. (2009) Functioning and disability in bipolar disorder: an extensive review. Psychother Psychosom 78:285–297.

Scott J, Paykel E, Morriss R, et al. (2006) Cognitive-behavioural therapy for severe and recurrent bipolar disorders—Randomised controlled trial. Br J Psychiatry 188:313–320.

Tabares-Seisdedos R, Balanza-Martinez V, Sanchez-Moreno J, et al. (2008) Neurocognitive and clinical predictors of functional outcome in patients with schizophrenia and bipolar I disorder at one-year follow-up. J Affect Disord 109(3):286–99.

Tohen M, Hennen J, Zarate CM Jr, et al. (2000) Two-year syndromal and functional recovery in 219 cases of first-episode major affective disorder with psychotic features. Am J Psychiatry 157:220–228.

Tohen M, Vieta E, Gonzalez-Pinto A, et al. (2010) Baseline characteristics and outcomes in patients with first episode or multiple episodes of acute mania. J Clin Psychiatry 71:255–261.

Torrent C, Del Mar Bonnin C, Martinez-Aran A, et al. (2013) Efficacy of functional remediation in bipolar disorder: a multicenter randomized controlled study. Am J Psychiatry 170(8):852–859.

Torres IJ, Defreitas VG, Defreitas CM, et al. (2010) Neurocognitive functioning in patients with bipolar I disorder recently recovered from a first manic episode. J Clin Psychiatry 71:1234–1242.

Ustun B and Kennedy C (2009) What is 'functional impairment'? Disentangling disability from clinical significance. World Psychiatry 8:82–85.

Vita A, De Peri L, and Sacchetti E (2009) Gray matter, white matter, brain, and intracranial volumes in first-episode bipolar disorder: a meta-analysis of magnetic resonance imaging studies. Bipolar Disord 11(8):807–814.

Wright JR Jr (2012) Albert C. Broders' paradigm shifts involving the prognostication and definition of cancer. Arch Pathol Lab Med 136:1437–1446.

Zarate CA Jr, Tohen M, Land M, et al. (2000) Functional impairment and cognition in bipolar disorder. Psychiatr Q 71:309–329.

Index

Printed in Great Britain
by Amazon

24124866R00203